Pregnancy After Assisted Reproductive Technology

Pregnancy After Assisted Reproductive Technology

Edited by
Eric R. M. Jauniaux
Professor of Obstetrics and Fetal Medicine at the UCL EGA Institute for Women's Health, University College London, London, UK

Botros R. M. B. Rizk
Professor of Obstetrics and Gynecology and Director of the Division of Reproductive Endocrinology and Infertility, University of South Alabama College of Medicine, Mobile, AL, USA

CAMBRIDGE
UNIVERSITY PRESS

CAMBRIDGE UNIVERSITY PRESS
Cambridge, New York, Melbourne, Madrid, Cape Town,
Singapore, São Paulo, Delhi, Tokyo, Mexico City

Cambridge University Press
The Edinburgh Building, Cambridge CB2 8RU, UK

Published in the United States of America by Cambridge University Press, New York

www.cambridge.org
Information on this title: www.cambridge.org/9781107006478

First published 2012

Printed and bound in the United Kingdom by the MPG Books Group

A catalogue record for this publication is available from the British Library

Library of Congress Cataloguing in Publication data
Pregnancy after assisted reproductive technology / edited by Eric R.M. Jauniaux,
Botros R.M.B. Rizk.
p. ; cm.
Includes bibliographical references and index.
ISBN 978-1-107-00647-8 (hardback)
I. Jauniaux, E. II. Rizk, Botros.
[DNLM: 1. Reproductive Techniques, Assisted. 2. Infertility. 3. Pregnancy
Complications. WQ 208]
616.6′92–dc23

2012013395

ISBN 978-1-107-00647-8 Hardback

Thank you to our families for their constant support during the production of this book.

Contents

Contributors *page* viii

1 **Introduction** 1
Eric R. M. Jauniaux and Botros R. M. B. Rizk

2 **Assisted reproductive technology pregnancies: the historical perspective** 4
Basil C. Tarlatzis, Dimitra S. Kyrou, and Eric R. M. Jauniaux

3 **The role of ultrasound in early pregnancy after assisted conception** 14
Andrea Day and Davor Jurkovic

4 **Pregnancy after ovarian hyperstimulation syndrome** 36
Botros R. M. B. Rizk and Raphael Ron-El

5 **Early pregnancy failure after assisted reproductive technology** 51
Sotirios H. Saravelos and Lesley Regan

6 **Singleton pregnancy after assisted reproductive technology: the obstetric perspective** 66
Annika K. Ludwig, Michael Ludwig, and Eric R. M. Jauniaux

7 **Early and late pregnancy and psychological complications after assisted reproductive technology** 72
Gamal I. Serour

8 **Multiple gestation pregnancy after assisted reproductive technology** 82
Eric R. M. Jauniaux

9 **Pregnancy after intracytoplasmic spermatozoon injection** 93
Willem Verpoest and Paul Devroey

10 **Pregnancy outcome after oocyte and embryo cryopreservation** 108
Eleonora Porcu and Antonia Bazzocchi

11 **Pregnancy after fertility preservation** 124
Ephia Yasmin and Melanie C. Davies

12 **Pregnancy after ovarian transplantation** 137
Sherman J. Silber

13 **Prenatal diagnosis after assisted reproductive technology** 149
Ido Ben-Ami and Ron Maymon

14 **Children born after assisted reproductive technology** 168
Alastair G. Sutcliffe and Tajinder Singhrao

15 **Ethical and legal perspectives of assisted reproductive technology pregnancies** 182
Françoise Shenfield

Index 193

The color plates can be found between pages 118 and 119.

Contributors

Antonia Bazzocchi
Infertility and IVF Center, University Hospital S. Orsola-Malpighi, University of Bologna, Bologna, Italy

Ido Ben-Ami
Department of Obstetrics and Gynecology, Assaf Harofeh Medical Center, Zerifin, Israel

Melanie C. Davies
Reproductive Medicine Unit, University College London Hospital, London, UK

Andrea Day
Gynaecology Diagnostic and Outpatient Treatment Unit, University College Hospital, London, UK

Paul Devroey
Department of Gynaecology and Reproductive Medicine, Universitair Ziekenhuis Brussel, Brussels, Belgium

Eric R. M. Jauniaux
Institute for Women's Health, Royal Free and University College London Medical School, London, UK

Davor Jurkovic
Gynaecology Diagnostic and Outpatient Treatment Unit, University College Hospital, London, UK

Dimitra S. Kyrou
Department of Obstetrics and Gynecology, Medical School, Aristotle University of Thessaloniki, Thessaloniki, Greece

Annika K. Ludwig
Amedes Group Hamburg, Hamburg, Germany

Michael Ludwig
Amedes Group Hamburg, Hamburg, Germany

Ron Maymon
Department of Obstetrics and Gynecology, Assaf Harofeh Medical Center, Zerifin, Israel

Eleonora Porcu
Infertility and IVF Center, University Hospital S. Orsola-Malpighi, University of Bologna, Bologna, Italy

Lesley Regan
Department of Obstetrics and Gynaecology, Imperial College London, St Mary's Campus, London, UK

Botros R. M. B. Rizk
Division of Reproductive Endocrinology and Infertility, University of South Alabama College of Medicine, Mobile, AL, USA

Raphael Ron-El
Infertility and IVF Unit, Assaf Harofeh Medical Center, Tel Aviv University, Tel Aviv, Israel

Sotirios H. Saravelos
Department of Obstetrics and Gynaecology, Imperial College London, St Mary's Campus, London, UK

Gamal I. Serour
Al Azhar University, The Egyptian IVF and ET Center, Maadi, Cairo, Egypt

Françoise Shenfield
Institute for Women's Health, Royal Free and University College London Medical School, London, UK

Sherman J. Silber
Infertility Center of St. Louis, St. Luke's Hospital, St. Louis, MO, USA and Academic Medical Center for Reproductive Medicine, Amsterdam, the Netherlands

Tajinder Singhrao
Institute of Child Health, University College London, London, UK

Alastair G. Sutcliffe
Institute of Child Health, University College London, London, UK

Basil C. Tarlatzis
Department of Obstetrics and Gynecology, Medical School, Aristotle University of Thessaloniki, Thessaloniki, Greece

Willem Verpoest
Centre for Reproductive Medicine, Universitair Ziekenhuis Brussel, Brussels, Belgium

Ephia Yasmin
Reproductive Medicine Unit, University College London Hospital, London, UK

Chapter 1

Introduction

Eric R. M. Jauniaux and Botros R. M. B. Rizk

Reproduction has been a major preoccupation since the dawn of human existence and treating infertility a medical objective for centuries. Since antiquity, written records indicate that most humans have been prolific, but difficulty with conception has been and remains a real problem for many couples around the world. In many cultures it has become a taboo, and as with a silent disease, is often not discussed. The inability to conceive continues to bear a stigma, and infertility may have a profound psychological and social impact resulting in marital discord, emotional stress, and depression. The lack of an heir in Royal and upper-class families can also have far-reaching political consequences [1]. Overall, there have been millions upon millions of couples that have had to cope with infertility throughout the ages [2]. In the U.K., fertility problems affect one in seven couples [3] whereas in the U.S., around 25% of married childless women 15–44 years of age have impaired fecundity [4]. It is estimated that four million modern couples have an infertility problem at any given time. Infertility and sterility now rank third among the most life-threatening diseases of the twenty-first century, according to the World Health Organization (WHO).

In ancient times, medicine was empirical and often based on magic. Physicians were commonly priests to a local deity who was responsible for the diseases and the gods played a fundamental role in the control of human reproduction and treatment of infertility. Some of the oldest written evidence for fertility tests dates back to ancient Egypt. In Egyptian society, women were equal to men, and difficulty with conception was not considered divine punishment but an illness that had to be diagnosed and treated. As far back as 1820 BCE, there are recorded documents discussing the treatment of gynecological disorders. For example, The Carlsberg IV (Copenhagen) and Kahum 28 (London) papyri describe a test to determine if a woman will bear children. The test was based on the use of an onion placed for the night until dawn inside her flesh (vagina). If the odor appeared in her mouth she was told that she would bear children; if not, she will never bear children [5].

The earliest known use of a modern artificial reproduction technique is the case of a couple treated by the famous Scottish surgeon John Hunter, probably in 1776 (reported by E. Home at the Royal Society in 1799). The husband, a linen draper, was suffering from hypospadias and Hunter advised the couple to have normal intercourse, then he collected the semen in a warmed syringe and injected it into the wife's vagina. The couple had their first baby within the following year [6]. The first published account of a successful human artificial insemination was performed by a doctor Girault in France on June 5, 1838. His patient, a young countess, gave birth to a normal son on March 1, 1839. This case was the first in a series of 12, which were recorded in a paper published in 1868 (*L'Abeille Medicale* **25**: 409–417) [7]. The American gynecologist Dr James Marion Sims (1813–1883) published his book on sterility, which included a chapter on artificial insemination. This book generated an extremely vigorous debate around the medical, moral, and ethical issues surrounding artificial insemination.

The first published reference to donor insemination was made by an Italian, Paolo Mantegazza, in 1887 [7]. With the exception of France, the wide acceptance of artificial insemination among the medical establishment took many decades. It was still extremely controversial in the U.S. in the 1940s; donor insemination was still quite controversial in Australia in the 1970s when the first spermatozoon banks and public hospital-based donor insemination programs were established. The use of donor spermatozoa or eggs is still forbidden by many religions.

Pregnancy After Assisted Reproductive Technology, ed. Eric R. M. Jauniaux and Botros R. M. B. Rizk. Published by Cambridge University Press.

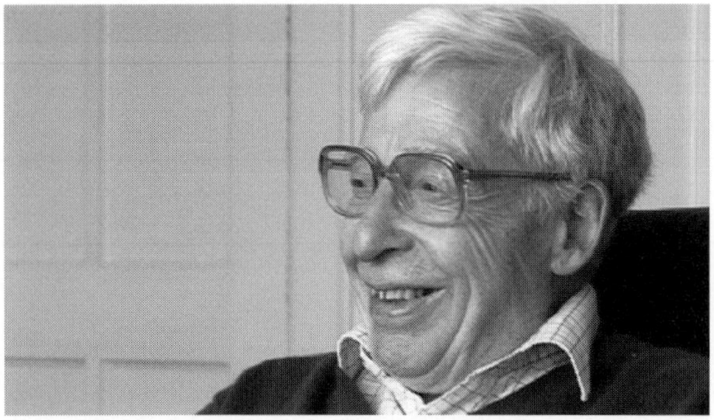

Figure 1.1. Photograph of Sir Professor Robert "Bob" Edwards in 2008 (Bourn Hall, E. Jauniaux).

Robert "Bob" Edwards (Figure 1.1) was awarded the Nobel prize in medicine in 2010 and a knighthood in 2011 for his pioneering work in the development of in vitro fertilization (IVF). Bob dedicated his career to helping couples overcome infertility and his IVF technique has touched millions of lives across the globe. He first established principles of early embryo development that served as the foundation for his later work. Louise Brown was born on July 25, 1978 at 23:47 GMT at Oldham General Hospital, Manchester, U.K. The world's first "test-tube baby" is the result of a decade of hard work and of an unusual collaboration between a scientist, Bob Edwards, and an obstetrician – gynecologist, Patrick Steptoe. This achievement is a landmark in not only the reproductive sciences but also the history of mankind's technological evolution. Steptoe had been facing considerable criticism over his use of laparoscopy, even being isolated at clinical meetings in London [8], yet he had done more than 1000 cases whereas committee members had not done any.

A decade later they made medical history but they also opened a new ethical and religious Pandora's box. Prominent ethicists, the Vatican, politicians, Nobel prize winners, and rigid protestants decried them, forecasting abnormal babies, a rumor that is still present in the collective mind of lay people today. They announced how IVF did not cure infertility, because women remained infertile after their IVF baby, and some labeled IVF as eugenic. The birth of the first IVF baby was snubbed by some clinicians now styled as "pioneers in artificial reproduction technologies" (ART), shouting that the test-tube claim was a fake! A grant application to the U.K. Medical Research Council for an IVF clinic in Newmarket, near Cambridge, U.K., was rejected because it was claimed that laparoscopy was dangerous and rhesus monkeys should have been used initially. Major ethical arguments in the press formed a constant background for more than a decade after Louise Brown's birth.

At some point, Bob Edwards had to issue eight libel actions in the High Court of London, U.K., on a single day, and many have continued to oppose what they saw to be interfering with nature. When interviewed on her 30th anniversary, Louise Brown said: "The children at school used to ask questions like 'how did you fit in a test tube?' and things like that, but they could see I was normal; they could see I was the same as them." The same year it was estimated that around three and a half million women worldwide had undergone IVF. In the U.K., birth country of the first IVF baby, it took more than 25 years before the government supported funding for IVF in the National Health Service (NHS), but four years down the line 94 % of trusts were still not providing the full three cycles recommended by the Department of Health guidelines [9]. Low-cost IVF programs are being developed for low-income countries to improve access to ART for infertile couples living in Africa [10], showing the universal desire of achieving a pregnancy and the worldwide contribution of IVF to the treatment of sterility.

When, on October 4, 2010, it was announced that Edwards had been awarded the 2010 Nobel prize in physiology or medicine for the development of in vitro fertilization, a Vatican official condemned the move as "completely out of order." Edwards' work not only provided the means to overcome many forms of infertility, but it also gave us a better understanding of the early stages of human embryonic development and preimplantation genetic diagnosis (PGD) [11,12]. His original IVF work has also opened up areas further from reproductive health such as human embryonic stem cell research. From the beginning of his career, Edwards realized the wide-ranging new therapeutic applications of embryos created in vitro for degenerative disorders and cancer [13–19], opening another ethical and philosophical Pandora's box and a new debate [20–23], which is going to carry on for many decades to come.

For decades, rumors were spread about the long-term health of children born following IVF and other ART. However, the most common complications associated with IVF treatment have remained indirect and technical, such as the failure of treatment, ovarian hyperstimulation syndrome, the surgical risks associated with egg collection, and the possibility of ectopic pregnancy. Probably the most controversial possible complications of IVF/ART are the risk associated with multiple pregnancies and the issue of birth defects following the use of newer ARTs such as intracytoplasmic spermatozoon injection (ICSI). These issues and other topics related to ART pregnancies are presented and discussed in this book, which we dedicate to Bob Edwards as a tribute to his constant support and friendship and to mark his unique contribution to medicine.

References

1. Poulakou-Rebelakou E, Tsiamis, Tompros N, Creatsas G. The lack of a child, the loss of a throne: the infertility of the first royal couple of Greece (1833–62). *J R Coll Physicians Edinb* 2011; **41**: 73–77.
2. Rutstein SO, Shah IH. Infecundity, infertility and childlessness in developing countries. DHS Comparative Reports, 9, *ORC Macro and WHO*, 2004.
3. National Institute for Health and Clinical Excellence (NICE). Fertility: assessment and treatment for people with fertility problems. *Clinical guideline* **11**. London, UK: NICE, 2004.
4. Chandra A, Martinez GM, Mosher WD, Abma JC, Jones J. Fertility, family planning, and reproductive health of US women: data from the 2002 National Survey of Family Growth, National Center for Health Statistics. *Vital Health Stat* 2005; **23**: 1–160.
5. Nunn JF. *Ancient Egyptian Medicine*. University of Okaloma, Norman, OK, 1996.
6. Moore W. *The Knife Man*. London, UK: Bantam, 2005.
7. Poynter FNL. Hunter, Spallanzani, and the history of artificial insemination. In: Stevenson LG, Multhauf RP, eds. *Medicine, Science and Culture*. Baltimore, MD: Johns Hopkins, 1968.
8. Edwards RG. The bumpy road to human in vitro fertilization. *Nat Med* 2001; **7**: 1091–1094.
9. Buxton J. Postcode lottery continues for infertile English couples. *Bionews* **464**, 2008.
10. Edwards RG. Changing genetic world of IVF, stem cells and PGD. C. Embryogenesis and the differentiation of the haemopoietic system. *Reprod Biomed Online* 2005; **11**: 777–785.
11. Murage A, Muteshi MC, Githae F. Assisted reproduction services provision in a developing country: time to act? *Fertil Steril* 2011; **96**: 966–968.
12. Gardner RL, Johnson MH. Bob Edwards and the first decade of Reproductive BioMedicine Online. *Reprod Biomed Online* 2011; **22**: 106–124.
13. Edwards RG. Embryonic stem cells. *Bone Marrow Transplant* 1992; **9**: 4–6.
14. Edwards RG. IVF and the history of stem cells. *Nature* 2001; **413**: 349–351.
15. Edwards RG. Personal pathways to embryonic stem cells. *Reprod Biomed Online* 2002; **4**: 263–278.
16. Edwards RG, Jauniaux E, Binns RM, et al. Induced tolerance and chimaerism in human fetuses using coelocentesis: a medical opportunity to avert genetic disease? *Hum Reprod Update* 1995; **1**: 419–427.
17. Edwards RG, Hollands P. Will stem cells in cord blood, amniotic fluid, bone marrow and peripheral blood soon be unnecessary in transplantation? *Reprod Biomed Online* 2007; **14**: 396–401.
18. Li J, Li M, Niu B, Gong J. Therapeutic potential of stem cell in liver regeneration. *Front Med* 2011; **5**: 26–32.
19. Yabut O, Bernstein HS. The promise of human embryonic stem cells in aging-associated diseases. *Aging* 2011; **3**: 494–508.
20. Edwards RG. A burgeoning science of embryological genetics demands a modern ethics. *Reprod Biomed Online* 2007; **15** : 34–40.
21. Sage WM. Will embryonic stem cells change health policy? *J Law Med Ethics* 2010; **38**: 342–351.
22. Power C, Rasko JE. Will cell reprogramming resolve the embryonic stem cell controversy? A narrative review. *Ann Intern Med* 2011; **155**: 114–121.
23. Ledford H. Hidden toll of embryo ethics war. *Nature* 2011; **471**: 279.

Chapter 2

Assisted reproductive technology pregnancies: the historical perspective

Basil C. Tarlatzis, Dimitra S. Kyrou, and Eric R. M. Jauniaux

Introduction

Since the birth of the world's first in vitro fertilization (IVF) baby in 1978, an estimated four million children have been born to date following artificial reproductive technology (ART) [1]. The first data on the number of ART births worldwide were collected in 1989. In that year, only about 30 000 babies were born following ART. Based on the most recent data from the International Committee for Monitoring Assisted Reproductive Technologies (ICMART) for the year 2002 collected from 53 participating countries, it has been estimated that ART now produced approximately 200 000 babies per year, representing an increase of 12% compared to the year 2000 [2]. This chapter reviews the history of ART starting with the first attempts at IVF in animals and presents the incredible journey taken by the pioneers to give us an efficient treatment for human infertility, culminating in 2010 with the award of the Nobel prize to Robert Edwards.

How did it all begin?

Probably one of the first unpublished attempts at IVF is that of the famous British surgeon John Hunter (1728–1793) (Figure 2.1), who in the summer of 1767 attempted to artificially impregnate silkworms. He kept a female moth in confinement until she laid some unfertilized eggs, dissected a male moth to collect a sample of semen, and then combined the two in a covered box. The experiment was successful, leading to eight of the eggs hatching at the same time. "Thus then I ascertained that the eggs could be impregnated by art [sic], after they were laid" Hunter recorded [3]. Hunter's scientific approach was ahead of its time, but if most of his numerous discoveries were presented at the Royal Society in London, they remain unpublished during his life. Furthermore, his discoveries on evolution, which were later to inspire Charles Darwin, challenging the traditional biblical story made him a pariah at the Royal Society.

Similarly, Anton Philips van Leeuwenhoek (1632–1723), who recorded the first microscopic observations of human spermatozoa in 1677, had a lot of trouble with his discoveries and in particular with Dutch theologists. Most of his microscopic observations were initially met with scepticism, including by the Royal Society. At around the same time (1779), Lazzaro Spallanzani (1729–1799), an Italian physiologist, described the role of semen in fertilization, and showed that spermatozoa have to make physical contact with the egg for fertilization to take place. He is also credited with having noted that frog oocytes only develop into tadpoles after contact with semen, with having performed the first artificial insemination of a mammal (dog), and with having attempted IVF in frogs. However, these early experiments were ignored by the scientific establishment, and before the nineteenth century, precisely how fertilization took place and the role played by the male and female gametes led to numerous fruitless debates among European scientific societies.

The first observation of spermatozoon penetration into an ovum was reported in a non-mammalian species (*Ascaris mystax*) by Henry Nelson at the Royal Society in 1851 and published the following year in the *Philosophical Transactions* [4]. Newport (1853) made similar observations in amphibians, and van Beneden (1854) and Hertwig (1876) are credited with the first observations on fertilization in mammals. In 1890, Walter Heape (1855–1929), who had performed research on reproduction in numerous animal species, became the first known scientist to successfully transfer embryos in a mammal (rabbit). In his first experiments, probably performed at a laboratory at his home in Manchester (U.K.), he flushed two embryos from the

Pregnancy After Assisted Reproductive Technology, ed. Eric R. M. Jauniaux and Botros R. M. B. Rizk. Published by Cambridge University Press.

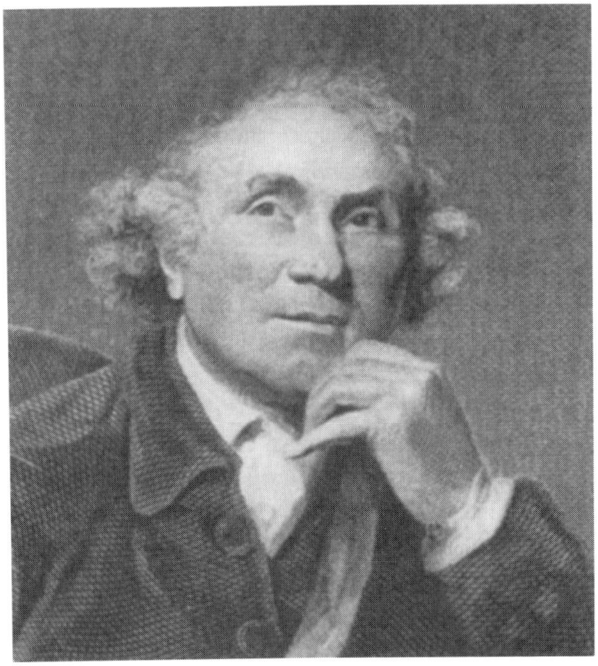

Figure 2.1. Extract of the portrait of John Hunter by Sir J Reynolds PRA, 1786.

Fallopian tubes of an Angora doe rabbit and placed them into the uterus of a recently mated Belgian hare doe, resulting in the birth of a litter of six young, four of them Belgians and two of them Angoras. His experiments proved conclusively that it was possible to transfer embryos to a gestational carrier without affecting their development [5]. In his book *The Breeding Industry* (Figure 2.2), published in 1906, he criticized the British Government for not supporting the scientific study of animal breeding and improvement [6]. The same criticism could be applied to the fact that it took nearly 30 years after the birth of the first IVF baby for the British Government to provide funding for IVF treatment within the National Health Service (NHS).

Many scientists, inspired by Heape's results, started culturing eggs and embryos in laboratories around the world. Gregory Pincus (1903–1967), working at Harvard University, was the first to show that eggs of various animals could be maturated when released from their follicles and cultured in vitro. In 1935 he described the first experimental condition that allowed rabbit oocytes to mature in culture, reaching the metaphase stage of meiosis II [7]. He claimed to have achieved successful mammal birth from the result of in vitro fertilization of rabbit eggs. As nobody could repeat his experiments at the time, doubts were cast over the authenticity of the claim. It was in 1959 that Min Chueh Chang (1908–1991), who was working at the Worcester Foundation for Experimental Biology in Shrewsbury, MA (U.S.) that Pincus co-founded in 1944, reported that in vitro-matured black rabbit oocytes could be fertilized in vitro and also give rise to viable embryos. Furthermore, when these embryos were transferred back to adult females, they resulted in viable offspring [8]. This was the sort of evidence attesting to the feasibility of in vitro fertilization (IVF) for which many scientists had been searching. In the years that followed, Chang and his colleagues conducted further research to determine specific conditions of successful IVF and performed the technique on other mammals such as hamsters, mice, and rats. It was on the basis of Chang's findings

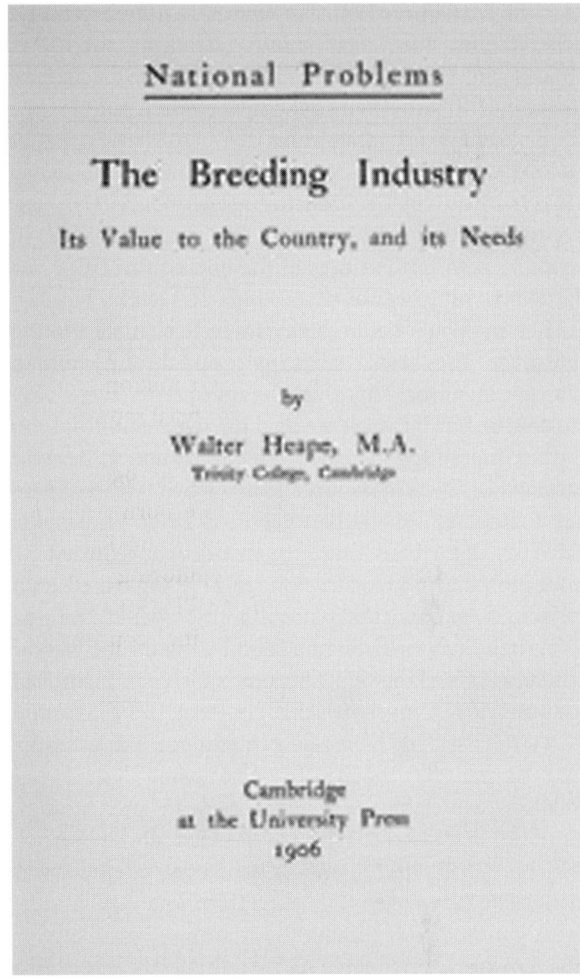

National Problems

The Breeding Industry

Its Value to the Country, and its Needs

by

Walter Heape, M.A.

Trinity College, Cambridge

Cambridge
at the University Press
1906

Figure 2.2. Front cover of Walter Heape's book *The Breeding Industry*, published in 1906.

that the first IVF of human eggs was done. As these experiments were very controversial at the time, Pincus and Chang remained best known for having invented the combined oral contraceptive pill.

Robert Edwards started his career studying genetics at Edinburgh University (U.K.), obtaining his PhD in 1956 for his work on inducing heteroploidy in mouse preimplantation embryos. He became interested in working with human eggs at the end of the 1950s. At the National Institute of Medical Research, London (U.K.) in 1960, he became interested in alleviating infertility and tried maturing animal and human oocytes in vitro. The animal experiments were very successful, but Edwards worked for two years trying to induce human egg maturation without success, because human eggs did not mature in vitro when released from the follicle, as Pincus had reported in 1939. Finally, Edwards discovered that human oocytes required 37 hours to polar body extrusion, and having timed each stage of human oocyte maturation, he opened the way to human IVF [9,10]. After a couple of years at Glasgow University, working on embryonic stem cells, he moved to Cambridge University (U.K.) in 1963. In 1968 he and Barry Bavister, his then research student, achieved the first human fertilization in vitro using a high-pH medium, which proved unnecessary in later studies. Reading the *Lancet*, Edwards learned about Patrick Steptoe (1913–1988) and laparoscopy. Steptoe was criticized for developing this technique by almost every gynecologists because they thought it was dangerous. Edwards and Steptoe set up a small laboratory in a room next to the operating theater in Oldham District General Hospital in the suburbs of Manchester, 180 miles from Cambridge. This meant that Edwards would have to travel three to four hours one way to get to collect oocytes retrieved by laparoscopy by Steptoe at Oldham. Women stimulated with low-dose human menopausal gonadotrophin/human chorionic gonadotrophin (HMG/hCG) ovulated at 37 hours post-hCG; thus Steptoe aspirated eggs at 35–36 hours to gain 5–6 provulatory oocytes on average before they ovulated [11–14]. Their attempts met significant hostility and opposition in the U.K. including a refusal by the British government (Medical Research Council) to fund their research because laparoscopy was considered too dangerous, and a number of lawsuits followed.

Having seen the results of Edwards and Steptoe's experiments, another research team followed their tracks and the first IVF pregnancy, which resulted in early miscarriage, was reported in 1973 by the Monash research team of Carl Wood in Melbourne (Australia) [15]. In 1976 Steptoe and Edwards published a case of an ectopic pregnancy following transfer of a human embryo at the early blastocyst stage [16]. After this adverse outcome, they decided to abandon ovarian stimulation and instead rely on the natural menstrual cycle of the patients. Based on the concentration of luteinizing hormones in the women's urine, they could predict when the maturing oocyte would reach the metaphase stage of meiosis II in vivo and then proceed to egg retrieval by laparoscopy before ovulation occurred. They managed to aspirate a single oocyte in a natural menstrual cycle without using any fertility medication. In addition, they proceeded to an earlier embryo transfer, at the eight-cell stage, in order to compensate for the inadequate culture conditions in vitro [17].

The birth of Louise Brown, the world's first "test tube baby," at 11:47 P.M. on July 25, 1978 at the Oldham General Hospital, Manchester (U.K.) made medical history (Figure 2.3). Her mother Lesley had failed to conceive over a nine-year period due to her

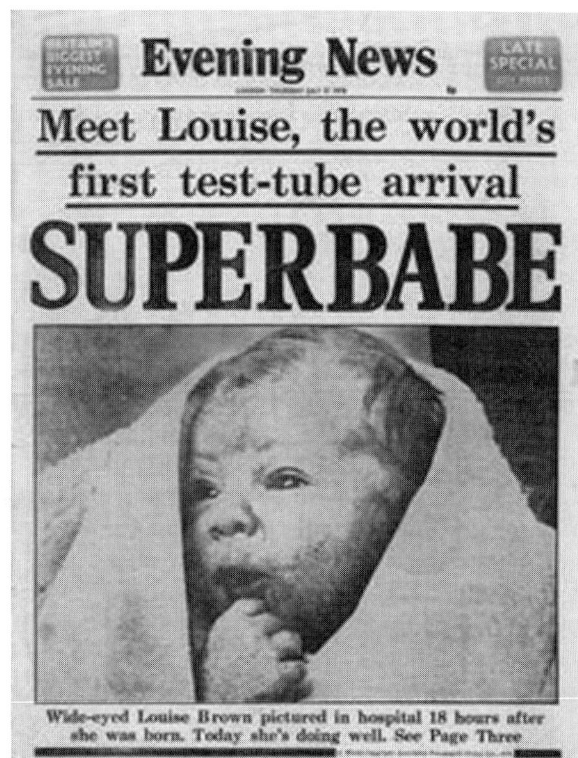
Evening News

Meet Louise, the world's first test-tube arrival

SUPERBABE

Wide-eyed Louise Brown pictured in hospital 18 hours after she was born. Today she's doing well. See Page Three

Figure 2.3. Front cover of the *Evening News* of July 27, 1978, two days after Louise Brown was born at Oldham General Hospital, Manchester, U.K.

bilateral Fallopian tube obstruction and had been referred to Steptoe in 1976. A single oocyte was aspirated from one of Lesley's ovaries during laparoscopy, fertilization in vitro was performed, and a few days later the developing embryo was transferred into Lesley's uterus [18].

On December 20, 2006, Louise gave birth to her own child, Cameron John Mullinder, without the need for IVF treatment. Following the birth of Louise Brown, Edwards and Steptoe founded an infertility clinic at Bourn Hall, in Cambridge, U.K. (Figure 2.4) where the second and third children in the world were born after IVF [19]. In 1984 Edwards was elected as a Fellow of the Royal Society (London), in 2001 he was awarded the Albert Lasker Clinical Medical Research Award by the Lasker Foundation (New York), and on October 4, 2010 it was announced that Edwards had been awarded the 2010 Nobel prize in physiology or medicine for the development of in vitro fertilization. A Vatican official condemned the move as "completely out of order."

The first IVF birth in Australia was achieved in 1980 by the Victorian Monash–Melbourne team, also using the natural cycle [20]. Nevertheless, the achievement of pregnancies was still sporadic, mainly due to the limitations of the natural cycle.

A major breakthrough that increased the achievement of pregnancies in a consistent way and led to the worldwide application of IVF was the re-introduction in 1981 of ovarian stimulation in IVF by Trounson et al. [21]. In vitro fertilization started to spread over the world and one year later the first IVF baby in the U.S. was announced by Howard and Georgianna Seegar Jones in Norfolk, VA [22]. In 1982, the first French IVF birth was reported in Clamart, Île-de-France, by Testart and Frydman [23]. The same year the first IVF birth was announced in Sweden [24] and in Austria [25]. By 1986 about 1000 additional births had been reported in different countries.

Further assisted reproductive technology developments and pregnancies

Gamete intra-Fallopian transfer and zygote intra-Fallopian transfer

Intratubal transfer procedures were attempted as an alternative to IVF. Although the technique of gamete intra-Fallopian transfer (GIFT) for all forms of non-tubal infertility was introduced in 1979 by Shettles [26], it was only four years later that the first pregnancy was reported by Tesarík et al. [27]. The original concept was that transferring gametes back into the Fallopian tube would benefit from the protective tubal environment. If fertilization occurred, transfer of embryos in the uterus would take place at a more appropriate time, and finally, the avoidance of uterine cavity trauma, which might occur during a transcervical intrauterine transfer procedure, would lead to higher implantation rates. However, the main disadvantage of the GIFT technique was the lack of control with regard to fertilization.

In 1986 zygote intra-Fallopian transfer (ZIFT), a technique in which pronuclear-stage embryos were transferred into the Fallopian tube, was introduced by Devroey et al. [28] and the first report of a pregnancy was announced the same year. Zygote intra-Fallopian transfer combined both the advantages of the GIFT

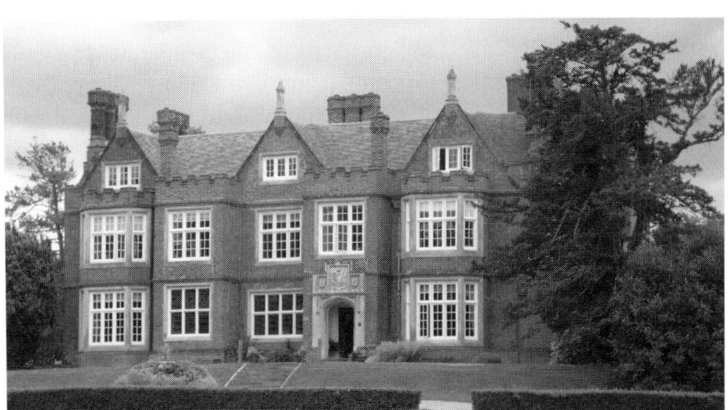

Figure 2.4. Outside view of Edwards and Steptoe's Bourn Hall infertility clinic.

technique with those of IVF, as normal fertilization could be confirmed, excluding polyploid embryos and incubating immature oocytes.

Intracytoplasmic spermatozoon injection

Although IVF had been successfully applied in couples with male infertility, it became apparent that the results of conventional IVF were significantly decreased when the semen characteristics of the male partner were well below the World Health Organization (WHO) criteria. This was due to the significantly lower percentage of oocytes than would normally have been fertilized, resulting in the formation of fewer embryos available for transfer [29]. Several procedures of assisted fertilization were developed and used in cases of severe semen deficiencies instead of conventional IVF, such as partial zona dissection (PZD) and subzonal insemination (SUZI). However, both were associated with low fertilization, pregnancy, and delivery rates that precluded their routine clinical use.

The first direct injection of a single spermatozoon into the ooplasm, after passage through the zona pellucida and the membrane of the oocyte, was reported by Lanzendorf et al. [30], but was abandoned because of disappointing results. However, the team at the Free University of Brussels (Belgium) continued to experiment with this technique and obtained the first successful fertilization and pregnancy, which was delivered on January 14, 1992. In 1992 Palermo et al. reported the first pregnancies obtained by this novel technique of assisted reproduction, which they called intracytoplasmic spermatozoon injection (ICSI), in couples with infertility caused by severely impaired spermatozoon characteristics and for which IVF and SUZI had failed [31]. Hence, from 47 metaphase-II oocytes, 38 oocytes remained intact after injection, 31 became fertilized, and finally, 15 embryos were transferred. After eight treatment cycles, four pregnancies occurred, two singletons and one twin pregnancy, that resulted in four healthy babies.

Spermatozoon recovery techniques and assisted conception for azoospermia

Various procedures for spermatozoon recovery have made it possible to help men with both obstructive and nonobstructive azoospermia to achieve genetic fatherhood. Human pregnancy by IVF using spermatozoa by percutaneous epididymal spermatozoon aspiration (PESA) was first reported in 1985 [32]. The first two babies born after microsurgical epididymal spermatozoon aspiration (MESA) from men with congenital bilateral absence of the vas deferens (CBAVD) were reported in 1988 [33]. However, the overall results of IVF and MESA in cases of obstructive azoospermia were poor, with low conception rates [34].

The introduction of ICSI not only significantly improved the fertility prospects after assisted reproduction by using spermatozoa recovered from the seminal tract, but has also allowed extension of the spectrum of recovery techniques. For example, in the case of obstructive azoospermia, it became possible to use not only spermatozoa obtained by MESA, but also spermatozoa obtained from the testicle by means of testicular biopsy (TESE), or spermatozoa percutaneously aspirated from the testicle/epididymis by minimally invasive techniques (TESA, PESA, FNA [fine needle aspiration]). Within this context, ICSI with epididymal or testicular spermatozoa has revolutionized the treatment of patients who were infertile because of congenital disorders causing obstruction of the excretory ducts. The first successful fertilization by testicular spermatozoa from a man with CBAVD and ICSI was in 1993 by Schoysman et al. [35], while the first pregnancies using TESE and ICSI were reported by Silber et al. [36] and Tournaye et al. [37] in 1994. The first pregnancies after TESE and ICSI in cases of nonobstructive azoospermia were reported by Devroey et al. in 1995 [38].

Embryo and oocyte cryopreservation

The introduction of superovulation treatment as part of ART usually results in the development of multiple embryos. Replacement of more than one embryo increases pregnancy rates to a certain extent, but at the same time leads to multiple pregnancies, with increased pre- and postnatal risks (see Chapter 8). In this respect, cryopreservation of human embryos has been considered as the method to reduce multiple pregnancy rates. Furthermore, success with frozen embryo transfer cycles increases the cumulative pregnancy rate per retrieval. The first report on human pregnancy following cryopreservation, thawing, and transfer of an eight-cell embryo was reported by Trounson and Mohr in 1983 [39], who used a slow freezing protocol with dimethyl sulfoxide (DMSO). Unfortunately, this pregnancy was terminated at 24 weeks' gestation, because of the development of a septic *Streptomyces agalactiae* chorioamnionitis after premature rupture of the membranes. The first live birth of twins following the transfer of intact frozen-thawed embryos was subsequently reported by Zeilmaker et al. in 1984 [40].

Although pregnancy rates related to the use of frozen-thawed oocytes are improving, they still remain well below those that can be achieved with established IVF procedures. The first successful attempt of deep freezing and thawing of a human oocyte was reported by Chen in 1986 [41], while a twin pregnancy was achieved after insemination and replacement in utero of frozen–thawed oocytes one year later by Van Uem et al. [42].

Slow-freeze protocols using controlled rate freezers that decrease the temperature to below −30°C have traditionally been used for embryo cryopreservation in the laboratory. Additionally, diverse cryoprotectant solutions have been used for embryo dehydration, depending on the cell stage. Recently, a lot of attention has been given to an ultra-rapid method of cryopreservation or vitrification, whereby the embryo is transitioned from 37°C to −196°C in less than 1 sec. Vitrification has shown great promise for cryopreservation of human embryos and oocytes, because it minimizes cryo-injuries by preventing the formation of intracellular ice crystals. The first successful human cleavage-stage embryo vitrification followed by a successful delivery was reported by Gordts et al. in 1990 [43], while the first live births after vitrification of oocytes from a stimulated IVF cycle were reported in 2003 by Yoon et al. [44].

Oocyte donation

The first successful delivery following oocyte donation was announced by Buster et al. in 1983 [45]. The original technique involved intracervical artificial insemination of a volunteer with spermatozoa from the partner of the infertile woman, uterine lavage during the preimplantation interval, and finally, transfer of the developed embryo to the uterus of the infertile woman, who received a hormone replacement regimen in order to synchronize endometrial and embryo development. The same year, the first pregnancy after ovum donation, IVF, and transfer in a woman without ovaries was reported by Trounson et al. [46]. Within a year, the first pregnancy resulting from oocyte donation in a woman with ovarian failure was also reported [47].

Preimplantation genetic diagnosis

When Robert Edwards moved to Cambridge (U.K.), he suggested to one of his students, Richard Gardner, that he follow-up on the Glasgow work on stem cells. Their first approach was to inject one or several mouse inner cellular mass cells or cultured embryo stem cells into the blastocoelic cavity of recipient blastocysts, using specific genetic markers for host and donor cells. The method worked as chimerism and was established in literally all tissues of many offspring. They also worked jointly to test if operations on rabbit blastocysts would permit the excision of a few cells, which could be used for establishing the gender ("sexing") by staining them for the sex chromatin body expressed in female but not male embryos. After transferring the "sexed" blastocysts to recipient females, all offspring were correctly sexed – the first example of preimplantation genetic diagnosis (PGD) [48].

Preimplantation genetic diagnosis was only introduced clinically at the beginning of the 1990s as an alternative to prenatal diagnosis, in order to select healthy embryos, thus reducing the risk of having a child affected by a sex-linked genetic disease. The first embryos obtained in vitro were tested to determine their gender, and only female embryos were transferred. Handyside et al. [49] were the first to describe pregnancies from biopsied human preimplantation embryos that were selected for gender by Y-specific DNA amplification in order to avoid the transmission of a sex-linked disease to boys, adrenoleukodystrophy, and X-linked mental retardation. Since then, techniques for genetic analysis at the single-cell level, involving assessment of first and second polar bodies, fluorescence *in situ* hybridization (FISH) for the analysis of chromosomes, and polymerase chain reaction (PCR) for the analysis of genes in cases of monogenic diseases, have been introduced. The first report on polar body biopsy, transfer of the embryo, and achievement of pregnancy was by Verlinsky et al. in 1990 [50]. Pregnancy after embryo biopsy and coamplification of DNA from X- and Y-chromosomes was reported by Grifo et al. [51]. Munné et al. published the first report of aneuploidy testing in 1995 [52]. The first live birth following blastocyst biopsy and PGD analysis was reported in 2002 by De Boer et al. [53]. The same year, the first clinical application of comparative genomic hybridization and polar body testing for PGD of aneuploidy was performed by Wells et al. [54]. The first clinical experience of preimplantation human leukocyte antigen (HLA) matching without PGD of a causative gene was reported by Verlinsky et al., demonstrating the feasibility of this novel approach for stem cell transplantation in siblings with bone marrow failure [55]. Recently, Fishel and colleagues from CARE Fertility, Nottingham (U.K.) reported a live birth after polar body array comparative genomic hybridization [56].

In vitro maturation

The application of IVF in combination with ovarian stimulation has proved to be a successful treatment for infertile couples. However, several drawbacks of this technique, for example, the risk of ovarian hyperstimulation syndrome, the high cost of medication, the inconvenience of daily gonadotropin injections, and their side effects, have stimulated researchers to develop new treatment strategies. The idea of retrieving immature oocytes from the unstimulated ovary, to mature them in vitro, and finally to fertilize the resulting mature oocytes in order to create multiple embryos seemed to be an attractive idea and a solution that could compensate for the disadvantages of IVF. The first human pregnancy following in vitro maturation (IVM) in an unstimulated cycle in a donor oocyte program was reported by Cha et al. [57], 13 years after the birth of Louise Brown. In 1994 the first live birth as a result of IVM in a polycystic ovarian syndrome (PCOS) patient following transvaginal ultrasound-guided oocyte collection was reported by Trounson et al. [58]. A first report of fertility preservation for cancer patients using IVM and oocyte vitrification was published by Rao et al. [59]. The team at McGill Reproductive Center (Canada) has reported a series of deliveries after transfer of human blastocysts derived from oocytes matured in vitro, showing an implantation rate of 26.8% and a clinical pregnancy rate of 51.9% [60].

Ovarian tissue cryopreservation

Cryopreservation of ovarian tissue is the only option available for prepubertal girls and women who have to undergo chemotherapy without delay and wish to preserve their fertility. Several attempts were made to cryopreserve ovarian cortex strips and reimplant them after thawing. With regards to autotransplantation, Oktay and Karlikaya were the first to report on ovarian tissue transplants after frozen storage [61]. However, the first pregnancy was reported a few years later by Donnez et al. [62]. In 1997, they took biopsy samples of ovarian cortex from a woman with stage IV Hodgkin's lymphoma, which were cryopreserved before chemotherapy was initiated. After her cancer treatment, the patient developed premature ovarian failure. In 2003, after thawing, orthotopic autotransplantation of the ovarian cortical tissue was realized by laparoscopy. Eleven months after reimplantation, a viable intrauterine pregnancy was confirmed, which resulted in a live birth. Since this first live birth after autotransplantation of cryopreserved ovarian tissue, orthotopic reimplantation has led to the birth of 13 healthy babies from cancer patients and women treated with high doses of chemotherapy for benign diseases [63]. Pregnancies have also been obtained after heterologous transplantation of fresh or cryopreserved ovarian cortical tissue between twins discordant for premature ovarian failure [64,65]. Despite the births from ovarian tissue transplantation, the overall success rate remains low and further research is needed in order to define the optimal conditions for ovarian tissue transplantation. Alternatives, such as whole ovary or isolated follicle transplantation, require further investigation but are likely to be successful in humans in the future.

Conclusion

The road to finding a cure to human infertility has been bumpy, but since the birth of Louise Brown, the first IVF baby, substantial progress has been made. As technology and outcomes improved, ART became a successful treatment for an increasing number of infertile couples worldwide. The advent of those techniques greatly contributed to the rise in the number of children born from ART. Robert Edwards forced the doors open but we are still at the end of the beginning of the development of ART.

References

1. Data presented at the 2010 Annual Conference of the European Society of Human Reproduction and Embryology in Rome, Italy, 2010.
2. International Committee Monitoring Assisted Reproductive Technologies (ICMART): de Mouzon J, Lancaster P, Nygren KG, et al. World collaborative report on assisted reproductive technology, 2002. *Hum Reprod* 2009; **24**: 2310–2320.
3. Hunter J. The Works, vol 4. Cited by Moore W in *The Knife Man*. London, UK: Bantam, 2005; 461–463.
4. Nelson H. The reproduction of the *Ascaris mystax*. *Phil Trans R Soc Lond* 1852; **142**: 563–594.

5. Heape W. Preliminary note on the transplantation and growth of mammalian ova within a uterine foster-mother. *Proc Roy Soc* 1891; **48**: 457–458.
6. Biggers JD. Walter Heape, FRS: a pioneer in reproductive biology. Centenary of his embryo transfer experiments. *J Reprod Fert* 1991; **93**: 173–186.
7. Pincus G, Enzmann EV. The comparative behavior of mammalian eggs in vivo and in vitro: I. The activation of ovarian eggs. *J Exp Med* 1935; **62**: 665–675.
8. Chang MC. Fertilization of rabbit ova in vitro. *Nature* 1959; **184**: 466–467.
9. Edwards RG, Fowler RE. The experimental induction of superfoetation in the mouse. *J Endocrin* 1958; **17**: 223–236.
10. Edwards RG, Gates AH. Timing of the stages of the maturation divisions, ovulation, fertilization and the first cleavage of eggs of adult mice treated with gonadotrophins. *J Endocrin* 1959; **18**: 292–304.
11. Edwards RG, Sirlin JL. Fate of spermatozoa penetrating into the tissues of the fallopian tube. *Nature* 1959; **183**: 1744–1745.
12. Edwards RG. Maturation in vitro of mouse, sheep, cow, pig, rhesus monkey and human ovarian oocytes. *Nature* 1965; **208**: 349–351.
13. Edwards RG. Maturation in vitro of human ovarian oocytes. *Lancet* 1965; **2**: 926–929.
14. Edwards RG, Bavister BD, Steptoe PC. Early stages of fertilization in vitro of human oocytes matured in vitro. *Nature* 1969; **221**: 632–635.
15. De Kretzer D, Dennis P, Hudson B, et al. Transfer of a human zygote. *Lancet* 1973; **29**: 728–729.
16. Steptoe PC, Edwards RG. Reimplantation of a human embryo with subsequent tubal pregnancy. *Lancet* 1976; **1**: 880–882.
17. Edwards RG, Steptoe PC, Purdy JM. Fertilization and cleavage in vitro of preovulator human oocytes. *Nature* 1970; **227**: 1307–1309.
18. Steptoe PC, Edwards RG. Birth after the reimplantation of a human embryo. *Lancet* 1978; **2**: 366.
19. Edwards RG, Steptoe PC, Purdy JM. Establishing full-term human pregnancies using cleaving embryos grown in vitro. *Br J Obstet Gynaecol* 1980; **87**: 737–756.
20. Lopata A, Johnston IW, Hoult IJ, Speirs AI. Pregnancy following intrauterine implantation of an embryo obtained by in vitro fertilization of a preovulatory egg. *Fertil Steril* 1980; **33**: 117–120.
21. Trounson AO, Leeton JF, Wood C, Webb J, Wood J. Pregnancies in humans by fertilization in vitro and embryo transfer in the controlled ovulatory cycle. *Science* 1981; **212**: 681–682.
22. Jones HW Jr, Jones GS, Andrews MC, et al. The program for in vitro fertilization at Norfolk. *Fertil Steril* 1982; **38**: 14–21.
23. Testart J, Frydman R. Full-term delivery after intrauterine implantation of an embryo obtained by in vitro fertilization. *J Gynecol Obstet Biol Reprod* 1982; **11**: 855–859.
24. Hamberger L, Wikland M, Nilsson L, et al. Methods for aspiration of human oocytes by various techniques. *Acta Med Rom* 1982; **20**: 370–378.
25. Feichtinger W, Szalay S, Kemeter P, Beck A, Janisch H. Twin pregnancy after laparoscopic oocyte recovery, in-vitro fertilization and embryo transfer. *Geburtshilfe Frauenheilkd* 1982; **42**: 197–199.
26. Shettles LB. Ova harvest with in vivo fertilization. *Am J Obstet Gynecol* 1979; **133**: 845.
27. Tesarík J, Pilka L, Dvorák M, Trávník P. Oocyte recovery, in vitro insemination, and transfer into the oviduct after its microsurgical repair at a single laparotomy. *Fertil Steril* 1983; **39**: 472–475.
28. Devroey P, Braeckmans P, Smitz J, et al. Pregnancy after translaparoscopic zygote intrafallopian transfer in a patient with sperm antibodies. *Lancet* 1986; **1**: 1329.
29. Tournaye H, Devroey P, Camus M, et al. Comparison of in-vitro fertilization in male and tubal infertility: a 3 year survey. *Hum Reprod* 1992; **7**: 218–222.
30. Lanzendorf SE, Maloney MK, Veeck LL, et al. A preclinical evaluation of pronuclear formation by microinjection of human spermatozoa into human oocytes. *Fertil Steril* 1988; **49**: 835–842.
31. Palermo G, Joris H, Devroey P, Van Steirteghem AC. Pregnancies after intracytoplasmic injection of single spermatozoon into an oocyte. *Lancet* 1992; **4**: 17–18.
32. Temple-Smith PD, Southwick GJ, Yates CA, Trounson AO, de Kretser DM. Human pregnancy by in vitro fertilization (IVF) using sperm aspirated from the epididymis. *J In Vitro Fert Embryo Transf* 1985; **2**: 119–122.
33. Patrizio P, Silber S, Ord T, Balmaceda JP, Asch RH. Two births after microsurgical sperm aspiration in congenital absence of vas deferens. *Lancet* 1988; **2**: 1364.
34. Silber SJ, Ord T, Borrero T, Balmaceda J, Asch R. New treatment for infertility due to congenital absence of the vas deferens. *Lancet* 1987; **2**: 850–851.
35. Schoysman R, Van der Zwalmen P, Nijs M, Segal-Bertin G, Van de Casseye M. Successful fertilization by testicular spermatozoa in an in-vitro fertilization programme. *Hum Reprod* 1993; **8**: 1339–1340.
36. Silber SJ, Nagy ZP, Liu J, et al. Conventional in-vitro fertilization versus intracytoplasmic sperm injection for patients requiring microsurgical sperm aspiration. *Hum Reprod* 1994; **9**: 1705–1709.

37. Tournaye H, Devroey P, Liu J, et al. Microsurgical epididymal sperm aspiration and intracytoplasmic sperm injection: a new effective approach to infertility as a result of congenital bilateral absence of vas deferens. *Fertil Steril* 1994; **61**: 1445–1450.

38. Devroey P, Liu J, Nagy Z, et al. Pregnancies after testicular sperm extraction and intracytoplasmic sperm injection in non-obstructive azoospermia. *Hum Reprod* 1995; **10**: 1457–1460.

39. Trounson A, Mohr L. Human pregnancy following cryopreservation, thawing and transfer of an eight-cell embryo. *Nature* 1983; **305**: 707–709.

40. Zeilmaker GH, Alberda AT, van Gent I, Rijkmans CM, Drogendijk AC. A report of pregnancy following transfer of intact frozen-thawed embryos. Two pregnancies following transfer of intact frozen-thawed embryos. *Fertil Steril* 1984; **42**: 293–296.

41. Chen C. Pregnancy after human oocyte cryopreservation. *Lancet* 1986; **1**: 884–886.

42. Van Uem JF, Siebzehnrübl ER, Schuh B, et al. Birth after cryopreservation of unfertilized oocytes. *Lancet* 1987; **329**: 752–753.

43. Gordts S, Roziers P, Campo R, Noto V. Survival and pregnancy outcome after ultrarapid freezing of human embryos. *Fertil Steril* 1990; **53**: 469–472.

44. Yoon TK, Kim TJ, Park SE, et al. Live births after vitrification of oocytes in a stimulated in vitro fertilization-embryo transfer program. *Fertil Steril* 2003; **79**: 1323–1326.

45. Buster JE, Bustillo M, Thorneycroft IH, et al. Non-surgical transfer of in vivo fertilized donated ova to five infertile women: report of two pregnancies. *Lancet* 1983; **2**: 223–224.

46. Trounson A, Leeton J, Besanko M, Wood C, Conti A. Pregnancy established in an infertile patient after transfer of a donated embryo fertilized in vitro. *BMJ* 1983; **286**: 835–838.

47. Lutjen P, Trounson A, Leeton J, et al. The establishment and maintenance of pregnancy using in vitro fertilization and embryo donation in a patient with primary ovarian failure. *Nature* 1984; **307**: 174–175.

48. Gardner RL, Edwards RG. Control of the sex ratio at full term in the rabbit by transferring sexed blastocysts. *Nature* 1968; **218**: 346–348.

49. Handyside AH, Kontogianni EH, Hardy K, Winston RM. Pregnancies from biopsied human preimplantation embryos sexed by Y-specific DNA amplification. *Nature* 1990; **344**: 768–770.

50. Verlinsky Y, Ginsberg N, Lifchez A, et al. Analysis of the first polar body: preconception genetic diagnosis. *Hum Reprod* 1990; **5**: 826–829.

51. Grifo JA, Tang YX, Cohen J, et al. Pregnancy after embryo biopsy and coamplification of DNA from X and Y chromosomes. *JAMA* 1992; **12**: 727–729.

52. Munné S, Sultan KM, Weier HU, et al. Assessment of numeric abnormalities of X, Y, 18, and 16 chromosomes in preimplantation human embryos before transfer. *Am J Obstet Gynecol* 1995; **172**: 1191–1199.

53. De Boer K, McArthur S, Murray C, Jansen R. First live birth following blastocyst biopsy and PGD analysis. *Reprod Biomed Online* 2002; **4**: 35.

54. Wells D, Escudero T, Levy B, et al. First clinical application of comparative genomic hybridization and polar body testing for preimplantation genetic diagnosis of aneuploidy. *Fertil Steril* 2002; **3**: 543–549.

55. Verlinsky Y, Rechitsky S, Sharapova T, et al. Preimplantation HLA testing. *JAMA* 2004; **17**: 2079–2085.

56. Fishel S, Gordon A, Lynch C, et al. Live birth after polar body array comparative genomic hybridization prediction of embryo ploidy – the future of IVF? *Fertil Steril* 2010; **93**: 1006.e7–e10.

57. Cha KY, Koo JJ, Choi DH, et al. Pregnancy after in vitro fertilization of human follicular oocytes collected from non stimulated cycles, their culture in vitro and their transfer in a donor oocyte program. *Fertil Steril* 1991; **55**: 109–113.

58. Trounson A, Wood C, Kausche A. In vitro maturation and the fertilization and developmental competence of oocytes recovered from untreated polycystic ovarian patients. *Fertil Steril* 1994; **62**: 353–362.

59. Rao GD, Chian RC, Son WS, Gilbert L, Tan SL. Fertility preservation in women undergoing cancer treatment. *Lancet* 2004; **363**: 1829–1830.

60. Son WY, Lee SY, Yoon SH, Lim JH. Pregnancies and deliveries after transfer of human blastocysts derived from in vitro matured oocytes in in vitro maturation cycles. *Fertil Steril* 2007; **6**: 1491–1493.

61. Oktay K, Karlikaya G. Ovarian function after transplantation of frozen, banked autologous ovarian tissue. *N Engl J Med* 2000; **342**: 1919.

62. Donnez J, Dolmans MM, Demylle D, et al. Live birth after orthotopic transplantation of cryopreserved ovarian tissue. *Lancet* 2004: **364**: 1405–1410.

63. Donnez J, Silber S, Andersen CY, et al. Children born after autotransplantation of cryopreserved ovarian tissue. A review of 13 live births. *Ann Med* 2011; **43**: 437–450.

64. Silber SJ, Lenahan KM, Levine DJ, et al. Ovarian transplantation between monozygotic twins discordant for premature ovarian failure. *N Engl J Med* 2005; **353**: 58–63.

65. Silber SJ, Gosden RG. Ovarian transplantation in a series of monozygotic twins discordant for ovarian failure. *N Engl J Med* 2007; **356**: 1382–1384.

Chapter 3

The role of ultrasound in early pregnancy after assisted conception

Andrea Day and Davor Jurkovic

Introduction

Ultrasound is currently considered the main diagnostic tool in obstetrics and gynecology. In assisted reproduction units, it is routinely used for the diagnosis and management of infertile women. Once pregnancy is achieved, transvaginal ultrasound is performed to locate the pregnancy, confirm viability, and monitor progress. Women who conceived by means of assisted reproductive technology (ART) tend to be older and are more likely to have uterine, tubal, or ovarian abnormalities, which increase their risk of early pregnancy complications such as ectopic pregnancy and miscarriage. In addition, assisted conception itself carries a risk of complications such as ovarian hyperstimulation and ovarian torsion. In order to provide women with high-quality care in their pregnancy, it is essential that clinicians are familiar with the ultrasound features of normal and abnormal pregnancy, as well as common gynecological abnormalities of the uterus and adnexa. If either ectopic pregnancy or miscarriage is diagnosed, ultrasound can also help in selecting women for different management options. This chapter describes ultrasound findings and management of early pregnancy and its complications, as well as uterine and adnexal pathologies frequently seen in these patients.

Normal pregnancy

Early pregnancy

In women who undergo assisted reproduction, the first confirmation of pregnancy is usually made by performing a urine pregnancy test or by measuring serum β-hCG (beta-human chorionic gonadotrophin) between days 14 and 17 after conception. The location of the gestation sac in a normal pregnancy can be reliably confirmed by ultrasound three weeks after conception (i.e., five weeks after the last menstrual period in a woman with a regular 28-day cycle). In practice, the first scan is usually scheduled for four to five weeks after conception when the embryonic heartbeat should also be visible. The transvaginal approach is more effective in early gestation and should be used in preference to transabdominal scanning. When assessing the uterus, the probe is moved in the transverse plane from the internal os to the fundus in search of an intrauterine pregnancy. The longitudinal view is then used to show the location of the gestational sac beneath the endometrial surface and to confirm its intrauterine location by demonstrating a communication between the cervical canal and the uterine cavity. If a gestational sac is not visible, the endometrial morphology and thickness need to be assessed. A thickened endometrium can be seen in early intrauterine pregnancy, in ectopic pregnancy (decidual reaction), or when retained products of conception (RPOC) are present, and therefore, measurements of endometrial thickness are not useful for differentiating these conditions [1]. Sweeping the probe both side-to-side and up-and-down will facilitate the assessment of the cervix, Cesarean section scar (if present), myometrium, and interstitial portion of the Fallopian tubes, to rule out unusual sites of ectopic pregnancy implantation.

In a normal pregnancy, the first structure to appear is the gestational sac, which becomes visible on a transvaginal scan at four weeks and three days of gestation. It usually appears as a circular structure, with a double echogenic rim surrounding a clear anechoic center, located below the midline echo, buried into the decidua (Table 3.1) (Figure 3.1(a)). Accumulation of blood within the uterine cavity can sometimes appear similar to an early gestational sac. This is described as a pseudosac, which is particularly common in ectopic

Pregnancy After Assisted Reproductive Technology, ed. Eric R. M. Jauniaux and Botros R. M. B. Rizk. Published by Cambridge University Press.

Table 3.1. Ultrasound differentiation between an early intrauterine gestational sac and a pseudosac

Ultrasound image / Characteristic	Early intrauterine pregnancy	Pseudosac
	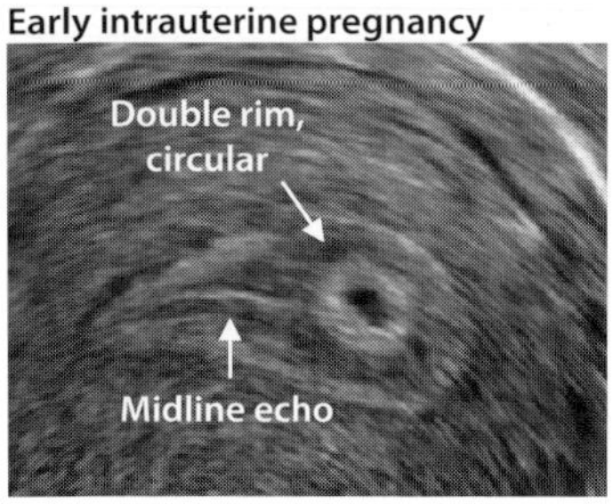	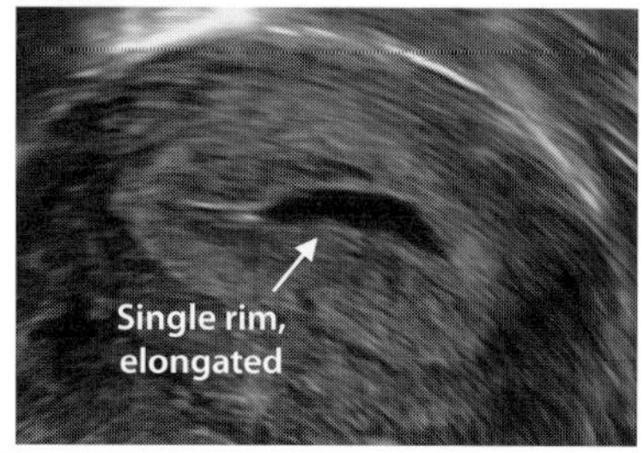
LOCATION	Below midline, buried into decidua	Midline, between endometrial layers
SHAPE	Circular and steady	Elongated, varies during scan
BORDER	Echogenic rim (double)	Single decidual layer
COLOR FLOW	High peripheral flow	Avascular

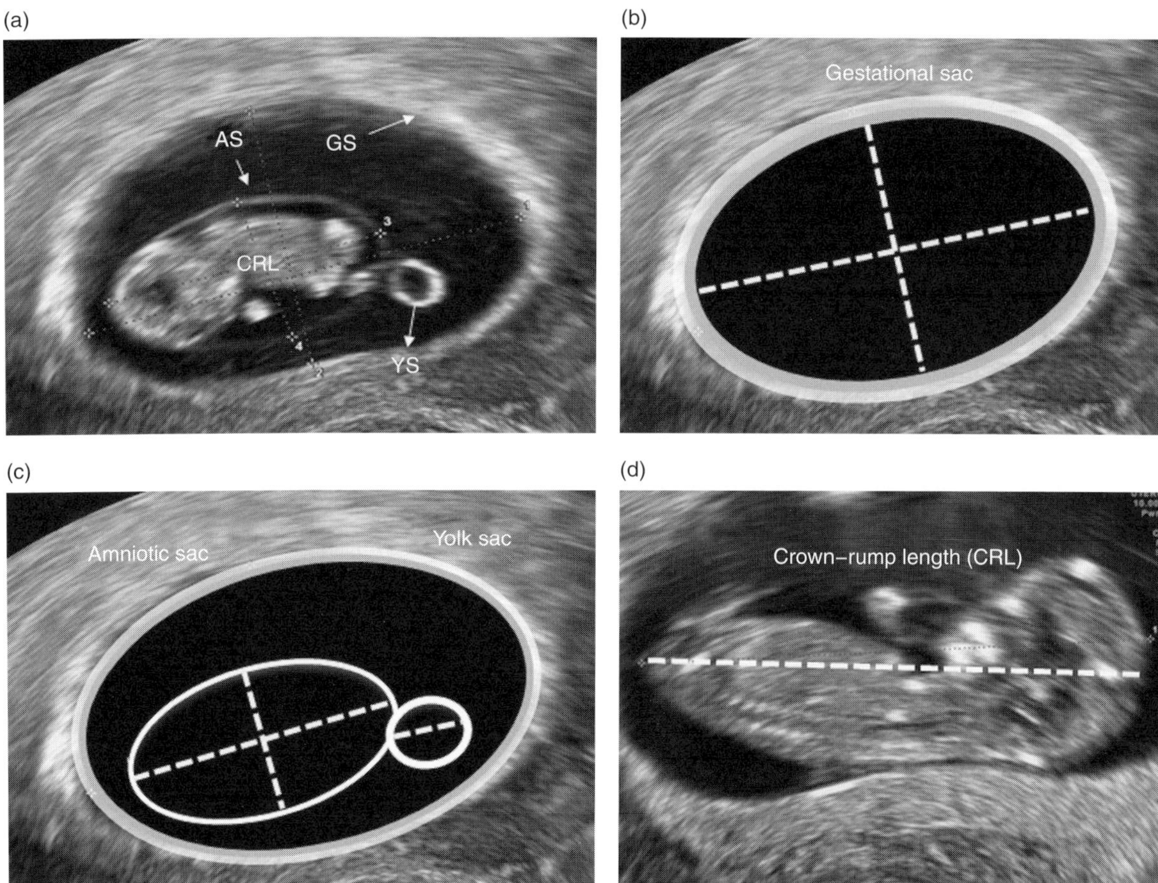

GS = gestational sac, YS = yolk sac, AS = amniotic sac, CRL = crown–rump length

Figure 3.1. Ultrasound structures measured in early pregnancy. (a): ultrasound findings in early pregnancy; (b): measurement of the gestational sac; (c): measurement of the yolk sac and amniotic sac; (d): measurement of crown–rump length (CRL).

pregnancy, and it should not be confused with an intrauterine gestation. A pseudosac appears like an elongated structure inside the cavity, surrounded by a single decidual layer (Table 3.1). This structure is avascular on color Doppler examination and may change in shape during the scan, while a normal pregnancy tends to have high peripheral blood flow and its shape is constant. The gestational sac is measured using the mean of three perpendicular diameters (Figure 3.1(b)). Growth rate in early gestation approximates 1 mm per day. A large, empty, and irregular gestational sac is suggestive of pregnancy failure (this will be discussed in more detail in the miscarriage section of this chapter).

The yolk sac becomes visible within the chorionic cavity from five weeks' gestation. The measurement technique is similar to that of the gestational sac, always including three perpendicular diameters from the center of the yolk sac wall (Figure 3.1(c)) [2]. If the yolk sac is large (>5.6 mm) [3] or not visible when the mean gestational sac diameter reaches >13 mm [4], repeated ultrasound a week later is advised as these findings are associated with early pregnancy failure.

Adjacent to the yolk sac, a linear structure becomes visible, which represents the embryonic pole and is measured by its greatest length. At six weeks' gestation, the embryo develops into a kidney-bean shape, with the yolk sac separated from the embryo by the vitelline duct. From seven weeks' gestation onwards, the crown (head) can be distinguished from the rump (trunk), and crown–rump length (CRL) should be measured from a sagittal section of the embryo, with care not to include the yolk sac inadvertently (Figure 3.1(d)) [5]. Three different images should be evaluated and the largest length should be recorded. If an embryo is not visible with a mean gestational sac diameter of >20 mm, the pregnancy is likely to be abnormal and another scan should be organized a week later. Close monitoring is also indicated if the embryo is smaller than expected for gestational age, as the date of oocyte retrieval and CRL are practically equivalent methods used to calculate gestational age [6] in patients undergoing assisted reproduction.

Viability is confirmed at around five weeks and three days of gestation, when the CRL measures 2–5 mm and cardiac activity can be seen. Background movement and maternal pulsation can sometimes be misinterpreted as embryonic cardiac activity. The heart rate should be measured using M-mode; pulsed Doppler examination produces high-energy acoustic outputs and should not be used in early first-trimester pregnancy [7]. It has been reported that rates below 100 beats per minute suggest a poor prognosis [8,9]. However, it is important to recognize that in very early normal gestations, the heart rate could be below 100 beats per minute, yet increase rapidly between six and nine weeks' gestation. Consequently, rate is a less reliable indicator than presence or absence of fetal heartbeat. If a heartbeat is not visible in a fetus measuring >10 mm, color Doppler may be useful to confirm a negative finding.

From seven weeks' gestation, the amniotic cavity becomes visible and should be measured in three dimensions (Figure 3.1(c)). In addition, the rhombencephalon and spine may be distinguished and the umbilical cord seen. At eight weeks' gestation, the forebrain, midbrain, hindbrain, and skull are apparent and limb buds start to grow. The amniotic cavity expands while the umbilical cord and vitelline duct lengthen and a midgut hernia appears. During seven to nine weeks' gestation, the amniotic and chorionic cavities are not fused and chorionicity and amnionicity of multiple pregnancies may be established.

Multiple pregnancy

The Human Fertilization and Embryology Authority (HFEA) monitors and regulates the number of embryos transferred, and currently in the U.K. no more than two embryos are transferred in a single treatment cycle in women less than 40 years of age, and no more than three embryos in women more than 40 years old who are using their own eggs [10]. Assisted reproductive technology enhances the rate of zygotic splitting, hence monozygotic twins sometimes occur after a single embryo transfer. The diagnosis of multiple pregnancy in the first trimester is essential, as determination of chorionicity and amnionicity is relatively simple, and women could be advised about the risk associated with different types of multiple pregnancies.

Dizygotic twins develop from two different oocytes fertilized by two different spermatozoa, and they implant separately. As a result, each embryo has its own gestational sac (chorion), amniotic sac (amnion), and placenta. Consequently, dizygotic twins are always dichorionic and diamniotic. Monozygotic twins arise from a single oocyte fertilized by one spermatozoon, which then divides. The stage of development at which it divides is what determines its chorionicity and amnionicity. If it divides prior to implantation, it results in a dichorionic and diamniotic pregnancy. If

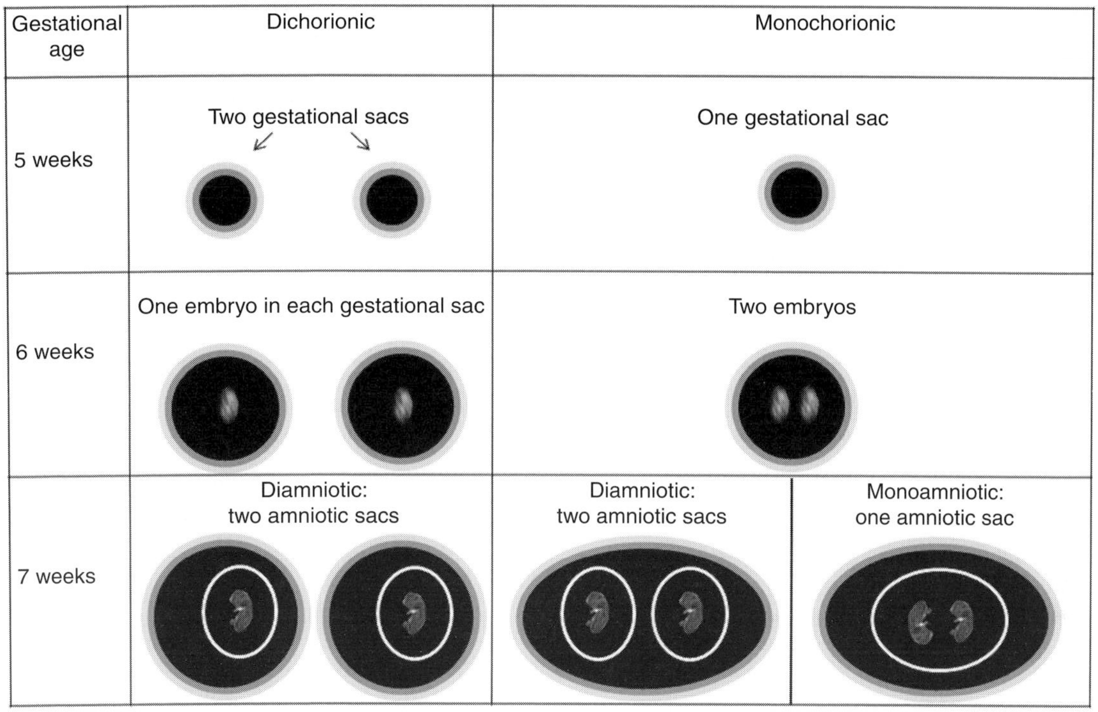

*Yolk sac not included the number is variable in monochorionic/monoamniotic twins

Figure 3.2. Schematic representation of ultrasound findings to determine amnionicity and chorionicity in early multiple pregnancy according to gestational week.

the division occurs after implantation, a single gestational sac is formed, hence pregnancy is monochorionic. Hereafter, if division occurs on day four to day eight of development, the pregnancy is monochorionic and diamniotic, and if it occurs on day nine to day thirteen of development, the pregnancy is monochorionic and monoamniotic.

On ultrasound scanning, the first clue to a multiple pregnancy is the presence of more than one gestational sac at around five weeks' gestation. The number of gestational sacs and yolk sacs may be variable and does not always correlate with the number of embryos in multiple pregnancies, and therefore, only the latter should be used to make the diagnosis. It is imperative to examine the entire chorionic cavity to make sure all embryos are seen when pregnancy progresses beyond six weeks' gestation. Figure 3.2 illustrates the ultrasound features for each type of multiple pregnancy according to gestational week. Amnionicity should be assessed at around seven weeks' gestation when the amnion is seen separate to the embryo. At this stage, the chorion and amnion are not fused, which facilitates determination of amnionicity and chorionicity (Figure 3.3). After the amnion and chorion are fused, the assessment of chorionicity becomes more difficult and it relies on the assessment of thickness of the dividing membrane and the shape of its junction with the uterine wall ("lambda" or "T" sign). If the dividing membrane between two embryos/fetuses within the same gestational sac is absent, the pregnancy is classified as monochorionic and monoamniotic (Figure 3.4). In the case of higher multiples, the same principles are applied.

Abnormal pregnancy

Miscarriage

Miscarriage is defined as a pregnancy failure occurring before the completion of twenty four weeks' gestation. Couples who have a history of infertility and conceive with assisted reproduction have a high risk of pregnancy (see Chapter 5) failure with an incidence of 15%–30% [11–13]. This is significantly higher if compared to the fertile population and could be attributed to higher maternal age at conception and early confirmation of pregnancy (see Chapter 5). In the U.K., the average age at which women undergo ART is 35 years

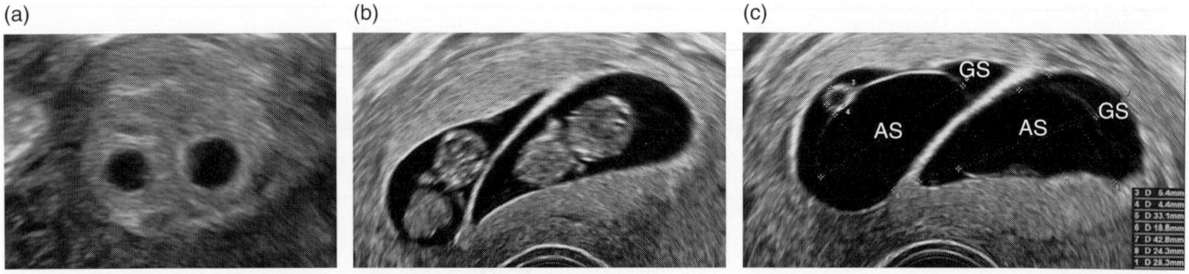

AS, amniotic sac; GS, gestational sac.

Figure 3.3. Ultrasound findings of a dichorionic and diamniotic pregnancy. (a): five weeks' gestation – two gestational sacs; (b): six weeks' gestation – two embryos; (c): seven weeks' gestation – two amniotic sacs.

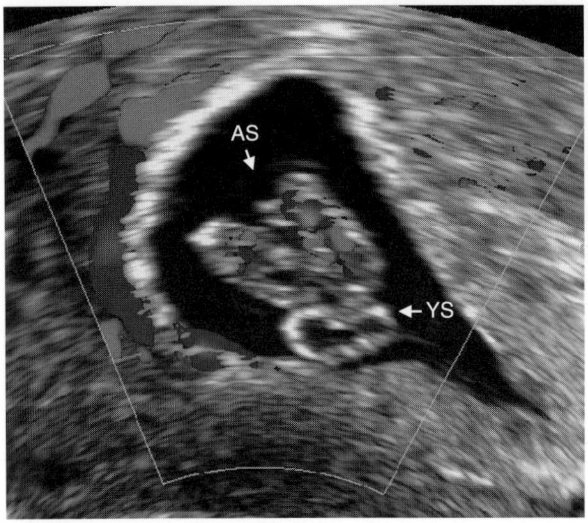

AS, amniotic sac; YS, yolk sac.

Figure 3.4. Ultrasound findings of a monochorionic and monoamniotic pregnancy: one gestational sac, one amniotic sac, one yolk sac, and two embryos. (See color plate section for colored image.)

old [14], and it is well known that from this age there is a significant increase in the rate of fetal death, with an odds ratio of 1.9 at 35 to 39 years old when compared with women less than 30 years of age [15]. Miscarriage can be suspected with the presence of abdominal pain or vaginal bleeding; however, ultrasound examination is the primary test to diagnose early pregnancy failure. Presence of an embryonic heartbeat at the time of the initial ultrasound scan does not always denote a normal pregnancy. Tummers et al. [11] looked at the risk of miscarriage in a group of patients who underwent in vitro fertilization (IVF) and intracytoplasmatic spermatozoon injection (ICSI) and reported a risk of miscarriage of 12.2 % after visualization of positive heart action in singleton pregnancies. Therefore, all pregnancy structures should be assessed as these will help predict outcome in potentially viable pregnancies. The risk of miscarriage gradually decreases with every subsequent week of gestation.

Table 3.2 lists the landmarks used for the diagnosis of miscarriage in early pregnancy. The presence of a large empty gestational sac (≥20 mm) or an embryo measuring 10 mm or more (CRL) without cardiac activity are suggestive of early pregnancy failure [16–19]. Diagnosis of miscarriage should only be made a week later and it should be confirmed by one additional independent operator. If the given criteria are not met (i.e., gestational sac <20 mm or CRL <10 mm), a repeat scan should be performed two weeks later, and if there is no significant change, a miscarriage can be diagnosed and should also be confirmed by an additional operator. Pregnancies achieved using ART have a certain date of fertilization, and theoretically failure to identify an embryonic heartbeat at six weeks' gestation could be used to diagnose a nonviable pregnancy. However, in some abnormal pregnancies the embryo develops more slowly and the cardiac activity may appear much later than expected. For that reason most units continue to follow the protocol shown in Table 3.2, established for the general population.

Other morphological features have been associated with a higher likelihood of miscarriage and may be used to initiate appropriate counseling and follow-up; however, these characteristics should not be used for the diagnosis of early embryonic demise. They include:

- Visualization of an amniotic and yolk sac without a viable embryo (Figure 3.5(a)).
- Irregular gestational sac with a thin trophoblastic reaction, which can demonstrate angular

Table 3.2. Criteria for the diagnosis of early embryonic demise

Landmark[17,18]	Ultrasound picture
GESTATIONAL SAC: Empty GS ≥ 20 mm, no change in 1 week Empty GS < 20 mm, no change in 2 weeks	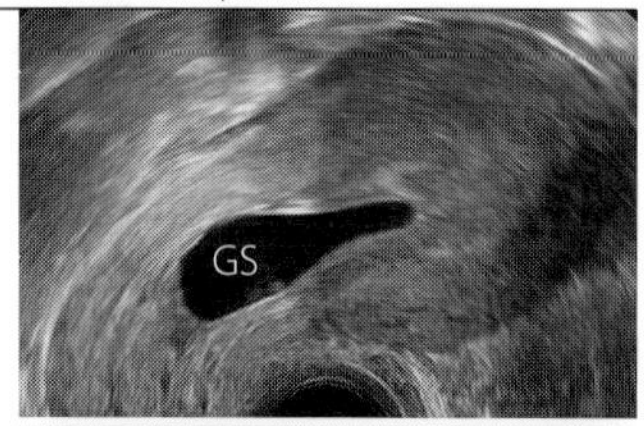
HEART ACTION: CRL ≥ 10mm without FH, no change in 1 week CRL < 10 mm without FH, no change in 2 weeks	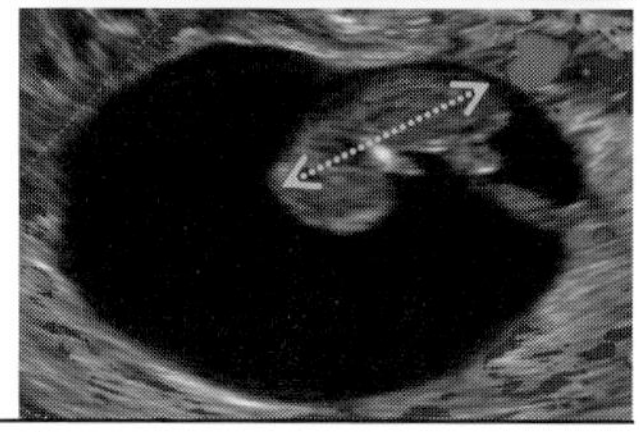

GS , gestational sac; CRL , crown–rump length; FH , fetal heartbeat.

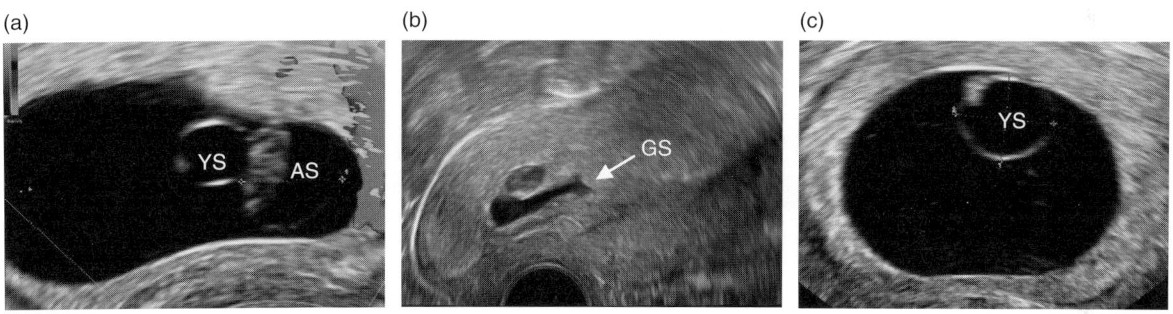

GS = gestational sac, YS = yolk sac, AS = amniotic sac

Figure 3.5. Ultrasound features associated with a higher likelihood of miscarriage. (a): yolk sac and amniotic sac without a viable embryo; (b): gestational sac located low in the uterine cavity; (c): large yolk sac. (See color plate section for colored image of Figure 3.5(a).)

appearance or be located low in the uterine cavity [20] (Figure 3.5(b)).

- Large yolk sac with a mean diameter >5.6 mm[3] (Figure 3.5(c)).
- Smaller than expected CRL, even with a normal heartbeat [21].
- Discrepancy between the sizes of the gestational sac and embryo, particularly if the mean gestational sac diameter minus CRL is <5 mm [22,23].
- Embryonic/fetal bradycardia (heart rate below the fifth percentile or <85 beats per minute [24]).

In multiple pregnancies, a significant discrepancy in CRL of twins may be associated with the loss of one twin [25]. Partial or complete reabsorption of an embryo may occur and is often described as "vanishing twin syndrome" [26,27]. This phenomenon was described mainly from transabdominal scans, which in itself might overestimate its true incidence as in some cases small subchorionic hematomas may be mistaken for a second gestational sac (see Chapter 8). The latest data published by HFEA report that in 2008 the loss of one twin occurred in 13% of patients and a miscarriage with loss of all embryos in 5% of cases (Figure 3.6) [28]. Similarly, in 2003 Benson et al. [29] reported a 12% loss of one twin and 9% loss of both. Patients may present with vaginal bleeding and ultrasound assessment is warranted.

Without a well-defined gestational sac, but given visible RPOC, an incomplete miscarriage can be diagnosed. The presence of blood clots may cause uncertainty and need differentiation. Retained products

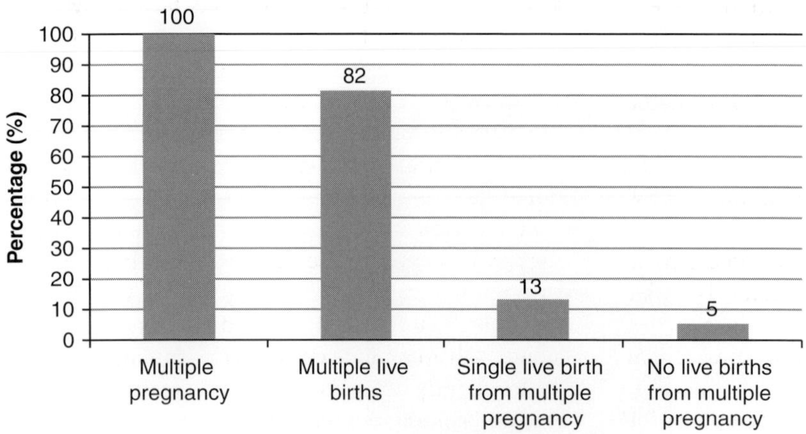

Figure 3.6. Outcomes of multiple pregnancies following assisted reproductive technology [HFEA 2008].

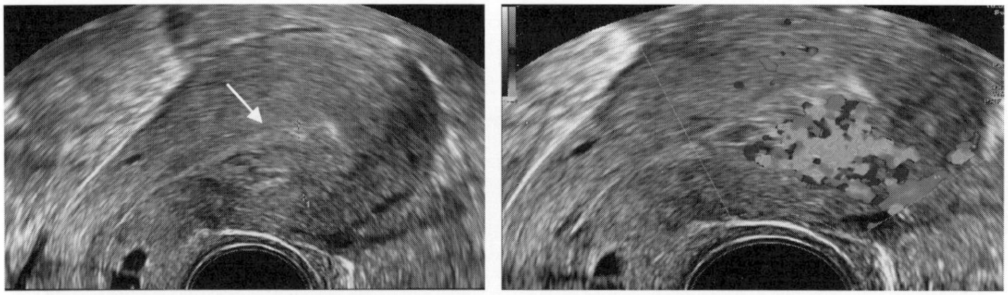

Figure 3.7. Ultrasound appearance of retained products of conception. (a): well-defined hyperechoic area (arrow); (b): high vascularity on Doppler examination. (See color plate section for colored image of Figure 3.7(b).)

are usually seen as a well-defined area of hyperechoic tissue within the endometrial cavity [30], and frequently demonstrate increased vascularity on color Doppler examination (Figure 3.7). Blood clots on the other hand are ill defined and avascular. The size of the RPOC should be measured using three perpendicular diameters. There is no correlation between the amount of products and the clinical picture, and therefore symptomatic women may be offered surgical removal of RPOC even if the amount of tissue appears to be very small on the ultrasound image [31].

Complete miscarriage is diagnosed only when ultrasound examination fails to identify any pregnancy tissue within the uterine cavity in women who had clear evidence of an intrauterine pregnancy on a previous ultrasound examination. If a woman did not attend for previous scans, the pregnancy should be described as a "pregnancy of unknown location" (PUL), and further investigations are required. Serum β-hCG and progesterone are the two most commonly used biochemical markers for pregnancy in women who, despite a positive pregnancy test, have no visible pregnancy on ultrasound examination. Serum β-hCG is produced by the trophoblast but has a long half-life (32–37 hours) in serum [32]. In practice, a decline in serum β-hCG by 13% or more over 48 hours suggests a failing pregnancy [33]. On the other hand, serum progesterone in early pregnancy is produced mainly by the corpus luteum and has a very short half-life. As a result, a single measurement of serum progesterone can be used instead of serial serum β-hCG assessments to diagnose early pregnancy failure. In patients undergoing ART, however, serum progesterone measurements are of less value, as the women often have multiple corpus lutea and the use of exogenous progesterone affects the accuracy of diagnosis. Biochemical markers must be assessed in conjunction with clinical and ultrasound information and should not be used alone as a diagnostic tool.

Management of miscarriage in women with a history of infertility and ART is, on the whole, not different to that of the general population. Urgent treatment such as evacuation of RPOC is only required in patients who are hemodynamically unstable due to heavy bleeding or in great pain. Patients who are stable or present with mild symptoms could be treated expectantly, medically, or with surgery. The type of miscarriage and presence of intravillous blood flow play a significant role in the effectiveness of expectant management. The presence of early embryonic demise [34] or of vascular products [35] on color Doppler examination predict a higher chance of failure, therefore patients with these findings may not benefit from conservative management.

Surgical treatment is the most effective option for management of miscarriage, with a 97% estimated rate of complete evacuation [36]. This procedure can also be carried out in the outpatient setting, under local anesthetic, avoiding the need for an operating theater [37]. Use of intraoperative ultrasound may prove useful and reduce the overall complication rate, especially in cases of acute uterine ante- or retroflexion or cervical stenosis [38]. It can also help ensure complete uterine evacuation. Cervical damage and uterine perforation are uncommon complications of surgery, with rates of 0.3% and 1.9% quoted [39]. Uterine perforation should be suspected in women who experience symptoms of shock postoperatively or develop acute abdominal pain or unexpected bleeding. Ultrasound findings in these cases show blood in the pouch of Douglas. More commonly, patients may have incomplete removal of tissue, which should be suspected in women who experience heavy bleeding, abdominal pain, or continue to bleed per vagina for more than two weeks after the procedure. In these cases, a repeat ultrasound scan is warranted.

Ectopic pregnancy

Prevalence of ectopic pregnancy is increasing with widening use of ART and better diagnosis due to ongoing improvements in ultrasound technology. In spite of this, the latest mortality rate was the lowest registered since 1988, with 1.65/10 000 deaths between 2006 and 2008 [40]. Women undergoing fertility treatment often have uterine or tubal pathology and possibly a history of previous ectopic pregnancy or tubal surgery, which are all considered risk factors for extrauterine implantation. The incidence of ectopic pregnancy in assisted conception is higher than when compared to the general population, ranging from 2% to 11% [41,42]. It is difficult to determine whether this increase is due to treatment or the cause of infertility itself. Furthermore, these patients are at particular risk of simultaneous occurrence of pregnancies on two or more implantation sites, with an incidence of 1/100 [43]. Figure 3.8 shows the most common sites of ectopic pregnancy. The difficulty with heterotopic pregnancy is that there usually is an intrauterine pregnancy, which gives false reassurance when initially identified on the scan, and diagnosis is usually late. As a result, a thorough ultrasound assessment is essential, not only to exclude extrauterine implantation, but also to identify ectopics early, so as to improve outcome and consequent fertility.

Transvaginal ultrasound is the gold standard for diagnosis of ectopic pregnancy and offers sensitivity of 87% and specificity of 94% [44]. Suspicion should arise if the uterine cavity appears empty. In 15% of cases of ectopic pregnancy, a pseudogestational sac may be present, which should not be misdiagnosed as an early intrauterine pregnancy. Table 3.1 describes the characteristics that differentiate these two structures. It is important to ensure that the entire uterine cavity has been assessed, including the cervical canal and interstitial portion of the tubes. For patients with a previous Cesarean section, the uterine scar should always be reviewed. Diagnosis of ectopic pregnancy should only be made if a gestational sac or RPOC are visualized outside the uterine cavity.

The Fallopian tube is the most common implantation site regardless of mode of conception. In assisted conception, tubal ectopics comprise around three quarters of all ectopics [45]. They are visualized on the scan as a mass in the adnexa, usually just above and medial to the ovary (Figure 3.9). Findings may include a live embryo, a clear gestational sac, perhaps with a yolk sac or a heterogeneous mass representing a tubal miscarriage. Diagnostic difficulties may arise if there is complex adnexal pathology, large tender stimulated ovaries, or a nonspecific adnexal mass made up of blood clots surrounding the ectopic gestation (Figure 3.10). The mass needs to move separately from the ovary and this is achieved using the non-scanning hand to apply mild pressure on the abdomen above the probe, eliciting the "sliding sign", which helps to distinguish it from a corpus luteum [46]. In addition, color Doppler can be useful both in identification of a mass and confirmation of trophoblastic flow within it. Corpus lutea demonstrate a vascular rim with the appearance of a "ring of fire" and should not be mistaken for an ectopic

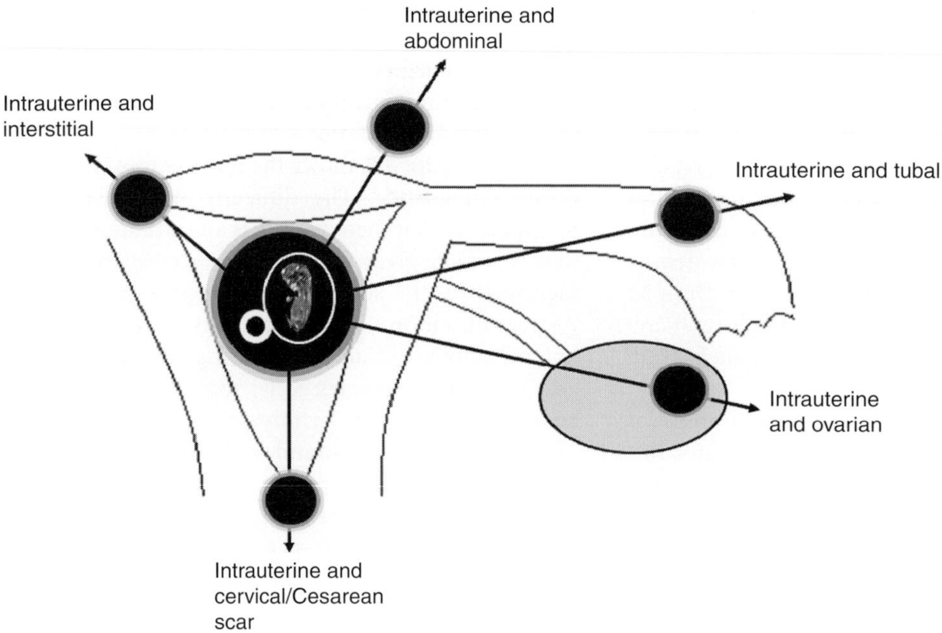

Figure 3.8. Schematic representation of concomitant ectopic pregnancy sites.

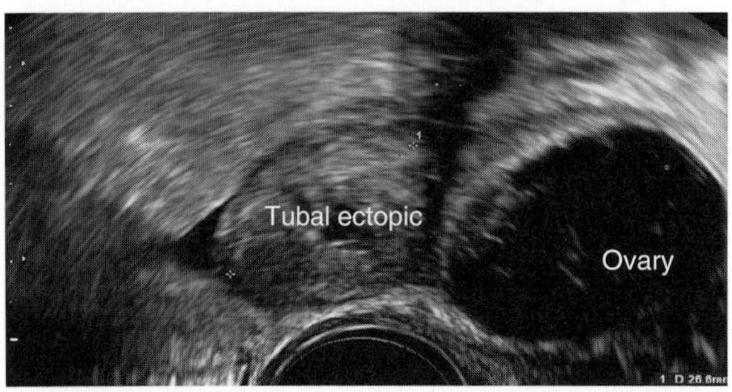

Figure 3.9. Ultrasound findings of a tubal ectopic pregnancy, demonstrating an echogenic mass medial to the ovary, which moves separately on palpation.

pregnancy (Figure 3.11). In spontaneous conceptions, the location of the corpus luteum is important as 78% of ectopics are ipsilateral to it [47]. However, in patients who undergo superovulation and assisted conception, identification of corpus lutea is only important in excluding an ovarian ectopic.

Non-tubal ectopics have significantly higher maternal morbidity and mortality usually due to delayed diagnosis. Interstitial ectopics occur when the gestational sac implants on the interstitial portion of the Fallopian tube. These patients remain asymptomatic longer because a thick myometrial layer surrounds the ectopic pregnancy, containing any bleeding and preventing early rupture. On ultrasound scanning, this is seen as myometrium from the uterine fundus enclosing the gestation. The most characteristic feature on the ultrasound image is visualization of the proximal interstitial tube communicating with the medial aspect of the ectopic gestation and the lateral aspect of the uterine cavity (Figure 3.12(a)). Three-dimensional ultrasound could be used to facilitate a correct diagnosis. Cornual ectopic pregnancy occurs only in patients with a unicornuate uterus where implantation takes place in the rudimentary horn. On the ultrasound scan the uterine shape is abnormal with a single interstitial tube and an ectopic gestation adjacent to the uterus. The rudimentary horn is usually mobile and enveloped in a continuous myometrial mantle (Figure 3.12(b)). Cervical and Cesarean scar pregnancies are caused by previous surgical trauma with implantation occurring in the myometrial defect. Patients typically present with painless vaginal bleeding. Cesarean scar pregnancies are located close to the internal os (Figure 3.12(c)), whereas cervical pregnancies tend to be located lower in the cervix (Figure 3.12(d)). Management is similar, thus differentiation is not essential. However, it is imperative to distinguish true extrauterine implantation from the cervical phase of a spontaneous intrauterine miscarriage or a low (isthmic) implantation. Visualization of the

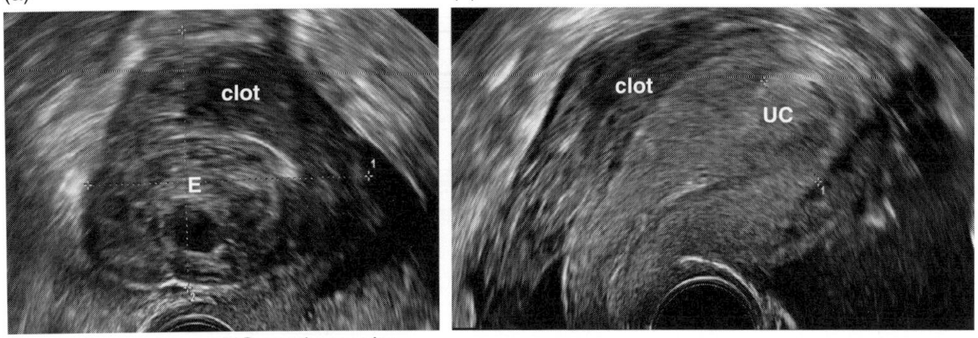

E, ectopic pregnancy; UC, uterine cavity.

Figure 3.10. Ultrasound scan showing a hemoperitoneum. (a): a blood clot surrounding an ectopic pregnancy; (b): a blood clot in the pouch of Douglas.

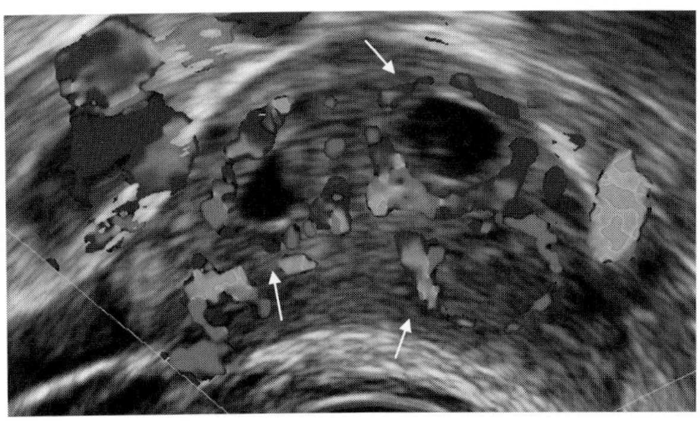

Figure 3.11. Doppler assessment demonstrates multiple "rings of fire" (arrows) surrounding four corpus lutea in an ovary. (See color plate section for colored image.)

insertion of the uterine artery may help determine the level of the internal os. In a miscarriage, the internal os might be open and gentle pressure with the probe may cause movement of the sac. Lack of peritrophoblastic blood flow also supports the diagnosis of a detached pregnancy retained in the cervical canal. Ovarian pregnancies are rare, characterized by the presence of a gestational sac surrounded by healthy ovarian tissue, where gentle palpation does not separate it from the ovary. The echogenicity and vascularity can be used to differentiate products of conception from a corpus luteum (Figure 3.12(e)). Abdominal pregnancies implant in the peritoneal cavity, and may result from primary implantation or be secondary to a tubal abortion with trophoblastic invasion and re-implantation. Diagnosis is made when the pregnancy is seen outside of the uterus, tubes, and ovaries.

Various amounts of clear anechoic fluid within the lesser pelvis are seen in the majority of pregnant women but only the presence of blood constitutes a significant finding (Figure 3.10). Blood clots appear hyperechoic and irregular on the scan and may be mistaken for bowel loops. Checking for the presence of peristalsis helps make the differential diagnosis. Blood clots are also usually covered with hypoechoic serum and appear jelly-like when gently pressed by the probe. In cases of severe intra-abdominal bleeding, blood can be seen in the upper abdomen below the liver; thus a transabdominal scan should also be performed in all cases of suspected ruptured ectopics.

In assisted conception, biochemical markers should be interpreted with caution as multiple pregnancy and molar pregnancy may elevate β-hCG; multiple corpus lutea and exogenous progesterone may raise serum progesterone. In pregnancies after ART, clinical and ultrasound findings should be the primary assessment tools to determine follow-up and management. Any patient who is hemodynamically unstable or has clinical or ultrasound evidence of intra-abdominal bleeding needs urgent surgical intervention, with consideration of an open procedure such as laparotomy if shock is present. To avoid adverse outcomes, surgery to achieve hemostasis should not be delayed. If the patient is stable, elective treatment can be considered and various options are possible, depending on the ectopic location, viability, initial serum β-hCG, or the presence of a concomitant intrauterine pregnancy.

Surgery remains the main therapeutic choice for the management of tubal ectopics. Indications for surgery include the presence of symptoms, a viable ectopic

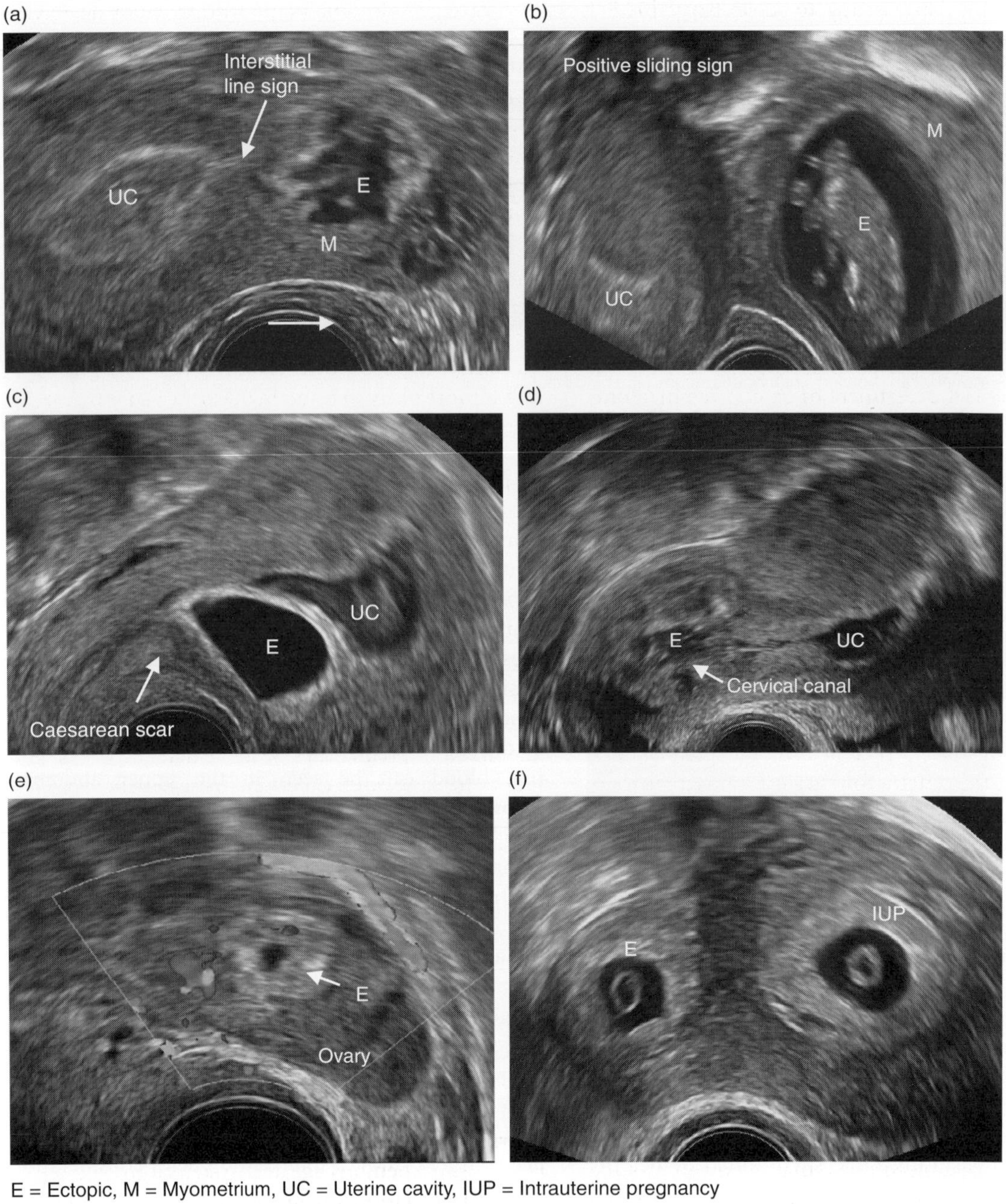

Figure 3.12. Ultrasound features of non-tubal ectopic pregnancy. (a): interstitial pregnancy; (b): cornual ectopic; (c): Cesarean scar ectopic; (d): cervical ectopic; (e): ovarian ectopic; (f): heterotopic (intrauterine and interstitial) pregnancy. (See color plate section for colored image of Figure 3.12(e).)

pregnancy, high serum β-hCG levels, a tubal heterotopic with a viable intrauterine pregnancy, and failure of conservative management. Minimally invasive surgery is widely used for this purpose as it has been demonstrated to have advantages such as less postoperative pain, shorter hospital stay, quicker recovery, and reduced costs [48,49]. In some cases, laparotomy is preferred due to severe abdominopelvic adhesions or the surgeon's inexperience. There does not seem to be a significant difference in the future reproductive outcome when comparing laparoscopy to laparotomy [50,51]. Salpingotomy has a high risk of residual trophoblastic tissue, with subsequent need of postoperative β-hCG monitoring and a higher chance of recurrence of ectopic pregnancy on the scarred tube [52]. On the other hand, a higher fertility outcome has been reported with salpingotomy in women with contralateral tubal pathology and previous infertility factors [53,54]. In practice, there is a general consensus that salpingotomy should only be attempted if the woman desires further pregnancies and there is evidence of contralateral tubal damage at the time of laparoscopy. In patients with a diagnosis of heterotopic tubal pregnancy, laparoscopic salpingectomy is the treatment of choice. Salpingotomy in these patients is not recommended as it involves considerable risk of persistent active trophoblast [55], and serial serum β-hCG measurements cannot be used to detect active residual trophoblast.

Medical management of tubal ectopics consists of the use of methotrexate, which is a folic acid antagonist that interferes with the synthesis of DNA and cell proliferation. As well as acting on the trophoblast, methotrexate has an effect on other body cells, hence causing adverse effects. It should not be used in the presence of a viable heterotopic intrauterine pregnancy due to the risk of teratogenicity. If a heterotopic pregnancy is excluded and the criteria for surgical management are not met, conservative management can be considered. Another option is expectant management. From the literature, it is difficult to reach a conclusion about the effectiveness of expectant management of tubal ectopic pregnancy, and the main limitations are its high failure rate and the inability to predict who is likely to fail with this method. The serum β-hCG level at presentation can be used to select patients for expectant management, with levels of <1500 IU/L reported to have a success rate of 60%–70% [56].

Interstitial pregnancy can be managed expectantly if the ectopic is nonviable, small, and solid because the risk of rupture and bleeding is small. In medium-sized interstitial pregnancies (<5 cm), conservative management is widely used. Methotrexate can be administered systemically or locally, but the failure rate is higher in women presenting with a β-hCG level of >10 000 IU/L. Evidence of intra-abdominal bleeding and concomitant intrauterine pregnancy are contraindications for medical treatment. Serial β-hCG measurements are continued until it becomes undetectable. Methotrexate is teratogenic, and therefore in viable heterotopic interstitial pregnancies a feticide with intracardiac injection of potassium chloride (KCl^-) into the ectopic can be performed with low risk of complications. Large interstitial ectopics (>5 cm in size) should be considered for surgery as the risk of rupture is increased and the time to pregnancy resolution is very long. A laparoscopy and partial excision of the Fallopian tube using the endoloop is preferable to laparotomy and cornual resection. Although there is a small risk of remaining trophoblast following partial salpingectomy, this is less likely to cause problems in interstitial compared to tubal pregnancies. Cornual resection is associated with a high risk of bleeding, requires extensive uterine manipulation, and is more likely to result in the loss of an intrauterine pregnancy in heterotopic pregnancies. This should only be considered in cornual ectopics, as they have a high risk of rupture and excision of the rudimentary horn is the treatment of choice.

The preferred management choice for the treatment of cervical and Cesarean scar pregnancy depends on symptoms, gestational age, presence of cardiac activity, and a coexisting viable intrauterine pregnancy. Surgical evacuation appears to be effective and safe in pregnancies of less than 14 weeks' gestation. The risk of severe bleeding and hemorrhage is very high if surgery is attempted in pregnancies of more than 14 weeks' gestation. In these cases, expectant management should be attempted in the hope that the pregnancy will continue until viability is reached. If a concomitant intrauterine pregnancy is present, both pregnancies are viable, and the diagnosis is early (<8 weeks' gestation), a feticide of the ectopic pregnancy is recommended in the same manner as described above (using KCl^-). If the pregnancy is of 8 weeks' gestation or longer, a termination of both pregnancies (ectopic and intrauterine pregnancy) should be considered as the risk of heavy vaginal bleeding is significant. Additional hemostatic measures such as insertion of a cervical suture, balloon tamponade, or arterial embolization may be necessary to reduce the risk of severe hemorrhage and hysterectomy.

Ovarian ectopic pregnancy is difficult to diagnose and manage. Surgical excision of trophoblastic tissue and ovarian conservation is the aim. However, if the ectopic pregnancy is large and the excision is complicated by severe bleeding, an ovarian wedge resection or oophorectomy may be necessary. Oophorectomy may also need to be considered in cases of a concomitant viable intrauterine pregnancy if the surgeon is not certain whether the ovarian ectopic has been completely excised.

The management of early (< 8 weeks' gestation) and nonviable abdominal pregnancy is relatively straightforward and can be done laparoscopically. The risk of hemorrhage increases with advanced gestation and after 8 weeks', the placenta is best left *in situ* to prevent intractable hemorrhage occurring during surgery. If the diagnosis is made after the pregnancy progresses beyond 18 weeks' gestation and there is a simultaneous viable intrauterine pregnancy, expectant management may be employed until both pregnancies reach the point of viability. A nonviable small heterotopic abdominal pregnancy may be managed expectantly, provided the woman is asymptomatic and there is no sign of intra-abdominal bleeding. In cases of live abdominal ectopics, the placenta should be left *in situ* as the likelihood of severe bleeding is high.

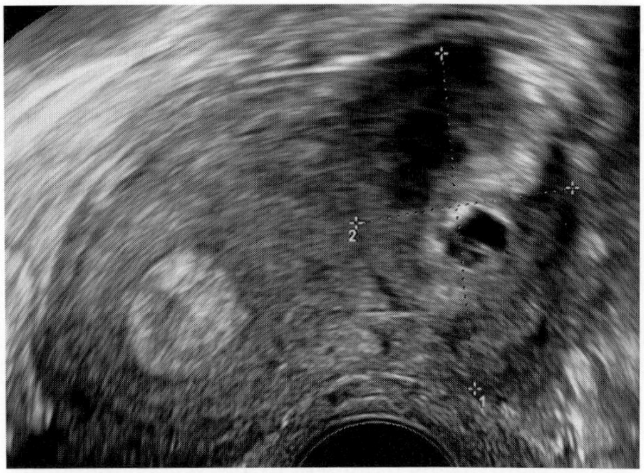

Figure 3.13. Ultrasound findings in fibroid degeneration showing central cystic changes with hypoechoic fluid.

Uterine pathology

The risk of miscarriage and preterm delivery is increased in some types of congenital uterine anomalies. During pregnancy it is very difficult to differentiate between arcuate, septate, and mild forms of bicornuate uterus, and it is best not to attempt to classify these anomalies until the pregnancy is completed. In cases of a unicornuate uterus and severe forms of bicornuate uterus the diagnosis can be made during pregnancy. In these cases, women should be warned about the increased risk of early delivery and the baby being breech. Antenatal care in these patients may involve serial measurements of cervical length during the second trimester of pregnancy and insertion of a cervical suture.

Uterine fibroids are very common, but they cause significant problems only in a small minority of women. Fibroids may increase rapidly in size during pregnancy and possibly cause pressure symptoms. Rapid growth sometimes outstrips the blood supply to the fibroid, which can result in ischemia and necrosis. The ultrasound appearance of fibroids varies, but usually they are seen as well-defined hypoechoic concentric rings representing muscle fibers and connective tissue, which commonly generate acoustic shadowing. Degeneration may appear as a central cystic area filled with hypoechoic fluid, septae, and possibly only peripheral blood flow on Doppler assessment (Figure 3.13). Clinically, women can experience severe pain, which may require hospitalization and analgesia. It is also important to determine the location of the fibroids in relation to the uterine cavity in early pregnancy. The risk of first-trimester miscarriage is increased in women with submucous fibroids. Most of these, however, are detected during routine fertility investigations and they are often removed prior to pregnancy using hysteroscopic resection. Very large fibroids that are located posteriorly and in the lower part of the uterus may obstruct the urethra and cause urinary retention. They are also associated with an increased risk of late miscarriage and preterm labor.

Tubo-ovarian pathology

Pelvic abnormalities such as endometriosis, pelvic inflammatory disease, ovarian tumors, and adhesions adversely affect fertility and are often the reason for a woman requiring assisted conception. Infertile women have extensive investigations to diagnose and treat pathology prior to treatment, with the aim of optimizing the success of each treatment cycle. It is therefore unusual to find neoplastic adnexal lesions in pregnancy following assisted conception. Functional cysts, however, are very common, which could be complicated by hemorrhage or torsion. Occasionally, subtle pelvic abnormalities such as hydrosalpinges and ovarian fibromas may be missed on prepregnancy scans, only to be identified on ultrasound images during the first trimester of pregnancy. Following ovarian puncture and egg retrieval, a pelvic hematoma or abscess may form, which could resemble true ovarian tumors or mimic pelvic malignancy. Diagnosis and management of tubo-ovarian pathology in pregnancy poses a challenge, and it is imperative that clinicians become familiar with the characteristics that discriminate between benign and malignant forms.

Table 3.3. Ultrasound characteristics used for assessing ovarian cysts

Characteristic	Ultrasound image	Definition
Size	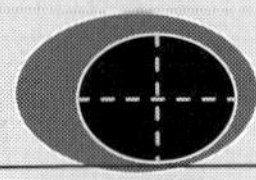	Measurement of three diameters (in mm) in two perpendicular planes of both ovary (with cyst) and cyst
Echogenicity	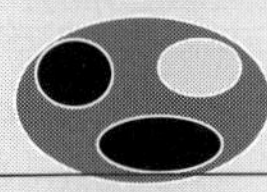	Dependent on cystic contents: anechoic (black), low level, "ground glass" (homogeneously dispersed echogenicity) or hyperechoic (white)
Septations	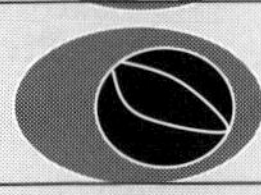	Thin strand of tissue running across cyst cavity from one surface to the contralateral side. Unilocular (no septum) or multilocular (at least one septum)
Solid papillary projections	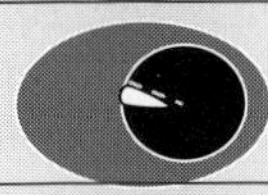	Solid projection into the cyst cavity arising from the cyst wall with a height of ≥3 mm.
Solid components	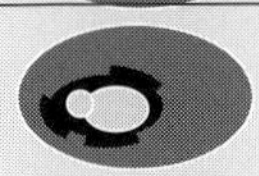	High echogenicity suggesting the presence of tissue
Ovarian crescent sign	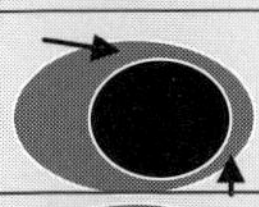	Presence of healthy ovarian tissue adjacent to the tumor enclosed within the ovarian capsule. Pressure with the probe should not separate this tissue from the cyst
Vascularity	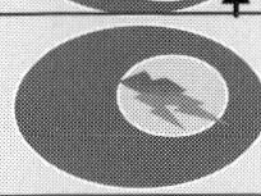	Doppler assessment of the tumor to establish blood flow
Mobility	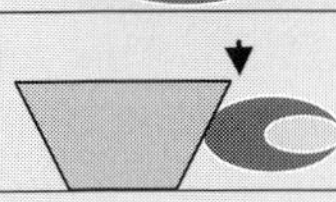	Examiner should apply pressure with the non-examining hand on the abdomen to assess for mobility

(Definitions adapted from Timmerman et al. [58])

(a) (b)

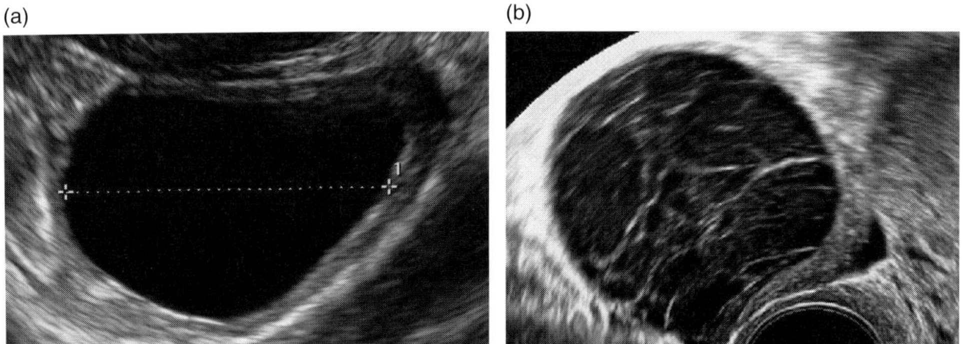

Figure 3.14. Functional ovarian cysts. (a): simple cyst appearing as round, anechoic, with smooth borders and surrounded by healthy ovarian tissue; (b): hemorrhagic cyst shown with mixed internal echoes representing old blood.

Evaluation of specific ultrasound characteristics, also called "pattern recognition," has been shown to be superior to all other methods in distinguishing between benign and malignant extrauterine pelvic masses [57]. Table 3.3 outlines the ultrasound characteristics that should be assessed (definitions adapted from Timmerman et al. [58]). Size, echogenicity, presence of septations, papillary projections, solid

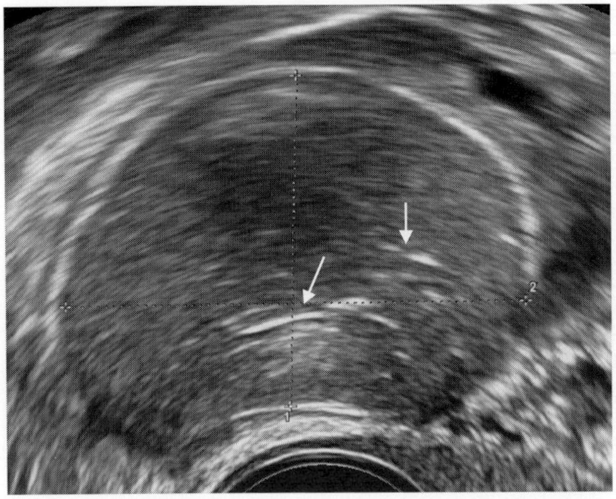

Figure 3.15. Ultrasound features of dermoid cysts, also showing long echogenic lines and bright prominent spots representing hair (arrows).

components, healthy ovarian tissue surrounding the cyst, vascularity, and mobility are all important features that will help predict not only the nature, but also the histological type of adnexal tumors.

Functional ovarian cysts are produced by sustained luteinizing hormone (LH) and/or follicle-stimulating hormone (FSH) secretion by the pituitary gland or exogenous administration during ovarian stimulation. They are common, benign, and resolve spontaneously. Their reported incidence in patients undergoing ART varies from 2% to 40% [59–62]. On ultrasound scanning, their appearance is usually rounded, unilocular, anechoic, with smooth thin internal borders (Figure 3.14(a)). They are surrounded by healthy ovarian tissue and are avascular on Doppler examination. Their size may vary and most resolve by 16 weeks' gestation [63]. The corpus luteum may be cystic or solid, or may contain mixed internal echoes, a fine "spider web" aspect, or a ground-glass appearance, which may represent hemorrhage within the cyst (Figure 3.14(b)). To distinguish the corpus luteum, Doppler examination may be used, demonstrating a "ring of fire" appearance surrounding the cyst (Figure 3.11).

Other benign tumors include dermoid cysts, serous cystadenomas, mucinous cystadenomas, and endometriomas. Small dermoid cysts are common and easy to recognize due to the presence of fat and hair, which produce a typical heterogenic appearance. Hair floating in the fluid is seen on ultrasound as long echogenic lines (Figure 3.15). Fat content may produce distal acoustic shadowing known as the "tip-of-the-iceberg" phenomenon, and is important as it may cause underestimation of size. In contrast, ultrasound characteristics of the different benign epithelial tumors are less characteristic and may overlap (Figure 3.16). Serous cystadenomas are generally unilocular, homogeneous, with thin walls, which could easily be confused with a functional cyst. Mucinous cystadenomas may be larger, unilocular or multilocular, containing thick cystic fluid with different echogenicities. Endometriomas are mostly unilocular, homogenous, well-circumscribed thick-walled cysts, with low level echoes that give it a ground-glass appearance (Figure 3.17(a)). This represents old blood and may contain some blood clots that are seen as small solid foci. It is important to increase the gain to be able to see the echogenic foci and septations. Decidualization during pregnancy can mimic a malignancy and should not be acted on immediately (Figure 3.17(b)). The background of endometriosis or additional ultrasound findings such as an endometriotic nodule should evoke this possibility. Regular follow-up scans may be required to confirm regression of the cyst and rule out malignancy.

Primary and metastatic malignant ovarian tumors rarely develop in pregnancy and account only for 1%–8% of all adnexal masses surgically removed in pregnancy [64–66]. Features suggestive of malignancy

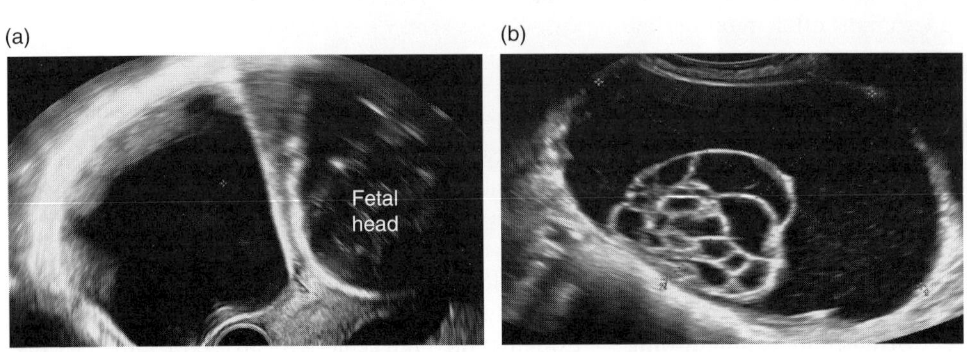

Figure 3.16. Ultrasound appearance of benign epithelial tumors. (a): cystadenoma in pregnancy; (b): borderline tumor.

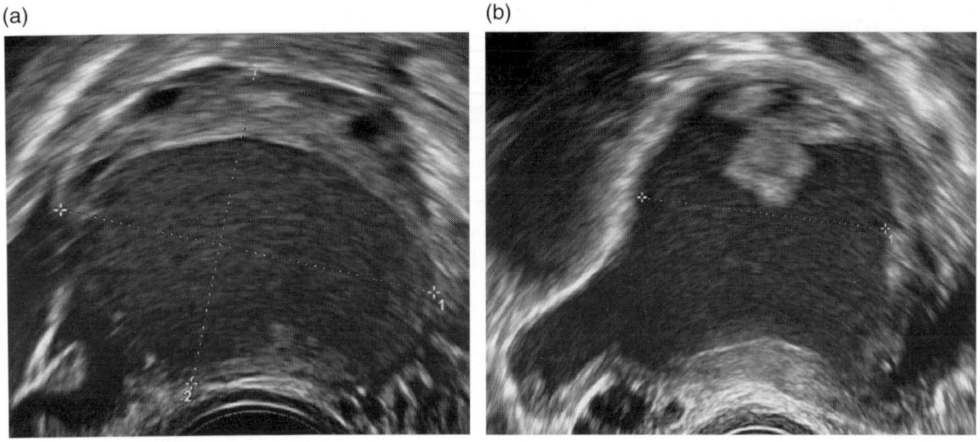

Figure 3.17. (a): ultrasound appearance of an endometrioma, a homogenous echogenic cyst; (b): decidualization of an endometrioma in pregnancy, causing thickening and irregularities of the inner cyst wall.

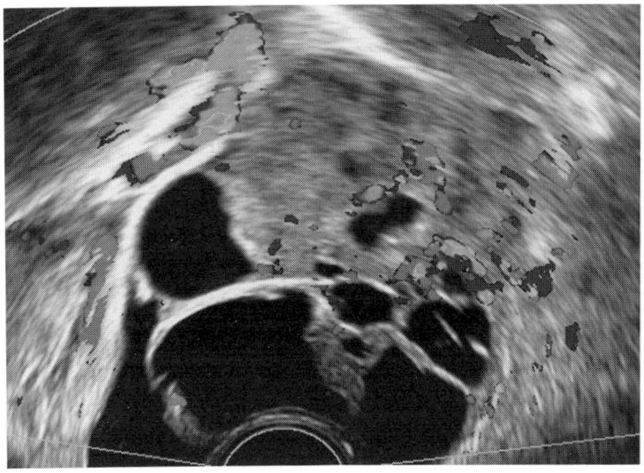

Figure 3.18. Ultrasound appearance of a malignant ovarian tumor. (See color plate section for colored image.)

include: older women (≥40 years of age), persistent large growing mass, irregularities in the cyst wall or ovarian surface, and solid components (Figure 3.18). Malignancy is also more likely in bilateral, predominately solid tumors with thick irregular septae. Papillary projections are seen most often in borderline tumors, but may also be present in benign cysts (particularly mucinous cystadenomas and adenofibromas) or malignant neoplasms. The presence of a rim of healthy ovarian tissue adjacent to the cyst wall is reassuring and makes the diagnosis of invasive malignancy unlikely [67]. All pelvic tumors tend to be more vascular in pregnant than non-pregnant women, which limits the value of Doppler studies of intratumoral blood flow. The presence of ascites should be noted, although it is not a particularly helpful sign following assisted conception. Tumor markers such as CA125, β-hCG, and α-fetoprotein are raised in pregnancy, and therefore are not useful for differential diagnosis [64,68–70]. Surgical intervention is required for any adnexal mass that is highly suspicious of malignancy. Benign cysts are best removed after pregnancy is completed unless they cause pain requiring intervention.

Complications

Ovarian hyperstimulation syndrome

In ART, gonadotrophins and anti-estrogens are used to stimulate the ovaries and maximize the release of oocytes for fertilization (see Chapter 4). The prolonged effect of β-hCG may cause excessive luteinization of ovaries with subsequent production of vasoactive mediators, which initiate fluid shifts from the intravascular space to extravascular areas (i.e., third-spacing). Consequently, the ovary becomes enlarged with multiple cysts, ascites starts to build up, and hypovolemia develops (Figure 3.19). This systemic condition secondary to superovulation is described as ovarian hyperstimulation syndrome (OHSS).

Ovarian hyperstimulation syndrome is usually mild and self-limiting, but in some cases, especially in advanced or multiple pregnancy, it can cause severe complications, which are associated with significant maternal morbidity and mortality. A detailed history should be taken and a physical examination performed with particular attention paid to the level of hydration, hemodynamic stability, presence of third-space fluid accumulation, and thromboembolism. Ultrasound examination is preferred to bimanual vaginal

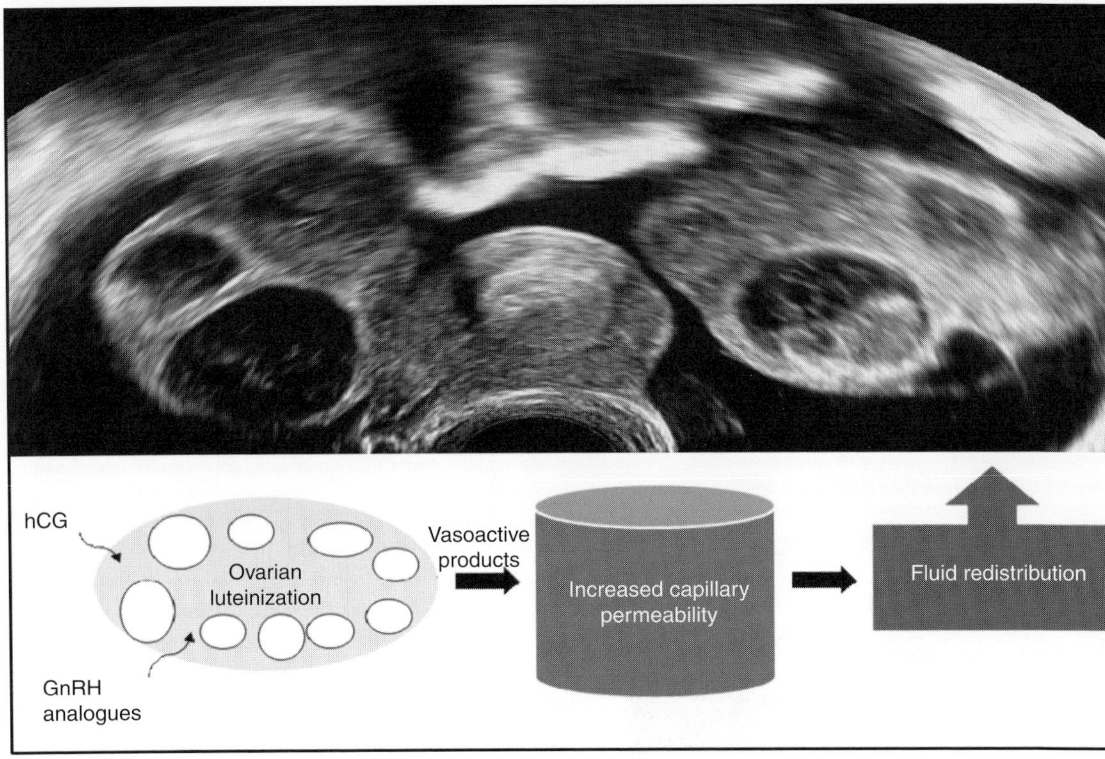

GnRH, gonadotrophin releasing hormone; hCG, human chorionic gonadotrophin.

Figure 3.19. Ovarian hyperstimulation syndrome (OHSS). Above: ultrasound image demonstrating bilateral ovarian enlargement, multiple follicles, and ascitis. Below: diagrammatic representation of the physiopathology of OHSS.

examination and is very useful in assessing ovarian volume and the amount of ascites. Ultrasound features of OHSS include: bilateral enlarged ovaries, multifollicular appearance, stromal edema, intra-ovarian hemorrhage, and ascites (Figure 3.20). In some cases, the ovaries cannot be fully visualized on transvaginal ultrasound, and therefore abdominal ultrasound examination may be necessary.

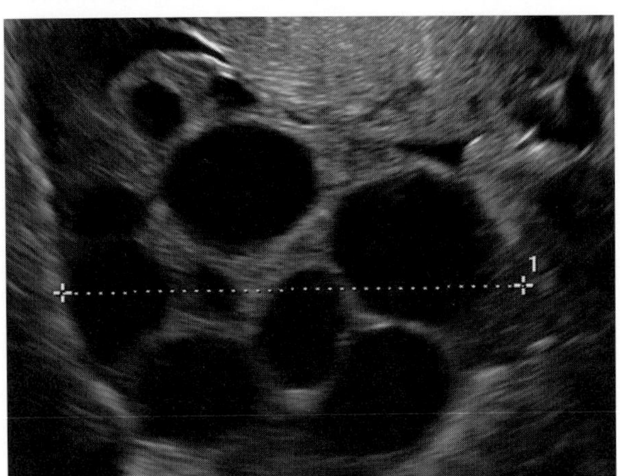

Figure 3.20. Ultrasound findings in ovarian hyperstimulation syndrome (OHSS) demonstating ovarian enlargement, multiple follicles, and ascites.

Clinical and ultrasound features can be used to classify this condition as mild, moderate, and severe (Table 3.4) [71]. Mild OHSS occurs in patients with enlarged ovaries (<8 cm) and symptoms of abdominal pain or bloating. Although some authors disregard this category because it occurs frequently (in 33% of in vitro fertilization patients [72]) and may have minimal clinical significance, it is important to recognize that even mild OHSS might worsen over time, and therefore needs monitoring. Moderate and severe forms of OHSS have an incidence of 3%–8% [72]. Moderate OHSS is characterized by the presence of ascites and larger ovaries (8–12 cm), and is upgraded to severe or critical when there are systemic effects. Clinical presentation and management of this condition is covered in Chapter 4, but it is important to

Table 3.4. Clinical, biochemical, and ultrasound features used to classify ovarian hyperstimulation syndrome by severity

Feature \ Severity	Mild	Moderate	Severe	Critical
Ovarian size (cm)*	<8	8–12	>12	Variable
Symptoms	Pain/bloating	Nausea +/- vomiting		
Ascitis	None	On USS	Clinical	Tense
Hydrothorax	None	None	Occasional	Large
Renal failure	None	None	Oliguria	Oligo/anuria
Hypoproteinemia	None	None	Present	Present
Hematocrit (%)	Normal	Normal	45–55	>55
White blood cells				>25 000
Thromboembolism	None	None	None	Present
ARDS	None	None	None	Present

*, ovarian size may not correlate with severity in assisted reproductive technology (follicular aspiration); ARDS, acute respiratory distress syndrome; USS, ultrasound scan. (Criteria according to Mathur et al., 1995 [71].)

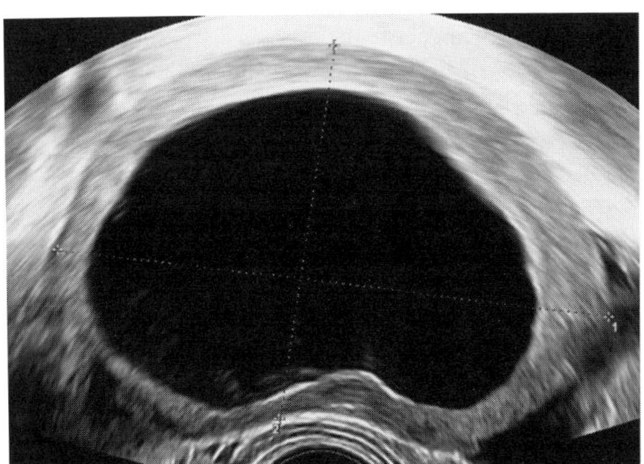

Figure 3.21. Ultrasound findings in ovarian torsion showing an enlarged and edematous ovary with hyperechoic edges.

highlight that paracentesis should only be considered in women who are uncomfortable because of abdominal distension or in whom oliguria persists despite adequate volume replacement. Paracentesis should be done under ultrasound guidance to avoid puncturing hyperstimulated ovaries.

Ovarian torsion

Heavy ovaries are prone to twisting with various degrees of vascular and lymphatic obstruction, causing ovarian congestion, edema and subsequent infarction. Pregnancy and ovarian stimulation are both risk factors for torsion and this represents the main complication of adnexal masses, especially in the first trimester. The incidence of torsion in pregnancies conceived using ovarian stimulation has been reported as 0.6% [73]. Size and contents of an ovarian lesion contribute to the risk and should always be considered. McWilliams et al. [74] found that the risk of torsion is highest when the lesion measures 8–12 mm. When considering the nature of the mass, endometriomas or invading tumors are less likely to undergo torsion due to the reduced mobility secondary to adhesions or invasion. Hyperstimulated ovaries on the other hand, are more likely to undergo tortion, with a rate reported to be as high as 7.5% [75].

The clinical picture is the main diagnostic measure and any woman with sudden onset of severe abdominal pain should be assessed promptly. On ultrasound scanning, the ovary appears enlarged and edematous; comparing it with the contralateral ovary may be useful (Figure 3.21). On the other hand, assessment of blood supply with Doppler ultrasound may not be helpful as the arterial perfusion can be maintained even in severe cases of torsion. Clinical findings should always prevail, and any patient with acute onset of unilateral abdominal pain associated with nausea and vomiting, suspected to have ovarian torsion, should be considered for surgery even if the ultrasound findings are normal.

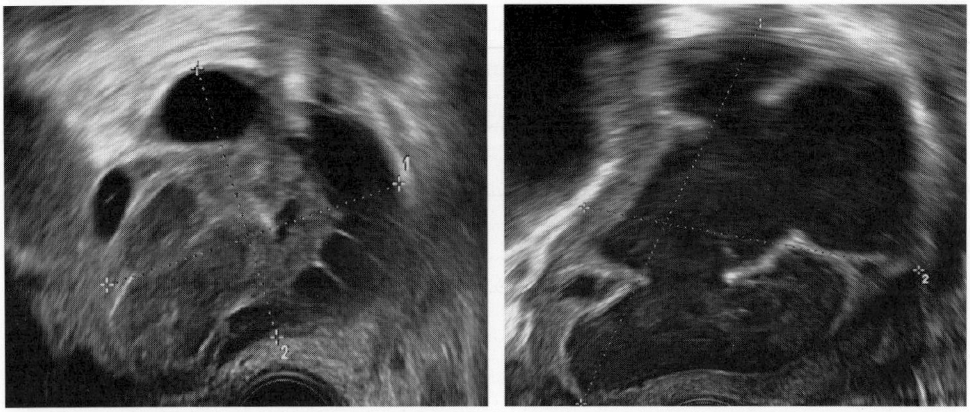

Figure 3.22. Ultrasound findings of a tubo-ovarian abscess showing (a): swollen walls (cyst and Fallopian tube) and containing homogenous echogenic material (pus); (b): an inflamed tube with swollen mucosal folds.

Traditionally, salpingo-oophorectomy was the treatment of choice for all patients with ovarian torsion because of the theoretical risk of thromboembolism secondary to ischemia. However, the latest literature review published in 2010 failed to find any study that reports an increase in thromboembolic morbidity associated with untwisting the adnexa as treatment of adnexal torsion [76]. Therefore, in patients who have a history of infertility and who conceived with assisted reproductive technology, conservative management should be considered, which consists of untwisting the adnexa even if it appears necrotic, and performing aspiration or cystectomy to avoid recurrence. Cohen et al. followed up 96 women who underwent detorsion of black-bluish ovaries sparing the affected ovary, and 93% had normal ovarian volume and follicular development on ultrasound imaging performed six weeks after discharge. Six of these patients who were followed up, underwent IVF, and authors report that oocytes retrieved from the spared ovaries were fertilized in all six patients. They conclude that ovarian torsion should be treated with conservative management, regardless of ovarian color [77].

Ruptured cysts

Ruptured hemorrhagic cysts can cause severe pain and mimic an acute abdomen. The pouch of Douglas should be assessed in all patients to identify the presence of blood, which appears hyperechoic on the ultrasound image. Surgical management should only be considered if the patient is hemodynamically unstable, there is active bleeding, or the diagnosis is uncertain.

Pelvic infection

The risk of pelvic infection following transvaginal ultrasound directed follicular aspiration has been reported to be very low (0.6%) with tubo-ovarian abscess formation in half of these cases [78]. The ultrasound appearance of an abscess is varied and may comprise a unilocular or multilocular, thick-walled cyst filled with homogeneous echogenic material (pus), or a complex solid richly vascularized mass (Figure 3.22(a)). The diagnosis is easier to make if there is an associated pyosalpinx, which has a more characteristic appearance (Figure 3.22(b)). Inflamed Fallopian tubes are seen as thick-walled sausage-shaped cystic structures filled with pus, with thick incomplete septations that give a "cog-wheel" appearance.

Conclusion

Management of pregnancy after ART is often complex and challenging. In comparison to the fertile population, women who conceive after fertility treatment tend to be older and they often suffer from other gynecological comorbidities. They are more likely to carry twins and higher multiple pregnancies, which are more difficult to diagnose and manage. Ectopic pregnancies are also more common and concomitant intrauterine and ectopic pregnancies are particularly common after ART. The presence of multiple pregnancies and frequent use of hormonal support in early pregnancy prevents the use of standard clinical diagnostic algorithms in women with early pregnancy complications after ART. This makes management more complex and it increases the risk of misdiagnosis and adverse outcomes.

Enlarged ovaries, functional cysts, and other pelvic pathology are also more common in women with pregnancies after ART, further complicating management of these women. In these circumstances, high quality of ultrasound examination is essential to overcome the diagnostic difficulties and ensure optimal management. Involvement of senior colleagues and careful assessment of clinical symptoms and diagnostic features are essential to achieve a right balance between diagnosing and treating serious conditions without delay, and avoiding unnecessary interventions with a potential risk of harming pregnancies achieved through complex and prolonged treatment.

References

1. Mehta T, Levine D, McArdle C. Lack of sensitivity of endometrial thickness in predicting the presence of an ectopic pregnancy. *J Ultrasound Med* 1999; **18**: 117–122.
2. Jauniaux E, Jurkovic D, Henriet Y, Rodesch F, Hustin J. Development of the secondary human yolk sac: correlation of sonographic and anatomical features. *Hum Reprod* 1991; **6**: 1160–1166.
3. Lindsay D, Lovett I, Lyons E, et al. Yolk sac diameter and shape at endovaginal US: predictors of pregnancy outcome in the first trimester. *Radiology* 1992; **183**: 115–118.
4. Rowling S, Langer J, Coleman B, et al. Sonography during early pregnancy: dependence of threshold and discriminatory values on transvaginal transducer frequency. *Am J Roentgenol* 1999; **172**: 983–988.
5. Robinson H, Fleming J. A critical evaluation of sonar crown-rump length measurement. *Br J Obstet Gynaecol* 1975; **82**: 702–710.
6. Gjerris A, Loft A, Pinborg A, Tabor A, Christiansen M. First-trimester screening in pregnancies conceived by assisted reproductive technology: significance of gestational dating by oocyte retrieval or sonographic measurement of crown–rump length. *Ultrasound Obstet Gynecol* 2008; **32**: 612–617.
7. ISOUG Bioeffects and Safety Committee. Safety Statement, 2000. Reconfirmed 2003. *Ultrasound Obstet Gynecol* 2003; **21**: 100.
8. Doubilet P, Benson C. Embryonic heart rate in the early first trimester: what rate is normal? *J Ultrasound Med* 1995; **14**: 431–434.
9. Schats R, Jansen CA, Wladimiroff JW. Embryonic heart activity: appearance and development in early human pregnancy. *Br J Obstet Gynaecol* 1990; **97**: 989–994.
10. Human Fertilisation and Embryology Authority (HFEA). *Code of Practice*, 8th edn (revised October 2011).
11. Tummers P, De Sutter Paul, Dhont M. Risk of spontaneous abortion in singleton and twin pregnancies after IVF/ICSI. *Hum Reprod* 2003; **18**: 1720–1723.
12. Ezra Y, Schenker J. Abortion in assisted reproduction – true increase? *Early Pregnancy* 1995: **1**: 171–175.
13. Edi-Osagie E, Hooper L, Seif M. The impact of assisted hatching on live birth rates and outcomes of assisted conception: a systematic review. *Hum Reprod* 2003; **18**: 1828–1835.
14. Human Fertilisation and Embryology Authority (HFEA). *Fertility Facts and Figures*, 2008.
15. Fretts R, Schmittdiel J, McLean F, Usher R, Goldman M. Increased maternal age and the risk of fetal death. *New Engl J Med* 1995; **333**: 953–957.
16. Pereira L, Reeves M. Ultrasound criteria for diagnosis of early pregnancy failure and ectopic pregnancy. *Semin Reprod Med* 2008; **26**: 373–382.
17. Hatley W, Case J, Campbell S. Establishing the death of an embryo by ultrasound: report of a public enquiry with recommendations. *Ultrasound Obset Gynecol* 1995; **5**: 353–357.
18. Ferrazzi E, Garbo S, Sulpizio P, et al. Miscarriage diagnosis and gestational age estimation in the early first trimester pregnancy: transabdominal versus transvaginal sonography. *Ultrasound Obstet Gynecol* 1993; **3**: 36–41.
19. McKenna K, Feldstein V, Goldstein R, Filly R. The empty amnion: a sign of early pregnancy failure. *J Ultrasound Med* 1995; **14**: 117–121.
20. Tongsong T, Wanapirak C, Srisomboon J, et al. Transvaginal ultrasound in threatened abortions with empty gestational sacs. *Int J Gynaecol Obstet* 1994; **46**: 297–301.
21. Reljic M. The significance of crown–rump length measurement for predicting adverse pregnancy outcome of threatened abortion. *Ultrasound Obstet Gynecol* 2001; **17**: 510–512.
22. Dickey R, Olar T, Taylor S, Curole D, Matulich E. Relationship of small gestational sac–crown-rump length differences to abortion and abortus karyotypes. *Obstet Gynecol* 1992; **79**: 554–557.
23. Nazari A, Check J, Epstein R, Dietterich C, Farzanfar S. Relationship of small-for-dates sac size to crown-rump length and spontaneous abortion in patients with a known date of ovulation. *Obstet Gynecol* 1991; **78**: 369–373.
24. Laboda L, Estroff J, Benacerraf B. First trimester bradycardia. A sign of impending fetal loss. *J Ultrasound Med* 1989; **8**: 561–563.

25. Bora S, Bourne T, Bottomley C, Kirk E, Papageorguiou AT. Twin growth discrepancy in early pregnancy. *Ultrasound Obstet Gynecol* 2009; **34**: 38–42.

26. Landy H, Weiner S, Corson S, Batzer F. The "vanishing twin": ultrasonographic assessment of fetal disappearance in the first trimester. *Am J Obstet Gynecol* 1986; **155**: 14–19.

27. Jauniaux E, Elkazen N, Leroy F, et al. Clinical and morphological aspects of the vanishing twin phenomenon. *Obstet Gynecol* 1988; **72**: 577–581.

28. Human Fertilisation and Embryology Authority (HFEA). *Improving outcomes for Fertility Patients: Multiple Pregnancy. A Statistical Report*, 2011.

29. Benson C, Doubilet P, Laks M. Outcome of twin gestations following sonographic demonstration of two heart beats in the first trimester. *Ultrasound Obstet Gynecol* 1993; **3**: 343–345.

30. Jurkovic D. Three-dimensional ultrasound in gynecology: a critical evaluation. *Ultrasound Obstet Gynecol* 2002; **19**: 109–117.

31. Sawyer E, Ofuasia E, Ofili-Yebovi D, et al. The value of measuring endometrial thickness and volume on transvaginal ultrasound scan for the diagnosis of incomplete miscarriage. *Ultrasound Obstet Gynecol* 2007; **23**: 205–209.

32. Elson J, Tailor A, Salim R, et al. Expectant management of miscarriage – prediction of outcome using ultrasound and novel biochemical markers. *Hum Reprod* 2005; **20**: 2330–2333.

33. Kirk E, Condous G, Van Calster B, et al. Rationalizing the follow-up of pregnancies of unknown location. *Hum Reprod* 2007; **22**: 1744–1750.

34. Condous G. The management of early pregnancy complications. *Best Pract Res Clin Obstet Gynaecol* 2004; **18**: 37–57.

35. Schwarzler P, Holden D, Nielsen S, et al. The conservative management of first-trimester miscarriages and the use of colour Doppler sonography for patient selection. *Hum Reprod* 1991; **14**: 1341–1345.

36. Trinder J, Brocklehurst P, Porter R, et al. Management of miscarriage: expectant, medical or surgical? Results of randomised controlled trial (miscarriage treatment [MIST] trial). *BMJ* 2006; **332**: 1235–1240.

37. Milingos D, Mathur M, Smith N, Ashok P. Manual vacuum aspiration: a safe alternative for the surgical management of early pregnancy loss. *BJOG* 2009; **116**: 1268–1271.

38. Goldenberg R, Davis R, Hill D. The use of real-time ultrasound as an aid during difficult therapeutic abortion procedures. *Am J Obstet Gynecol* 1984; **148**: 826–827.

39. Chung T, Lee D, Cheung L, Haines C, Chang A. Spontaneous abortion: a randomized, controlled trial comparing surgical evacuation with conservative management using misoprostol. *Fertility Steril* 1999; **71**: 1054–1059.

40. Wilkinson H, Trustees and Medical Advisers. Saving Mothers' Lives: reviewing maternal deaths to make motherhood safer: 2006–2008. *BJOG* 2011; **118**: 1402–1403.

41. Ng E, Yeung W, So W, Ho P. An analysis of ectopic pregnancies following in vitro fertilisation treatment in a 10-year period. *J Obstet Gynaecol* 1998; **18**: 359–364.

42. Dubuisson J, Aubriot F, Mathieu L, et al. Risk factors for ectopic pregnancy in 556 pregnancies after in vitro fertilization: implications for preventive management. *Fertil Steril* 1991; **56**: 686–690.

43. Tal J, Haddad S, Gordon N, Timor-Tritsch I. Heterotopic pregnancy after ovulation induction and assisted reproductive technologies: a literature review from 1971 to 1993. *Fertil Steril* 1996; **66**: 1–12.

44. Shalev E, Yarom I, Bustan M, Weiner E, Ben-Shlomo I. Transvaginal sonography as the ultimate diagnostic tool for the management of ectopic pregnancy: experience with 840 cases. *Fertil Steril* 1998; **69**: 62–65.

45. Marcus S, Brinsden P. Analysis of incidence and risk factors associated with ectopic pregnancy following in-vitro fertilization and embryo transfer. *Hum Reprod* 1995; **10**: 199–203.

46. Timor-Tritsch I, Yeh M, Peisner D, Lesser K, Slavik T. The use of transvaginal ultrasonography in the diagnosis of ectopic pregnancy. *Am J Obstet Gynecol* 1989; **161**: 157–161.

47. Jurkovic D, Bourne T, Jauniaux E, Campbell S, Collins W. Transvaginal color Doppler study of blood flow in ectopic pregnancies. *Fertil Steril* 1992; **57**: 68–73.

48. Gray D, Thorburn J, Lundorff P, Strandell A, Lindblom B. A cost-effectiveness study of a randomised trial of laparoscopy versus laparotomy for ectopic pregnancy. *Lancet* 1995; **345**: 1139–1143.

49. Lundorff P, Thorburn J, Hahlin M, Kallfelt B, Lindblom B. Laparoscopic surgery in ectopic pregnancy. A randomized trial versus laparotomy. *Acta Obstet Gynecol Scand* 1991; **70**: 343–348.

50. Vermesh M, Presser S. Reproductive outcome after linear salpingostomy for ectopic gestation: a prospective 3-year follow-up. *Fertil Steril* 1992; **57**: 682–684.

51. Lundorff P, Thorburn J, Lindblom B. Fertility outcome after conservative surgical treatment of ectopic pregnancy evaluated in a randomized trial. *Fertil Steril* 1992; **57**: 998–1002.

52. Hajenius PJ, Mol F, Mol BW, et al. Interventions for tubal ectopic pregnancy. *Cochrane Database Syst Rev* 2007; **24**: CD000324.

53. Mol B, Matthijsse H, Tinga D, et al. Fertility after conservative and radical surgery for tubal pregnancy. *Hum Reprod* 1998; **13**: 1804–1809.

54. Bouyer J, Job-Spira N, Pouly JL, et al. Fertility following radical, conservative-surgical or medical treatment for tubal pregnancy: a population-based study. *BJOG* 2000; **107**: 714–721.

55. Lundorff P, Hahlin M, Sjöblom P, Lindblom B. Persistent trophoblast after conservative treatment of tubal pregnancy: prediction and detection. *Obstet Gynecol* 1991; **77**: 129–133.

56. Elson J, Tailor A, Banerjee S, et al. Expectant management of tubal ectopic pregnancy: prediction of successful outcome using decision tree analysis. *Ultrasound Obstet Gynecol* 2004; **23**: 552–556.

57. Valentin L. Prospective cross-validation of Doppler ultrasound examination and gray-scale ultrasound imaging for discrimination of benign and malignant pelvic masses. *Ultrasound Obstet Gynecol* 1999; **14**: 273–283.

58. Timmerman D, Valentin L, Bourne T, et al. Terms, definitions and measurements to describe the sonographic features of adnexal tumors: a consensus opinion from the International Ovarian Tumor Analysis (IOTA) Group. *Ultrasound Obstet Gynecol* 2000; **16**: 500–505.

59. Lockwood G, Pinkerton S, Barlow D. A prospective randomised single-blinded comparative trial of nafarelin acetate with buserelin in long-protocol gonadotrophin-releasing hormone analogue controlled in-vitro fertilization cycles. *Hum Reprod* 1995; **10**: 293–298.

60. Jenkins J, Davies D, Anthony F, et al. The detrimental influence of functional ovarian cysts during in-vitro fertilization cycles. *Hum Reprod* 1992; **7**: 776–780.

61. Meldrum D, Wisot A, Hamilton F, et al. Timing of initiation and dose schedule of leuprolide influence the time course of ovarian suppression. *Fertil Steril* 1988; **50**: 400–402.

62. Sampaio M, Serra V, Miro F, et al. Development of ovarian cysts during gonadotrophin-releasing hormone agonists (GnRHa) administration. *Hum Reprod* 1991; **6**: 194–197.

63. Fleischer A, Shah D, Entman S. Sonographic evaluation of maternal disorders during pregnancy. *Radiol Clin North Am* 1990; **28**: 51–58.

64. Leiserowitz G. Managing ovarian masses during pregnancy. *Obstet Gynecol Surv* 2006; **61**: 463–470.

65. Schmeler K, Mayo-Smith W, Peipert J, et al. Adnexal masses in pregnancy: surgery compared with observation. *Obstet Gynecol* 2005; **105**: 1098–1103.

66. Whitecar P, Turner S, Higby K. Adnexal masses in pregnancy: a review of 130 cases undergoing surgical management. *Am J Obstet Gynecol* 1999; **181**: 19–24.

67. Hillaby K, Aslam N, Salim R, et al. The value of detection of normal ovarian tissue (the 'ovarian crescent sign') in the differential diagnosis of adnexal masses. *Ultrasound Obstet Gynecol* 2004; **23**: 63–67.

68. Barrett R, Harper M, Marshall R. Tuboovarian pregnancy associated with elevated maternal serum alpha-fetoprotein. A case report. *J Reprod Med* 1990; **35**: 277–280.

69. Sarandakou A, Protonotariou E, Rizos D. Tumor markers in biological fluids associated with pregnancy. *Crit Rev Clin Lab Sci* 2007; **44**: 151–178.

70. McDonald J, Doran S, DeSimone C, et al. Predicting risk of malignancy in adnexal masses. *Obstet Gynecol* 2010; **115**: 687–694.

71. Mathur R, Joels L, Jenkins J. Ovarian hyperstimulation syndrome may be more likely if multiple pregnancy occurs following assisted conception. *Acta Genet Med Gemellol (Roma)* 1995; **44**: 233–235.

72. Delvigne A, Rozenberg S. Epidemiology and prevention of ovarian hyperstimulation syndrome (OHSS): a review. *Hum Reprod Update* 2002; **8**: 559–577.

73. Kemmann E, Ghazi D, Corsan G. Adnexal torsion in menotropin-induced pregnancies. *Obstet Gynecol* 1990; **76**: 403–406.

74. McWilliams G, Hill M, Dietrich C. Gynecologic emergencies. *Surg Clin North Am* 2008; **111**: 1313–1319.

75. Mashiach S, Bider D, Moran O, Goldenberg M, Ben-Rafael Z. Adnexal torsion of hyperstimulated ovaries in pregnancies after gonadotropin therapy. *Fertil Steril* 1999; **5**: 76–80.

76. Huchon C, Fauconnier A. Adnexal torsion: a literature review. *Eur J Obstet Gynecol Reprod Biol* 2010; **150**: 8–12.

77. Cohen S, Wattiez A, Seidman D, et al. Laparoscopy versus laparotomy for detorsion and sparing of twisted ischemic adnexa. *JSLS* 2003; **7**: 295–299.

78. Bennett S, Waterstone J, Cheng W, Parsons J. Complications of transvaginal ultrasound-directed follicle aspiration: a review of 2670 consecutive procedures. *J Assist Reprod Genet* 1993; **10**: 72–77.

Chapter 4

Pregnancy after ovarian hyperstimulation syndrome

Botros R. M. B. Rizk and Raphael Ron-El

Introduction

Ovarian hyperstimulation syndrome (OHSS) is a potentially life-threatening iatrogenic complication of ovulation induction, occurring during the luteal phase or during early pregnancy [1–5]. The incidence of severe OHSS, as calculated by the World Health Organization (WHO), is 0.2%–1% of all stimulation cycles in assisted reproduction. Ovarian hyperstimulation syndrome may involve, according to its grade of severity, major electrolytic imbalances, changes in hemodynamic and fluid metabolism, liver and pulmonary dysfunction, as well as increased coagulation with subsequent thromboembolism. Severe OHSS is characterized by bilateral cystic ovarian enlargement (Figures 4.1–4.3) and third-space shift of fluids resulting in pleural effusion and ascites (Figures 4.4–4.6). It often requires hospitalization, and in critical situations may require admission to the intensive care unit [6–9].

Raziel et al. [10] hypothesized that hospitalized patients with severe OHSS are exposed to several insults that could have an impact on the outcome of the pregnancy. These factors include OHSS itself, hemodynamic instability, increased vascular permeability, hemoconcentration, hypoxia, and liver and renal dysfunction (Figure 4.7). Furthermore, in early pregnancy following OHSS, there is exposure to high concentrations of endogenous estrogens, cytokines, renin, angiotensin, and prostaglandins [10–13], which could have an impact on placentation and subsequent placental and fetal development.

There is limited data on the relation of OHSS and pregnancy complications and the influence of OHSS on the pregnancy rate. It has been suggested that the incidence of multiple gestation pregnancy (MGP), early pregnancy failure, adnexal torsion, gestational diabetes mellitus, placental abruption, preterm birth (PTB), pregnancy-induced hypertension (PIH), and low birthweight (LBW) is higher in pregnancies subsequent to severe OHSS. However, most studies do not always use the same definition for the degree of severity of the OHSS and do not agree on the outcome of pregnancy following OHSS, and hence this interesting controversy remains with us. We present, in this chapter, the effect of OHSS on pregnancy outcome along with the pregnancy course and management of clinical complications.

Pregnancy rate in ovarian hyperstimulation syndrome

High pregnancy rates, ranging between 34% and 88%, have been reported in women with OHSS (Table 4.1). In 1967, Rabau et al. were among the first to report a 42% pregnancy rate in patients with OHSS [1], which was confirmed subsequently by most authors who found higher pregnancy rates in in vitro fertilization (IVF) patients in whom OHSS developed compared to IVF patients that did not develop OHSS [14,15]. The largest difference for pregnancy rates between OHSS patients and non-OHSS patients is 73% versus 14%, reported by Raziel et al. [10]. The authors concluded that the severity of OHSS is related to the probability of conception and with a higher rate of MGP.

Early-onset and late-onset ovarian hyperstimulation syndrome

Severe early-onset OHSS is defined as the onset of OHSS within three to seven days of initial human chorionic gonadotropin (hCG) exposure and relates to excessive preovulatory response to stimulation [16,17]. Late-onset OHSS is defined as the onset of OHSS within twelve to seventeen days of hCG administration that depends on the occurrence of pregnancy. Papanikolaou et al. [18] have investigated the

Pregnancy After Assisted Reproductive Technology, ed. Eric R. M. Jauniaux and Botros R. M. B. Rizk. Published by Cambridge University Press.

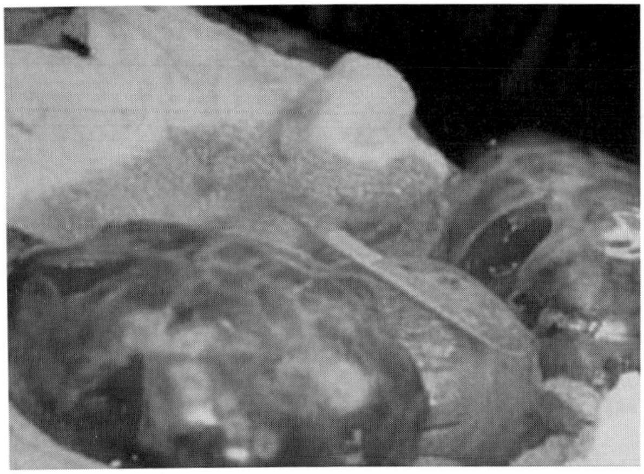

Figure 4.1. Hyperstimulated ovaries. (Reproduced with permission from Serour G. In: Gerris J, Delvigne A, Olivennes F, eds. *Ovarian Hyperstimulation Syndrome*. London, UK: Informa Press, 2006.) (See color plate section for colored image.)

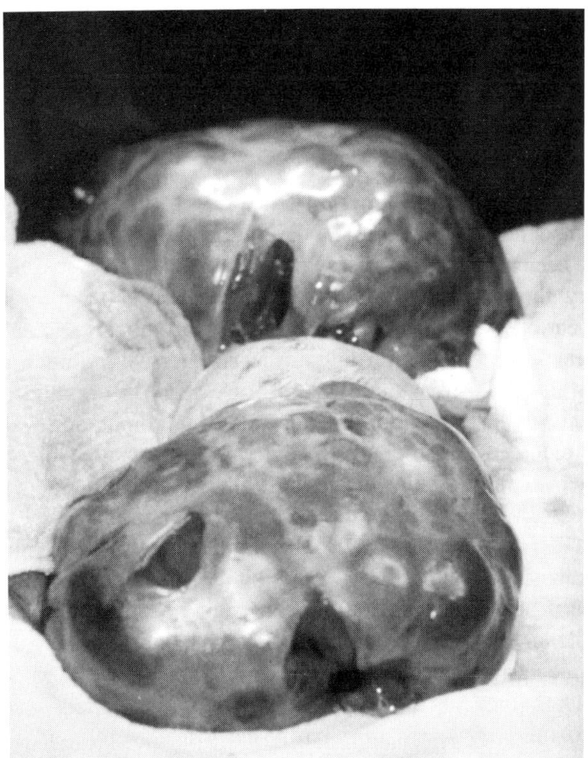

Figure 4.2. Hyperstimulated ovaries. (Reproduced with permission from Schenker JG. In: Zacur H, ed. *Reproductive Medicine and Surgery*. Baltimore, MD: Mosby, 1995.)

pregnancy outcome in early- and late-onset OHSS. Ovarian hyperstimulation syndrome occurred in 2.6% of the IVF cycles (113/4376). Early-onset OHSS occurred in 53 patients and late-onset OHSS in the remaining 60 patients (Table 4.2). Polycystic ovarian syndrome was diagnosed in 18.5% of patients who developed early-onset OHSS versus 11.5% of patients who developed late-onset OHSS ($P<0.05$). A total of 96.7% of the late OHSS cases occurred in a pregnancy cycle. Late-onset cases are more likely to be severe than the early-onset cases, resulting in longer hospital stays of 7.9 days versus 4.6 days ($P<0.05$). However, in the early OHSS group the biochemical pregnancy rate in early onset is 41.1% but the clinical pregnancy rate fell to 28% due to the increased rate of pregnancy loss compared with the non-OHSS patients. In late-onset OHSS, the clinical pregnancy rates and ongoing pregnancy rates are 92% and 88%, respectively. The multiple pregnancy rate did not differ significantly between early and late OHSS, 40% and 45%, respectively. However, comparing late OHSS with non-OHSS patients, there was a statistically significant difference in multiple pregnancy rates, 45% versus 29%. Papanikolaou et al. [18] concluded that early OHSS is associated with exongenously administered hCG and a higher risk of preclinical miscarriage whereas late OHSS is closely associated with the conception cycles, especially multiple pregnancies, and is more likely to be severe.

Ovarian hyperstimulation syndrome and early and late pregnancy outcome

Mathur and Jenkins [19] debated whether OHSS was associated with a poor obstetric outcome and reviewed forty-one IVF pregnancies complicated by moderate or severe OHSS, from the University of Bristol, U.K., over a three-year period. They observed no difference in the miscarriage rates between the pregnant OHSS patients and the group of 501 contemporary clinical pregnant patients resulting from IVF procedures without OHSS. They suggest that the higher miscarriage rate other studies report might be attributed to a higher incidence of MGP or greater severity of OHSS (Tables 4.3, 4.4).

Miscarriage rates in pregnancies following ovarian hyperstimulation syndrome

The risk of miscarriage is apparently higher in patients with severe OHSS than in IVF patients without OHSS (see Chapter 5). Most authors have found miscarriage rates in women with OHSS ranging between 27% and

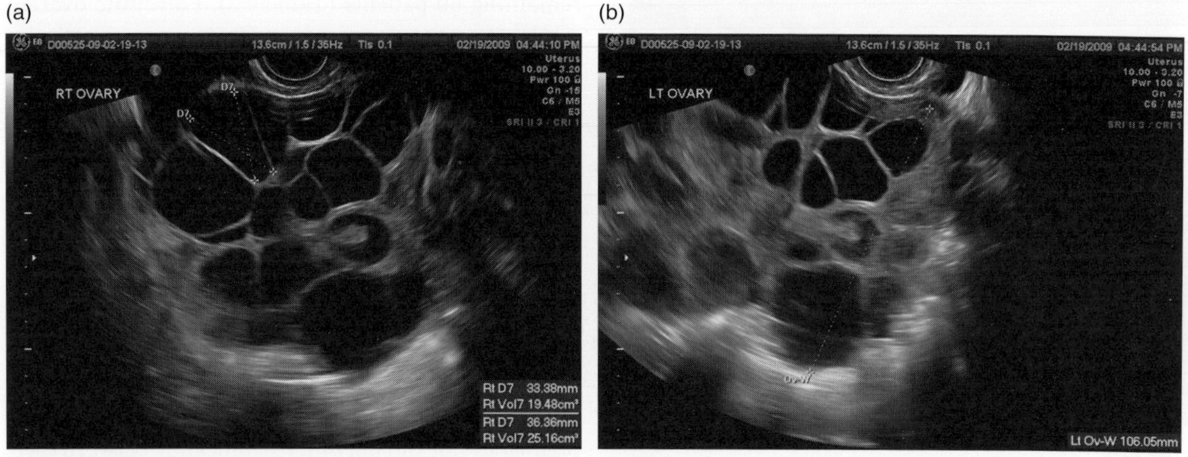

Figure 4.3. (a), (b): multiple ovarian cysts in a pregnant patient with ovarian hyperstimulation syndrome.

40% [20–22], with only a few authors finding no difference [16]. These high miscarriage rates are thought to have been caused by the excessively high serum estradiol levels, high cytokine production, and excessive renin–angiotensin activity, which are all characteristic of OHSS.

One of the largest studies is that of Raziel et al. [10], who found an increased early pregnancy loss of 38% in IVF patients who developed severe OHSS compared with 15% of IVF patients who did not develop OHSS. In an analysis of 104 IVF patients hospitalized for severe and critical OHSS over a six-year period, the same group of authors [11] compared the characteristics of pregnant and non-pregnant patients with severe OHSS and those who aborted compared with those with ongoing pregnancies. One of their main findings is that there was a prominent decline in severe and critical OHSS cases after IVF from 6.4% to 1.5% over the last three years of their study. They also found that pregnancy was achieved in 60 of the 104 patients (58%) with severe OHSS while pregnancy continued until delivery in 37 of the 60 patients (62%) and miscarriage occurred in 38%, including early miscarriage in 83% and late miscarriage in 17% of their cases.

Obstetric outcome after ovarian hyperstimulation syndrome

One of the largest studies on pregnancy outcome after OHSS is that of Abramov et al. [13], who reviewed all patients hospitalized between 1987 and 1996 in a multicenter study in Israel. Overall they found higher pregnancy rates, miscarriages, MGP, gestational diabetes, placental abruption, PTB, and LBW in IVF patients with OHSS compared with IVF patients without OHSS (Table 4.5). A high number (2902) of their patients were hospitalized for OHSS management and of these patients, 209 were severe or critical and 163 were IVF patients. Most were young (mean age: 29 years) and healthy women with a mean of 4.4 years of infertility duration. Anovulation was the most common indication for IVF (13%). The clinical pregnancy rate was 73% including 42% singletons, 34% twins, 17% triplets, and 7% quadruplets. The pregnancy loss rate was 30%, of which 25% were early pregnancy losses and 4.8% were late miscarriages. Fetal reduction was performed in 25% of MGP in addition to the occurrence of spontaneous reduction or vanishing twins in 18%, with threatened miscarriage in 18%. Premature rupture of membranes (PROM) occurred in 18% of patients compared with 5% occurrence in other IVF patients. Pregnancy-induced hypertension occurred in 13% of OHSS patients compared with 6% in the general IVF population, and gestational diabetes occurred in 6% versus 0.8%. The mean gestational age was 37 weeks for singletons, 35 for twins, and 34 for triplets (Table 4.6). Preterm birth occurred in 28% of the singleton pregnancies, 50% of the twin pregnancies, and 100% of triplet pregnancies. Spina bifida and truncus arteriosis were found in two fetuses of the study group with no other major malformations reported in the rest of pregnancies investigated. The rate of Cesarean section delivery was 44%.

More recently, Wiser et al. [23] evaluated the second and third trimester morbidity of patients who conceived and developed OHSS, and compared these

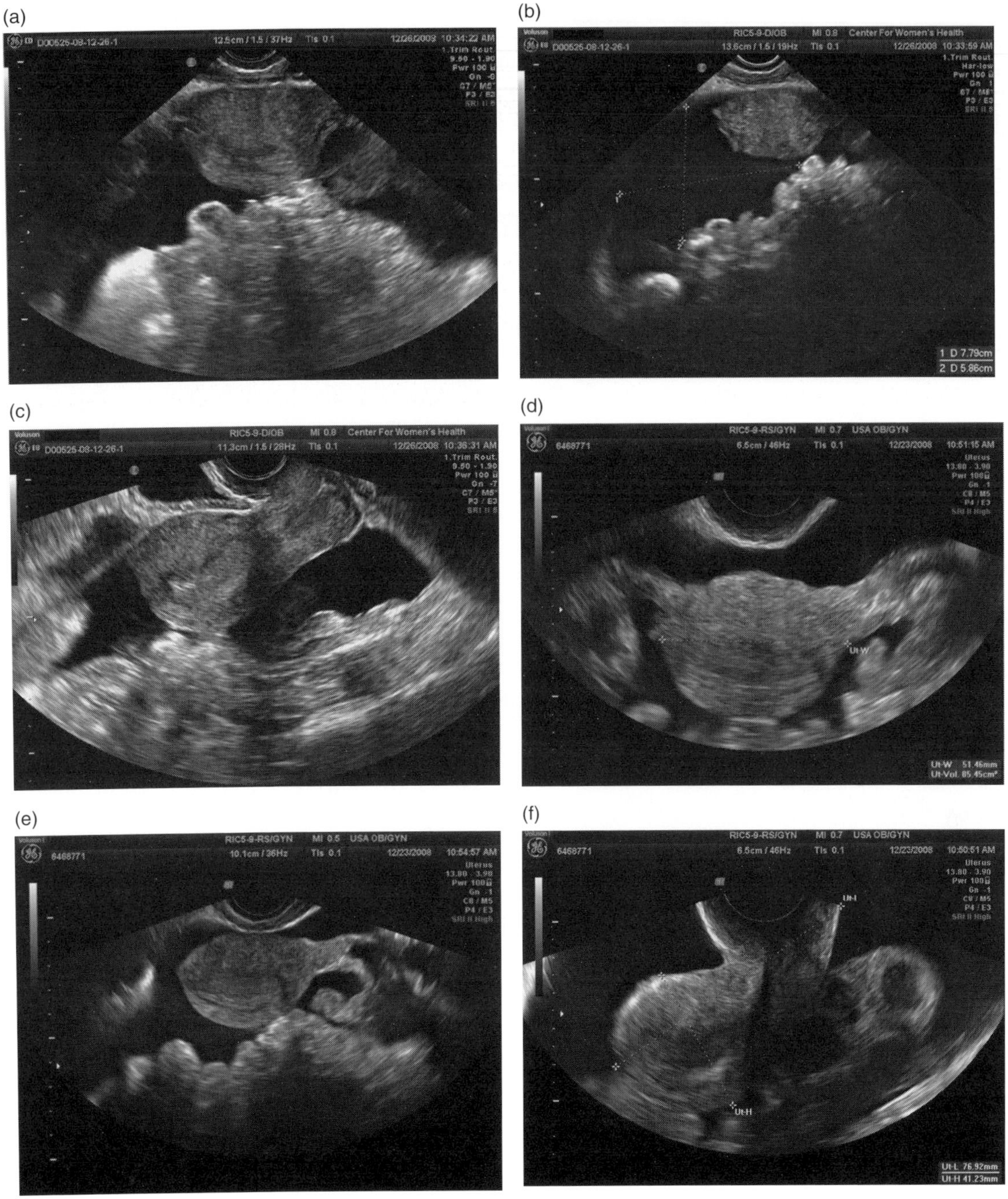

Figure 4.4. (a)–(f): ascites.

results with those of patients who conceived after IVF without OHSS (Tables 4.7,4.8). They evaluated 165 patients with OHSS, 101 singletons and 64 twins, and 156 IVF control patients, 85 singletons and 71 twins. Gestational diabetes and PIH were observed in both groups but at a similar rate. In particular, gestational diabetes presented with an incidence of 9.9% for singletons and 9.4% for twins in the OHSS group, and

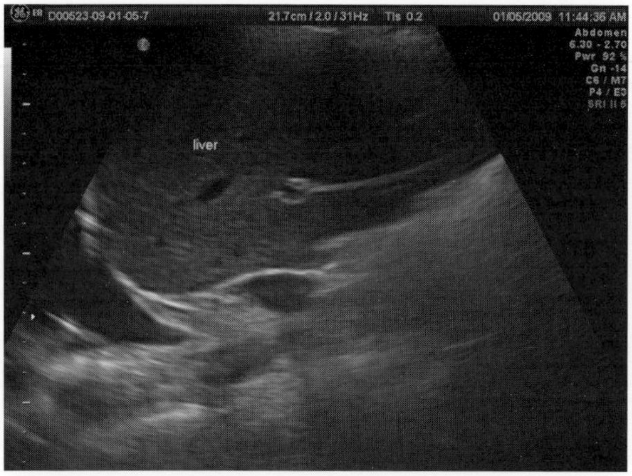

Figure 4.5. Right pleural effusion in a pregnant patient with ovarian hyperstimulation syndrome. (Reproduced with permission from Rizk B, ed *Ultrasonography in Reproductive Medicine and Infertility.* Cambridge, UK: Cambridge Univesity Press, 2010; 302.)

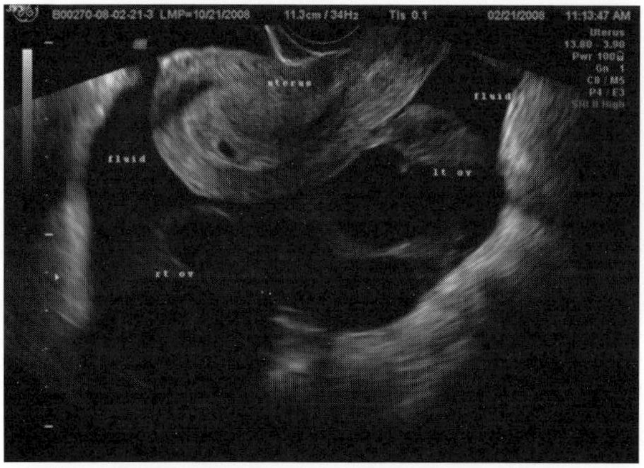

Figure 4.6. Ascites in a patient with moderate ovarian hyperstimulation syndrome in early pregnancy. (Reproduced with permission from Rizk B ed. *Ultrasonography in Reproductive Medicine and Infertility.* Cambridge, UK: Cambridge Univesity Press, 2010; 306.)

12.9% for singletons and 7.0% for twins in the non-OHSS group, whereas PIH presented in 6.9% of singleton pregnancies and 10.9% for twins, and 8.2% in singleton pregnancies and 7.0% in twin pregnancies in the non-OHSS group (Figure 4.8).

Medical treatment of severe ovarian hyperstimulation syndrome

Outpatient management is recommended for women with mild and moderate OHSS. By contrast, patients with severe OHSS should be evaluated to determine if they meet the criteria for admission to the hospital, in particular if they present with shortness of breath or diminished urine output or abdominal pain (Table 4.9). The medical management relies on the restoration of the intravascular volume to assist with renal perfusion as well as preventing thromboembolism. Critical OHSS should be managed by a multidisciplinary team, according to the end organ affected.

Correction of circulatory volume

The main line of treatment is correction of the circulatory volume and electrolyte imbalance. Several authors have described fluid management protocol for patient presenting with severe OHSS. At the Johns Hopkins Hospital, all the patients admitted with OHSS are initially treated with 1L of normal saline over one hour [24]. Lactated Ringer solution (Hopkins protocol) is not recommended because many of the OHSS patients tend to be hyponatremic. If the patient has a satisfactory urine output in response to the fluid bolus, at least 50 mL over the hour after the fluid bolus, an IV fluid maintenance protocol is initiated. Typically 5% dextrose in normal

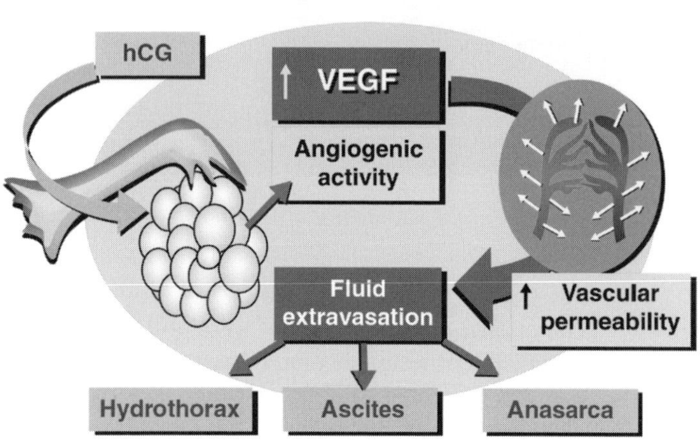

Figure 4.7. Diagrammatic representation of increased vascular permeability and ascites formation in ovarian hyperstimulation syndrome. (Reproduced with permission from Rizk B, ed. *Ultrasonography in Reproductive Medicine and Infertility.* Cambridge, UK: Cambridge University Press, 2010; 306.) (See color plate section for colored image.)

Table 4.1. Incidence of pregnancy in patients with ovarian hyperstimulation syndrome (1967–1992)

Reference	Year	Incidence %	Number of patients	Multiple pregnancies
Rabau et al.	1967	42	6/14	2/6
Schenker and Weinstein	1978	40	10/25	5/10
Tulandi et al.	1984	34.6	10/29	4/10
Golan et al.	1988	91	10/11	1/10
Borenstein et al.	1989	35	14/39	3/14
Herman et al.	1990	80	4/5	1/4
Forman et al.	1990	88	7/8	2/7
Smitz et al.	1990	70	7/10	3/7
Rizk et al.	1991	57	12/21	5/12

(Modified from Rizk 1994 [9].)

Table 4.2. Outcome of pregnancies following in vitro fertilization in patients with early-onset and late-onset severe ovarian hyperstimulation syndrome

Authors	Year	Number of OHSS patients	Clinical pregnancy rate per transfer (%)	Clinical miscarriage rate	Gestational age at birth (weeks, mean +/−SD)	C-section (%)
Abramov et al.	1998	163	41.7	Early-onset OHSS: 25	All births: 37 +/−3.2	44
				Late-onset OHSS: 4.8		
				Total: 29.8		
Mathur et al.	2000	41	No data	12.2	No data	No data
Raziel et al.	2002	104	58	Early-onset OHSS: 18.3	No data	No data
				Late-onset OHSS: 3.8		
				Total: 22.1		
Wiser et al.	2005	145	No data	(Only pregnancies beyond the first trimester included.)	All births: 35.3+/−3.2	No data
					Singleton: 35.3+/−3.4	
					Twins: 35.7+/−3.2	
Papanikolaou et al.	2005	113	Early-onset OHSS: 28.3	Early-onset OHSS: 6.6	No data	No data
			Late-onset OHSS: 91.8	Late-onset OHSS: 3.6		
			Total: 62	Total: 4.3		

OHSS, ovarian hyperstimulation syndrome; C, Cesarean. (Modified from Raziel et al., 2009 [10].)

Table 4.3. Pregnancy wastage in ovarian hyperstimulation syndrome and control pregnancies

	Mathur and Jenkins		Chen et al.		Abramov et al.
	OHSS pregnancies (n = 41)	Control pregnancies (n = 501)	OHSS pregnancies (n = 15)	Control pregnancies (n = 110)	OHSS pregnancies (n = 104)
Miscarriage	5 (12.2%)	84 (16.8%)	4 (26.6%)	19 (17.2%)	31 (29.8%)
≤12 weeks	5 (12.2%)	72 (14.4%)	–	–	26 (25%)
>12weeks	0	12 (2.4%)	–	–	5 (4.8%)
Spontaneous reduction	2/17 (11.7%)	29/172 (16.8%)	–	–	11/60 (18.3%)
Multiple pregnancies	17 (41.4%)	172 (34.3%)	7 (46.6%)	36 (32.7%)	60 (57.7%)

OHSS, ovarian hyperstimulation syndrome.
(Modified from Mathur and Jenkins, 2000 [19]; Abramov et al., 1998 [13]; Chen et al., 1997 [20].)

Table 4.4. Obstetric outcome of ovarian hyperstimulation syndrome and control pregnancies resulting in deliveries

	Mathur and Jenkins		Abramov et al.
	OHSS pregnancies (n = 36)	Control pregnancies (n = 444)	OHSS pregnancies (n = 68)
Multiple pregnancies	13 (36.1%)	122 (27.4%)	39 (59.5%)
Preterm deliveries	9 (25%)	88 (19.8%)	30 (44.1%)
Low birthweight*	26 (50%)	164 (28.5%)**	72 (64.3%)
Birthweight (g)	2455 (820–3940)	2940 (540–4730)**	2221 (252)
Singleton birthweight (g)	3230 (820–3940)	3320 (650–4730)	2785 (356)

OHSS, ovarian hyperstimulation syndrome;
*, <2500 g;
**, significant difference (P=0.002). (Modified from Mathur and Jenkins, 2000 [19]; Abramov et al., 1998 [13].)

saline is infused at 125–150 mL per hour and urine output is assessed every four hours. Hematocrit is determined four to six hours after the start of IV hydration to insure that hemoconcentration is corrected. If there is inadequate response in the urine output from the initial 1L fluid bolus, IV crystalloid fluids are stopped and a regimen of low volume hyperosmolar IV therapy is begun. An IV infusion of 200 mL of 25% albumin solution is given over four hours and the hematocrit is rechecked until it is 36%–38%. In the U.K., most IVF centers do not use IV crystalloids and only colloids are used for the fluid management of patients with severe OHSS; the crystalloid management protocol is typically criticized because it does not maintain intravascular fluid volume.

Albumin, dextran, mannitol, fresh frozen plasma, and hydroxyethyl starch have been used for the management of severe OHSS [25]. Hydroxyethyl starch has

Table 4.5. Outcome of in vitro fertilization pregnancies in different countries compared with pregnancies complicated by severe ovarian hyperstimulation syndrome

Outcome of IVF pregnancy	France	U.S.	U.K.	Australia and New Zealand	Israel	Severe OHSS [13]
Miscarriage	18	19	–	22	–	30
Ectopic pregnancy	5	6	–	6	–	2
Multiple pregnancy	27	22	23	22	24	58
Twins	22	19	19	19	19	34
Triplets and higher	4	3	4	3	5	24
Preterm rate	29	–	24	27	28	44
Singletons	9	–	13	17	–	28
Twins	43	–	57	56	50	50
Triplets and higher	90	–	95	97	100	100
Low birth weight	36	–	32	34	62	62
Singletons	11	–	12	15	35	35
Twins	60	–	55	56	64	64
Triplets and higher	95	–	94	94	100	100
C-section rate	43	–	–	–	44	44
Singletons	26	–	–	–	24	24
Twins	57	–	–	–	53	53
Triplets and higher	88	–	–	–	100	100
Fetal malformations	2.8	2.0	2.2	2.2	2.2	1.9

IVF, in vitro fertilization; OHSS, ovarian hyperstimulation syndrome; C, Cesarean. (Modified from Abramov et al., 1998 [13].)

the advantage of a non-biological origin and a high molecular weight of 200–1000 Kda versus 69 Kda for albumin. Abramov et al. [26] compared the efficacy of hydroxyethyl starch with albumin in 16 patients with severe OHSS. They observed higher urine output, fewer paracenteses, and shorter hospital stays with hydroxyethyl starch (Table 4.10). Gamzu et al. [27] compared hydroxyethyl starch (10%) and Haemaccel and found no clinical advantage for the hydroxyethyl starch.

Hyponatremia and hyperkalemia

Electrolyte imbalances are frequently encountered in cases of severe OHSS. Appropriate electrolyte solutions should be used and restriction of salt and water is not recommended [9]. Hyperkalemia may be associated with cardiac arrhythmias, and thus acute management may involve treatment that transfers potassium into the intracellular space such as with insulin, glucose, and sodium bicarbonate, and to protect the heart from elevated potassium levels such as with calcium gluconate, as recommended by the ASRM Practice Committee [28]. Electrocardiagraphic manifestations of cardiac arrhythmias include prolonged PR and QRS intervals, ST segment depression, and tall peak T waves. These indicate the immediate need for treatment with calcium gluconate. Cation exchange such as K Exalayte removes potassium from the body but its onset of action is one to two hours. It may be administered orally, or rectally as a retention enema.

Table 4.6. Early pregnancy outcome in early and late ovarian hyperstimulation syndrome

	Early n = 53	Late n = 60	Total n = 113	Non-OHSS n = 4263	SS early vs. late	SS early vs. non-OHSS
Pregnant	22	58	80	1401	<0.001	ns
(% per cycle)	(41.5%)	(96.7%)	(70.8%)	(32.8%)		
(% per ET)	(50.0)	(96.7%)	(76.9%)	(36.9%)		
Preclinical miscarriages	7 (31.8%)	3 (5.2%)	10 (12.5%)**	210 (14.4%)	0.01	<0.05
Clinical pregnancies	15	55	70	1187	0.01	ns
(% per cycle)	(28.3%)	(91.8%)	(61.8%)	(27.9%)		
(% per ET)	(34.1%)	(91.8%)	(66.9%)	(31.3%)		
Clinical miscarriages	1 (6.6%)	2 (3.6%)	3 (4.3%)	126 (10.5%)	ns	ns
Ongoing pregnancies	14	53	67	1061	0.01	ns
(% per cycle)	(26.4%)	(88.3%)	(64.4%)	(24.9%)		
(% per ET)	(31.8%)	(88.3%)	(64.4%)	(28.0%)		
Initial multiple pregnancy rate	6/15 (40%)	25/55* (45.5%)	30/70 (44.3%)	345/1187 (29.1%)	ns	ns

OHSS, ovarian hyperstimulation syndrome; SS, statistical significance; ET, embryo transfer; ns, not statistically significant;
*, P=0.02 (late- vs. non-OHSS);
**, P>0.05 (total OHSS vs. non-OHSS). (Papanikolaou et al., 2005 [18].)

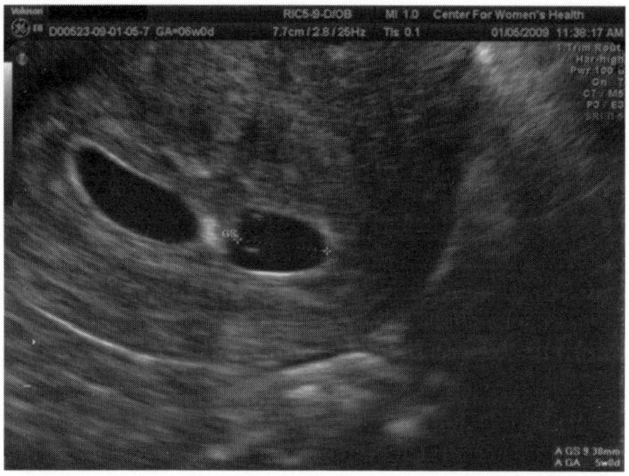

Figure 4.8. Twin pregnancies in a patient with ovarian hyperstimulation syndrome after in vitro fertilization. (Reproduced with permission from Rizk B, ed. *Ultrasonography in Reproductive Medicine and Infertility*. Cambridge, UK: Cambridge Univesity Press, 2010; 306.)

Diuretics

Diuretic therapy without prior volume expansion may precipitate intravascular coagulation. Lasix is used in patients with pulmonary edema. Some authors have recommended albumin/Lasix chase for the management of patients with severe OHSS [4].

Dopamine

Dopamine used in oliguric patients with severe OHSS results in significant improvement in renal function [29]. Dopamine produces its renal effect by increasing renal blood flow and glomerular filtration. Dopamine therapy should be given cautiously and under strict observation. In one report, intravenous dopamine (4.32 mg/kg per 24 hr) was administered to seven patients hospitalized with severe OHSS following gonadotrophin stimulation for IVF or gamete intra-Fallopian transfer (GIFT), beginning within 10 hours of admission [30]. Additional treatment included: bedrest, restriction of fluid intake to 500 mL/day, daily monitoring of urine output, and measurement of abdominal girth and weight. Biochemical and hematological clotting factors were measured daily in the pregnant women. Serum hCG should be measured every two days and the patients should be given a

Table 4.7. Maternal morbidity in singleton in vitro fertilization pregnancies complicated by ovarian hyperstimulation syndrome compared to singleton in vitro fertilization pregnancies without ovarian hyperstimulation syndrome

	Singleton IVF pregnancies with OHSS (n = 101)	Singleton IVF pregnancies without OHSS (n = 85)
Age (years)a	30.7+/−4.5	32.4+/−5.1
GDM (n (%))	10 (9.9)	11 (12.9)
PIH (n (%))	7 (6.9)	7 (8.2)
Hospitalization (days)	4.5+/−2.9	–
Week of delivery	39+/−1.9	39+/−1.9
Babies' weight at delivery	3045+/−544	3082+/−557
Cesarean section (n (%))	24 (24)	18 (21.1)

IVF, in vitro fertilization; OHSS, ovarian hyperstimulation syndrome; a, statistical significance at P <0.05 (from twins); GDM, gestational diabetes mellitus; PIH, pregnancy-induced hypertension. (Modified from Wiser et al., 2005 [23].)

Table 4.8. Comparison between the delivery outcomes in patients with twin in vitro fertilization pregnancies with and without ovarian hyperstimulation syndrome

	Twin IVF pregnancies with OHSS (n = 64)	Twin IVF pregnancies without OHSS (n = 71)
Age (years)a	29.0+/−4.2	30.8+/−4.4
GDM (n (%))	6 (9.4)	5 (7.0)
PIH (n (%))	7 (10.9)	5 (7.0)
Hospitalization (days)	6.2+/−3.8	
Week of delivery	35.3+/−4.3	35.7+/−3.2
Babies' weight at delivery	2148+/−607	2259+/−501
Cesarean section (n (%))	35 (54.6)	40 (56.3)

IVF, in vitro fertilization; OHSS, ovarian hyperstimulation syndrome; a statistical significance at P<0.05; GDM, gestational diabetes mellitus; PIH, pregnancy-induced hypertension. (Modified from Wiser et al., 2005 [23].)

protein- and salt-rich diet in order to increase the oncotic and osmotic blood pressure. Dopamine treatment can be continued until there is complete resolution of ascites. In the five patients who were pregnant, dopamine treatment was required for 9 to 22 days. The duration of treatment can be related to the magnitude of the increase of hCG with the longest (18–22 days) in patients with triplets, shortest (9–10 days) in patients with a singleton pregnancy, and intermediate (14 days) for patients with twins. In the two non-pregnant women, dopamine was only required for seven days [30]. It is also suggested that a 750 mg tablet of docarpamine (Dostinex) can be taken orally every eight hours in cases of OHSS refractory to the initial therapy with intravenous albumin [30]. Clinical symptoms associated with ascites gradually improved in these patients with this treatment, with no major adverse effects.

Thrombophilia and ovarian hyperstimulation syndrome

In 1999, Dulitzky et al. [31] found that 17 of their 20 patients with severe OHSS (85%) and 11 of 41

Table 4.9. Medical indications for hospitalization of patients with severe ovarian hyperstimulation syndrome

1. Severe abdominal pain or peritoneal signs
2. Intractable nausea and vomiting that prevents ingestion of food and adequate fluids
3. Severe oliguria or anuria
4. Tense ascites
5. Dyspnea or tachypnea
6. Hypotension (relative to baseline), dizziness, or syncope
7. Severe electrolyte imbalance (hyponatremia, hyperkalemia)

(Reproduced with permission from Rizk B, ed. In: *Ovarian Hyperstimulation Syndrome: Epidemiology, Prevention and Management*. Cambridge, UK: Cambridge University Press, 2006; Chapter 8.)

Table 4.10. Controlled cohort study to compare the efficacy of 6% human hydroxyethyl starch and human albumin for treatment of severe ovarian hyperstimulation syndrome

Variable	Human albumin group (n = 10)	Hydroxyethyl starch group (n = 6)
Baseline characteristics		
Age (years)	28.1+/−8.9	29.4+/−7.4
Estradiol level on day of hCG (pg/mL)	6164+/−1418	9080+/−2450
Ascites (%)	10 (100)	6 (100)
Pleural effusion (%)	2 (20)	1 (17)
Gastrointestinal symptoms (%)	4 (40)	6 (100)
Ovarian diameter	10.7+/−3.4	10.5+/−3.8
Oliguria (%)	1 (10)	1 (17)
Hematocrit (%)	42+/−3.6	43+/−7
Daily fluid intake (mL)*	3300+/−310	3150+/−2170
Patient outcome		
Daily urine output**	2557+/−1032	3580+/−1780
Abdominal paracentesis (%)	8 (80)	2 (33)
Total fluid aspirated per patient (mL)	2300+/−230	1930
Pleurocentesis (%)	2 (20)	0
Hospital stay (days)	19+/−8.2	15.7+/−5.7
Conception	7 (70)	4 (67)
Miscarriage	2 (20)	1 (17)
Congenital malformation	0	0

Values are means+/−SD or percentages of patients; *, including oral and intravenous hydration; **, during the first five days of hospitalization. (Reproduced with permission from Abramov et al., 2001 [26].)

controls (26.8%) had one or more positive markers of thrombophilia. Of the women with severe OHSS, six had a decreased antithrombin level, eight had decreased levels of protein S, seven were homozygous for the MTHFR 677T mutation, one was heterozygous for the factor V Leiden mutation, and five had antiphospholipid antibodies. Furthermore, eight of the women investigated and presenting with OHSS and no controls had more than one positive marker of thrombophilia. They concluded that the prevalence of thrombophilia is increased in women with severe OHSS and that prophylactic screening for this disorder and possible use of heparin prophylaxis for thromboembolic phenomena should be considered in these patients. Raziel et al. [12] postulated that the high prevalence of positive thrombolic markers may shed new light on the pathophysiology of OHSS. In particular, the high prevalence of thrombophilic markers in severe OHSS may be the explanation for the increased rate of pregnancy loss [32].

Thromboembolism and ovarian hyperstimulation syndrome

Thromboembolism is the most dangerous complication of OHSS [5–9,33,34]. The majority of thromboembolic cases are venous in origin (deep leg veins, internal jugular vein, subclavian vein, and inferior vena cava). Most of the serious complications, however, arise from arterial thromboses (middle cerebral artery, anterior cerebral artery, internal carotid artery, vertebral artery, humeral artery, femoral artery, mesenteric artery, aorta, and subclavian artery). The timing of arterial and venous thrombosis in OHSS patients differed. Arterial events usually occurred concurrently with the onset of OHSS whereas venous thromboses may occur several weeks after the clinical resolution of OHSS.

A systematic review found 96 cases of thrombotic complications following treatment with assisted reproductive technology (ART) [33]. Of these, 35 were arterial in nature and 61 were venous events. Of the 35 cases that resulted in arterial thrombosis, 21 cases were cerebrovascular accidents (60%), six cases involved the extremities (17%), and four cases were myocardial infarctions (11%). Two of the women who developed arterial strokes and one woman who had mesenteric infarction died from complications, representing 9% mortality among the reported cases. The predominant sites for venous thromboses were in the veins of the neck and upper extremities, that is, 49/61 cases (80%). There were no mortality cases reported among the venous thrombotic events. Pregnancy was reported in 74 cases (77%). Pregnancy was reported in 46% of women with arterial thromboses and 97% of women with venous thromboses. Ovarian hyperstimulation syndrome was reported in 27/31 (87%) women with arterial thrombosis and in 47/60 (78%) women with venous thrombosis.

Patients with severe OHSS should be started on subcutaneous heparin, 5000 units twice daily, or Lovenox, 40 mg subcutaneously, immediately on admission to the hospital and this regimen should continue throughout the hospital stay [28,33,34]. Prophylactic doses of anticoagulants should also be considered for patients who develop moderate and severe OHSS even if they are treated as outpatients [33]. This treatment should be maintained for an extended period of one to two months beyond the clinical resolution of OHSS. Patients with inherited thrombophilia should also receive thromboprophylaxis while undergoing ART.

Paracentesis

Ultrasound-guided paracentesis is indicated for patients with ascites that causes pain, compromised pulmonary function, oliguria, and anuria that does not respond to fluid management. A transvaginal or transabdominal approach may be used under ultrasound guidance. Aboulghar et al. [35] demonstrated that transvaginal aspiration of as little as 800 mL of ascitic fluid results in significant improvement of renal function and relief of abdominal discomfort. Serial paracentesis may be required to maintain adequate renal and pulmonary function. Severe ascites may be associated with hydrothorax, most commonly on the right side, as a result of transfer of ascetic fluid to the chest by a thoracic duct. Paracentesis will be effective in resolving hydrothorax and thoracocentesis is reserved for patients with bilateral or severe pulmonary effusions that persist [36].

Surgical treatment of severe ovarian hyperstimulation syndrome

Surgery is infrequently needed, but if required can be a challenge for the anesthesiologist (Table 4.11). Careful positioning of patients during surgery is important as the Trendelenberg position may further compromise the residual pulmonary functional capacity. Establishment of access lines may be necessary in patients with

Table 4.11. Challenges to the anesthesiologist in ovarian hyperstimulation syndrome

• Pulmonary compromise
• Severe hemoconcentration
• Pleural effusions
• Restricted IV access
• Infections and febrile morbidity
• Difficult positioning in surgery
• Thrombophlebitis
• Pelvic masses
• Ascites
• Electrolyte disturbances

(Reproduced with permission from Rizk B, ed. In: *Ovarian Hyperstimulation Syndrome: Epidemiology, Prevention and Management.* Cambridge, UK: Cambridge University Press, 2006; Chapter 8.)

contracted vascular volume. Drainage of pleural effusions may assist in improving pulmonary status.

Surgery for ruptured cysts

Laparotomy, in general, should be avoided in OHSS. If deemed necessary, as in cases of hemorrhagic ovarian cysts, it should be performed by an experienced gynecologist and only hemostatic measures undertaken so as to preserve the ovaries.

Ovarian torsion

Ovarian torsion (Figure 4.9) is an infrequent complication of ovulation induction, which if unrecognized and untreated, results in loss of one or both ovaries [26]. Presenting symptoms are severe unilateral adenexal pain in a patient with enlarged ovaries due to ovarian stimulation or with multiple pregnancy. Sonography with Doppler flow analysis can be diagnostic, but a finding of apparently normal blood flow does not completely rule out ovarian torsion [26].

Ovarian torsion (Figure 4.9) in patients with OHSS has varied in incidence between 3% in non-pregnant patients [37] and 16% in pregnant patients with OHSS [38]. Preservation of the ovary is very important in young and fertile women. Prompt and early diagnosis with laparoscopic unwinding can increase the likelihood of a viable ovary, thus resulting in a successful outcome.

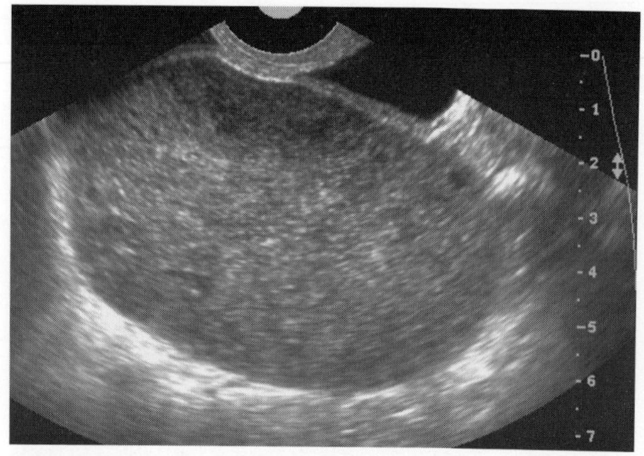

Figure 4.9. Ovarian torsion. (Reproduced with permission from Eyvazadeh and Levine. Acute pelvic pain. In: Rizk B, ed. *Ultrasonography in Reproductive Medicine and Infertility.* Cambridge, UK: Cambridge University Press, 2010; 178.)

Wiser et al. [23] observed a relatively high incidence of ovarian torsion in OHSS patients that required laparoscopy. The clinical decision to operate was based on clinical judgment, with laparoscopy being performed on 13 of the 165 IVF patients with OHSS. Ovarian detorsion was required in ten patients. Twin pregnancies were involved 3.5 times more than singletons. Successful outcomes were achieved in all the patients and their pregnancies continued without complications related to torsion.

In a review of 77 cases of ovarian torsion at a single hospital, Doppler flow sonography was performed preoperatively in 90% of cases but demonstrated compromised blood flow in only 29% of those scanned [39]. Of these, 30 (51%) required oophorectomy. Ovarian torsion followed ovulation induction in 21 of the 77 cases, and of these only one required oophorectomy possibly because of earlier diagnosis. Twenty-four patients were pregnant, two-thirds as a result of ovulation induction. The mean gestational age was 10.4 weeks (range 4–28 weeks) at the time of ovarian torsion. Although the adnexa usually appears dark, hemorrhagic, and ischemic, they can be saved, if the diagnosis is made soon enough, by simply unwinding, often as a laparoscopic procedure.

Surgery for ectopic pregnancy associated with ovarian hyperstimulation syndrome

The association between OHSS and ectopic pregnancy is not commonly encountered. Diagnosis of tubal pregnancy by vaginal ultrasound examination at this stage is not always possible. The presence of large ovaries filling the pelvis makes ultrasound scanning of other structures difficult. Fluid in the pouch of Douglas is of limited diagnostic importance in the presence of ascites.

Conclusion

Women with severe and critical OHSS should be managed by intravenous hydration and anticoagulation. Complications requiring surgery could present anesthetic challenges, and operations on women with OHSS should only be performed in units with expertise in OHSS. Early pregnancy losses are more common in early OHSS compared with late-onset OHSS. Patients may rarely develop late OHSS, even if they are not pregnant, if they have received hCG for luteal phase support. Overall, pregnancies following OHSS should be considered as high-risk pregnancies, in particular regarding the risks of early and late miscarriages probably linked to the high prevalence of thrombophilia in that population. Thromboembolism is the most dangerous complication of OHSS, and prophylactic doses of anticoagulants should be considered for patients who develop moderate and severe OHSS even if they are treated on an outpatient basis. All patients admitted for severe and critical OHSS should receive thromboprophylaxis. As prevention is the best treatment for OHSS, this may imply the need for more patient-friendly or mild stimulation protocols. Properly conducted studies including large numbers of patients are required in order to determine the best method of prevention and management.

References

1. Rabau E, David A, Serr DM, Mashiach S, Lunenfeld B. Human menopausal gonadotrophins for anovulation and sterility. Results of 7 years of treatment. *Am J Obstet Gynecol* 1967; **98**: 92–98.
2. Schenker JG, Weinstein D. Ovarian hyperstimulation syndrome (a current survey). *Fertil Steril* 1978; **30**: 255–268.
3. Golan A, Ron-El R, Herman A, et al. Ovarian hyperstimulation syndrome: an update review. *Obstet Gynecol Surv* 1989; **44**: 430–440.
4. Navot D, Bergh PA, Laufer N. Ovarian hyperstimulation syndrome in novel reproductive technologies: prevention and treatment. *Fertil Steril* 1993; **58**: 249–261.
5. Rizk B, Aboulghar MA. Classification, pathophysiology and management of ovarian hyperstimulation syndrome. In: Brinsden P ed. *Textbook of In-vitro Fertilization and Assisted Reproduction.* 2nd edn. Canforth, UK: Parthenon, 1999; 131–155.
6. Rizk B, Meagher S, Fisher AM. Ovarian hyperstimulation syndrome and cerebrovascular accidents. *Hum Reprod* 1990; **5**: 697–698.
7. Rizk B, Aboulghar M. Modern management of ovarian hyperstimulation syndrome. *Hum Reprod* 1991; 6: 1191–1198.
8. Rizk B, Aboulghar MA, Smitz J, Ron-El R. The role of vascular endothelial growth factor and interleukins in the pathogenesis of severe ovarian hyperstimulation syndrome. *Hum Reprod Update* 1997: **3**: 255–266.
9. Rizk B. Ovarian hyperstimulation syndrome. In: Studd JWW ed. *Progress in Obstetrics and Gynecology.* Edinburgh, UK: Churchill Livingstone, 1994; vol. **11**, ch. 8, 311–349.
10. Raziel A, Schacter M, Friedler S, Ron-El R. Outcome of IVF pregnancies following severe OHSS. *Reprod Biomed Online* 2009; **19**: 61–65.
11. Raziel A, Friedler S, Schachter S, et al. Increased early pregnancy loss in IVF patients with severe ovarian hyperstimulation syndrome. *Hum Reprod* 2002; **17**: 107–110.
12. Raziel A, Friedler S, Schachter M, et al. Hypercoaguable thrombophilic defects and hyperhomocysteinemia in patients with recurrent pregnancy loss. *Am J Reprod Immunol* 2001; **45**: 65–71.
13. Abramov Y, Elchalal U, Schenker JG. Obstetric outcome of in-vitro fertilized pregnancies complicated by severe ovarian hyperstimulation syndrome: a multicenter study. *Fertil Steril* 1998; **70**: 1070–1075.
14. Golan A, Ron-El R, Herman A, et al. Ovarian hyperstimulation syndrome following D-Trp-6 luteinizing hormone-releasing hormone microcapsules and nemotropins for in-vitro fertilization. *Fertil Steril* 1988; **50**: 912–916.
15. Delvigne A, Demoulin A, Smitz J, et al. The ovarian hyperstimulation syndrome in in-vitro fertilization: a Belgian multicentric study. I. Clinical and biological features. *Hum Reprod* 1993; **8**: 1353–1360.
16. Mathur R, Akande A, Keay SD, Hunt LP, Jenkins JM. Distinction between early and late ovarian hyperstimulation syndrome. *Fertil Steril* 2000; **73**: 901–907.
17. Lyons CA, Wheeler CA, Frishman GN, et al. Early and late presentation of the ovarian hyperstimulation syndrome: two distinct entities with different risk factors. *Hum Reprod* 1994; **9**: 792–799.
18. Papanikolaou EH, Tournaye H, Verpoest W, et al. Early and late ovarian hyperstimulation syndrome:

early pregnancy outcome and profile. *Hum Reprod* 2005; **20**: 636–641.

19. Mathur RS, Jenkins JM. Is ovarian hyperstimulation syndrome associated with a poor obstetric outcome? *Brit J Obstet Gynaecol* 2000; **107**: 943–946.
20. Chen CD, Wu MY, Chao KH, et al.. Serum estradiol level and oocyte number in predicting severe ovarian hyperstimulation syndrome. *J Formos Med Assoc* 1997; **96**: 829–834.
21. Macdougall MJ, Tan SL, Jacobs HS. In-vitro fertilization and the ovarian hyperstimulation syndrome. *Hum Reprod* 1992; **8**: 60–64.
22. Schenker JG, Polishuk WZ. The role of prostaglandins in ovarian hyperstimulation syndrome. *Eur J Obstet Gynecol* 1976; **6**: 47–52.
23. Wiser A, Levron J, Kreizer D, et al. Outcome of pregnancies complicated by severe ovarian hyperstimulation syndrome (OHSS): a follow-up beyond the second trimester. *Hum Reprod* 2005; **20**: 910–914.
24. Whelan JG, Vlahos NF. The ovarian hyperstimulation syndrome. *Fertil Steril* 2000; **73**: 883–896.
25. Badawy SZA, Rizk B. Controlled ovarian stimulation in difficult cases. *Sex Reprod Menopause* 2011; **9**: 17–23.
26. Abramov Y, Fatum M, Abrahamov D, Schenker JG. Hydroxyethylstarch versus human albumin for the treatment of severe ovarian hyperstimulation syndrome: a preliminary report. *Fertil Steril* 2001; **75**: 1228–1230.
27. Gamzu R, Almog B, Levin Y, et al. Efficacy of hydroxyethyl starch and Haemaccel for the treatment of severe ovarian hyperstimulation syndrome. *Fertil Steril* 2002; **77**: 1302–1303.
28. The Practice Committee of the American Society of Reproductive Medicine. Ovarian hyperstimulation syndrome. *Fertil Steril* 2008; **90**: S188–S193.
29. Ferraretti AP, Gianaroli L, Diotalleve L, Festi C, Trouson A. Dopamine treatment for severe hyperstimulation syndrome. *Hum Reprod* 1992; **7**: 180–183.
30. Tsunoda T, Shibahara H, Hirano Y, et al. Treatment for ovarian hyperstimulation syndrome using an oral dopamine prodrug, docarpamine. *Gynecol Endocrinol* 2003; **17**: 281–286.
31. Dulitzky M, Cohen SB, Inbal A, et al. Increased prevalence of thrombophilia among women with severe ovarian hyperstimulation syndrome. *Fertil Steril* 2002; **77**: 463–467.
32. Mikhail S, Rizk B, Nawar MG, Rizk CB. Thrombophilia and implantation failure. In: Rizk B, Garcia-Velasco J, Sallam H, Magrikiannakis A, eds. *Infertility and Assisted Reproduction*,. New York, NY: Cambridge University Press, 2008; 407–416.
33. Chan WS. The 'ART' of thrombosis: a review of arterial and venous thrombosis in assisted reproductive technology. *Curr Opin Obstet Gynecol* 2009; **21**: 207–218.
34. Shmorgun D, Claman P. The diagnosis and management of ovarian hyperstimulation syndrome. *J Obstet Gynaecol Can* 2011; **33**: 1156–1162.
35. Aboulghar MA, Mansour RT, Serour GI, Amin Y. Ultrasonically guided vaginal aspiration of ascites in the treatment of severe ovarian hyperstimulation syndrome. *Fertil Steril* 1990; **53**: 933–935.
36. Rinaldi MI, Spirtos NJ. Chest tube drainage of pleural effusion correcting abdominal ascites in a patient with severe ovarian hyperstimulation syndrome: a case report. *Fertil Steril* 1995; **63**: 1114–1117.
37. Gorkemli H, Camus M, Clasen K. Adnexal torsion after gonadotrophin ovulation induction for IVF or ICSI and its conservative treatment. *Arch Gynecol Obstet* 2002; **267**: 4–6.
38. Mashiach S, Bider D, Moran O, Goldenberg M, Ben-Rafael Z. Adnexal torsion of hyperstimulated ovaries in pregnancies after gonadotropin therapy. *Fertil Steril* 1990; **53**: 76–80.
39. Eyvazzadeh AD, Ryley DA, Khachadoorian HR, Alper MM, Reindollar RH. Adnexal torsion: a review of 80 cases. *Fertil Steril* 2005; **84**: S163–S164.

Chapter 5

Early pregnancy failure after assisted reproductive technology

Sotirios H. Saravelos and Lesley Regan

Placing early pregnancy failure in perspective: pathology or natural selection?

Pregnancy covers a wide and diverse spectrum of development starting with fertilization and ending in birth. Pregnancy failure, otherwise termed as pregnancy loss or miscarriage, can occur at different stages during this process and many different pathophysiological mechanisms may be implicated. Because this is a spectrum of development, defining the individual stages of pregnancy can be quite challenging. Nevertheless, early pregnancy commonly refers to the pregnancy stage following implantation and during the first trimester. This can be divided further into: (i) preclinical (or biochemical) pregnancies that are only identifiable by raised serial beta human chorionic gonadotrophin (β-hCG) measurements, and (ii) clinical pregnancies for which ultrasound or histological evidence of a gestation can be demonstrated.

In the past, focus was given primarily to those pregnancy failures occurring after a clinically recognized gestation, as preclinical pregnancy losses would commonly go unnoticed or present merely as a late period. However, with the development of over-the-counter pregnancy testing kits for early pregnancy recognition, and the widespread use of assisted reproductive technology (ART), the focus of interest in pregnancy failure has gradually shifted to the earlier stages of gestation. As a result, it has become increasingly evident that even women with normal fertility appear to have a large number of pregnancy losses occurring at a very early gestational stage.

Roberts and Lowe (1975) were among the first to demonstrate the scale of early pregnancy wastage, by using the registered number of births in England and estimating the number of fertile ovulatory cycles in married couples having unprotected intercourse. They calculated that only 22% of cycles exposed to the risk of pregnancy actually resulted in a live birth [1]. Because the sporadic miscarriage rate of pregnancies is far less than 78%, this finding implied that the vast majority of pregnancies were being lost at a very early gestational stage, before they were clinically recognized. In fact, a review of the literature suggests that of all pregnancies, approximately 30% fail prior to implantation, a further 30% fail following implantation but prior to clinical evidence of pregnancy, and about 10% suffer clinical miscarriages. This means that only 30% of all conceptions in fertile women will result in a live birth (Figure 5.1) [2].

The degree of magnitude of this vast pregnancy loss implies that our species is highly inefficient in terms of reproductive performance. Interestingly, other species do not seem to share this reproductive characteristic, and the underlying reasons and mechanisms for this interspecies difference are poorly understood. One possible explanation is that humans have a far higher occurrence of meiotic non-disjunction compared to other organisms (ranging from yeasts to mammals) [2], which is a significant cause of pregnancy failure. Furthermore, many mammals are capable of embryonic "diapause," which means that they can suspend embryonic development until the endometrium signals the presence of optimal metabolic and hormonal conditions for implantation. As there is no evidence of an embryonic diapause in humans, this suggests that a significant proportion of human embryos may attempt to implant at a time when the endometrium is suboptimal [3].

The understanding that profound early pregnancy wastage is a natural characteristic of the human species should offer some comfort to clinicians and their patients who are faced with relatively low pregnancy and live birth rates following ART. It also raises the

Pregnancy After Assisted Reproductive Technology, ed. Eric R. M. Jauniaux and Botros R. M. B. Rizk. Published by Cambridge University Press.

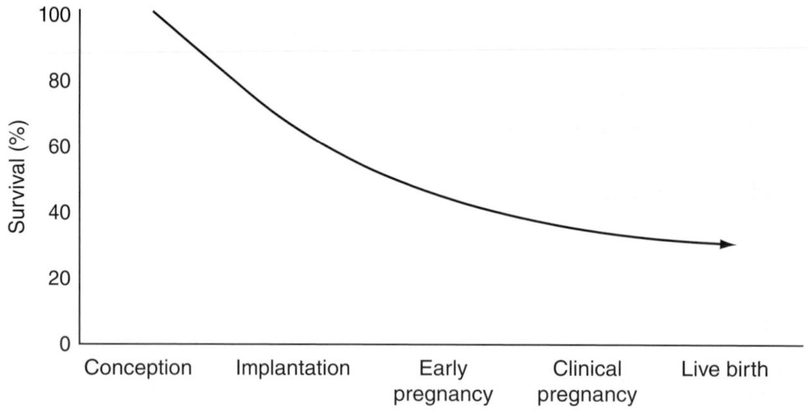

Figure 5.1. Human reproductive losses from conception to live birth.

possibility that the majority of early pregnancy failures following ART are the result of natural selection rather than being due to additional pathology.

Incidence of early pregnancy failure: is it higher following assisted reproductive technology?

In order to establish whether early pregnancy failure following ART is pathological or physiological, a group of women with subfertility undergoing ART would need to be compared to women with normal fertility not undergoing ART and women with subfertility also not undergoing ART. Comparing the rates of early pregnancy failure would answer the following questions: (i) is the incidence of early pregnancy failure in women undergoing ART higher? and (ii) if so, is this due to the underlying subfertility or due to the ART treatment itself?

Accurate comparison of early pregnancy failure rates in these patient groups is very difficult to achieve because of the marked difference in the intensity of surveillance they undergo. Women having ART routinely undergo serial β-hCG monitoring two weeks following oocyte retrieval, which identifies practically all biochemical failures. By contrast, women not undergoing ART would not be offered such intense surveillance, and therefore their preclinical pregnancy losses may go unnoticed and be consequently underestimated. The second reason is that women undergoing ART by default may have an increased risk of early pregnancy failure due to confounding factors such as increased age. This may give a false impression that the ART is to blame for the high rates of pregnancy failure, whereas in fact this may be entirely due to large differences in patient characteristics. The importance of controlling for such confounders cannot be overestimated; indeed, unselected women in their 30s have almost double the risk of pregnancy loss compared to women in their 20s [4].

In an attempt to answer the question of whether women undergoing ART experience more pregnancy failures compared to women in the general population, Wang et al. compared the early pregnancy loss rate in their cohort of women undergoing ART (n = 1945) to a previously published cohort study at the same center of women (n = 549) with normal fertility achieving natural conception [5,6], who had undergone similar surveillance in terms of β-hCG and ultrasound monitoring. The two study groups were heterogeneous, but nevertheless the authors found a small yet significant increase in the first-trimester pregnancy loss rate of women undergoing ART versus fertile women conceiving naturally (16.5% versus 14%; $P < 0.05$).

However, larger epidemiological surveys have refuted this finding, reporting that pregnancy loss rates are comparable in women undergoing ART and fertile women conceiving naturally. Data from the Society for Assisted Reproductive Technology Clinic Outcomes Reporting System (SART CORS), which includes 62 228 pregnancies, found that the pregnancy loss rate ranged from 14%–26% for ages 20–40 years, respectively (Figure 5.2), which was directly comparable to the 14%–28% pregnancy loss rate of women conceiving naturally, in matching age groups, as recorded by the National Survey of Family Growth [7].

Interestingly, a smaller study (n=500) found that the pregnancy loss rates tended to be higher in subfertile women who managed to conceive naturally versus subfertile women who conceived with ART

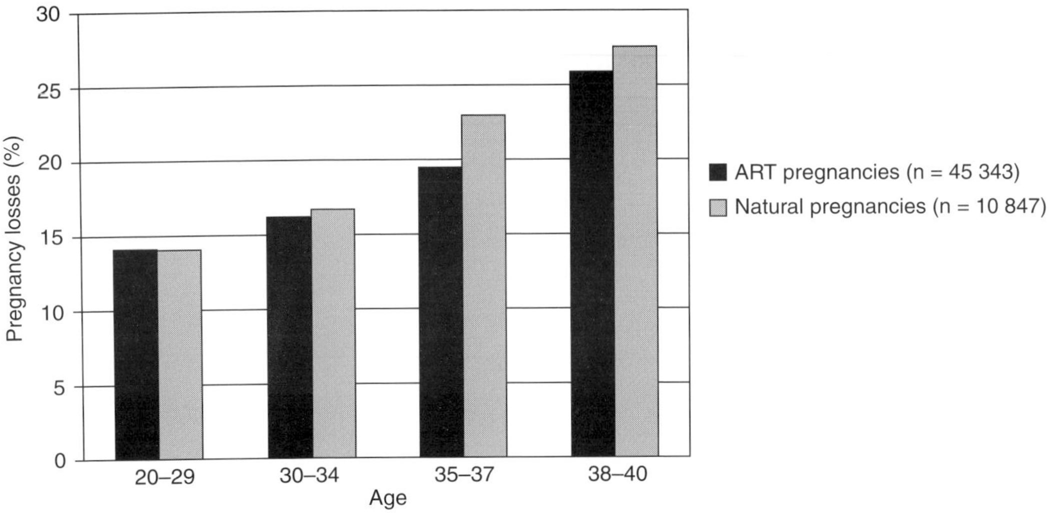

Figure 5.2. Clinical pregnancy losses in the United States – assisted reproductive technology versus natural pregnancies (data from SART CORS and the National Survey of Family Growth).

(26.2% versus 19.8%), although this did not reach statistical significance [8].

Overall, it appears that the incidence of early pregnancy failure is not significantly increased in women undergoing ART compared to women with or without subfertility conceiving naturally. This is reassuring for patients and clinicians and highlights the futility of promoting non-evidence-based therapies for women undergoing ART.

Early pregnancy failure: patient-dependent factors (Table 5.1)

Chromosomal abnormalities and maternal age

As previously noted, human embryos are more prone to chromosomal abnormalities when compared to other species [2,9]. This makes embryonic aneuploidy the leading cause of early pregnancy failure in humans. It is estimated that approximately 50% of clinically recognized pregnancy losses have a chromosomal abnormality, and this figure increases to 70% for women of advanced age undergoing ART [10]. Because karyotyping of products of conception cannot be performed for preclinical pregnancies, the true rate of human aneuploidy may be even higher.

Maternal age is the most important predictor of early pregnancy failure in women conceiving naturally and those undergoing ART. This is predominantly due to the effect of maternal age on the rate of chromosomal anomaly within the oocytes, which is thought to result from stages I and II meiotic errors, resulting in aneuploid embryos and early pregnancy failure in humans. Aneuploidy is present in approximately 47% of oocytes of women undergoing preimplantation genetic testing [11]. In contrast, aneuploidy in spermatozoa is thought to affect less than 10% of cells [2] and has not been shown in preliminary studies to vary drastically with age [12]. Hence, it appears that the rate of pregnancy failure is directly correlated to maternal age but a similar correlation with paternal age is not present [13]. More importantly, ART cycles using donor oocytes show that the pregnancy failure is affected by the age of the oocyte donor, but not by the age of the woman receiving the donor oocytes (Figure 5.3) [7].

Subfertility diagnosis

Any potential associations between the different diagnoses of subfertility and early pregnancy failure are difficult to examine as the underlying cause of subfertility may determine the choice of ART method, which also may affect the subsequent implantation/pregnancy rate.

Overall, data from national and regional registries analyzed by multivariate logistic regression indicate that although some diagnostic categories of subfertility, such as male factor infertility, may be associated with different rates of early pregnancy failure, there are

Table 5.1. The effect of patient-dependent factors on early pregnancy failure in women undergoing assisted reproduction

Factor	Effect on early pregnancy failure	Comment
1. Maternal age	↑	Oocyte aging/meiotic errors
2. Infertility diagnosis		
Endometriosis	?	Conflicting evidence
Male factor	↓	Absence of oocyte abnormalities
Uterine	↑	Mainly septate uterus and submucosal fibroids
PCOS	↑	Exact pathology unclear
3. Other diagnoses		
Thrombophilia/APS	?	Known cause of recurrent miscarriage
Antispermatozoon antibodies	None	Does not affect pregnancy rates
Thyroid antibodies	↑	Exact pathology unknown
High NK cells	?	Limited evidence
4. General risk factors		
Ethnic minorities	↑	Several confounding variables
Abnormal BMI	↑	U-shaped association
Smoking	↑	Multiple pathological mechanisms
Anxiety	None	Supportive care implicated in RM

PCOS, polycystic ovarian syndrome; APS, Antiphospholipid syndrome; BMI, body mass index; NK, natural killer; RM, recurrent miscarriage.

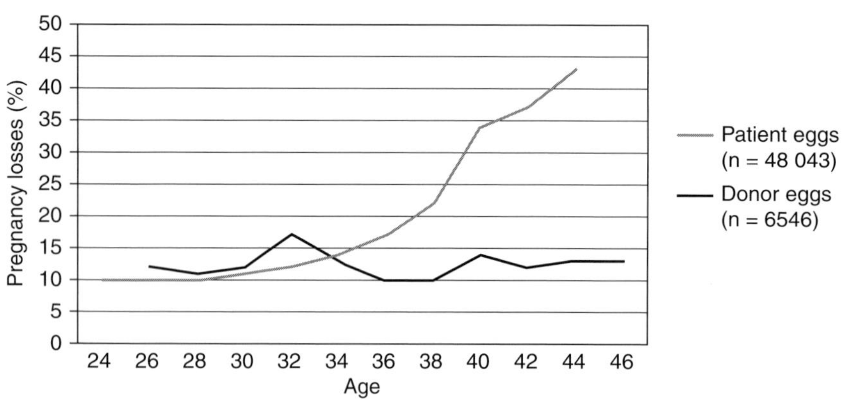

Figure 5.3. Clinical pregnancy loss rates for assisted reproductive technology pregnancies conceived with freshly fertilized donor oocytes versus patients' own oocytes. (Adopted from Schieve et al., 2003. [7])

no consistent differences demonstrated between most other diagnostic categories of subfertility (tubal pathology, endometriosis, ovulatory dysfunction, uterine factor, others less common, and unexplained) [7,14,15].

Endometriosis

Endometriosis has traditionally been thought to affect fertility via the presence of inflammatory factors that may induce negative effects on the quality of follicles, oocytes, and embryos, although this has not been substantiated in recent preliminary data [16]. The exact effect of endometriosis and its treatment on pregnancy rate and pregnancy failure remain highly debatable, with a meta-analysis suggesting that endometriosis results in significantly lower pregnancy rates [17], while data from the U.S. SART CORS register indicate that endometriosis is associated with higher live birth rates overall when compared to other causes of subfertility [7].

Male factor subfertility

Severe male factor infertility compared to other diagnoses has been shown to be associated with increased ongoing pregnancy rates in a national Dutch prospective cohort study of 4928 couples. One explanation is that improved outcomes may be associated with use of intracytoplasmic spermatozoon injection (ICSI) versus in vitro fertilization (IVF). An alternative explanation is that couples with severe male factor subfertility have oocytes of better quality compared to couples where a significant female factor is present, thereby leading to fewer pregnancy failures due to aneuploid embryos.

Uterine anomalies

Uterine abnormalities have been implicated in the etiology of sporadic and recurrent miscarriage but have not been associated with a significant increase in pregnancy loss following ART. The prevalence of a septate uterus is increased in the infertile and recurrent miscarriage population, suggesting that impaired implantation and subsequent embryonic growth at the site of the relatively avascular septum may be causal [18]. A similar mechanism has been proposed to explain the increase in implantation failure and pregnancy loss following ART in women with submucosal and intramural fibroids [19]. Hence, hysteroscopic surgical correction of the anomaly may be justified in women with a septate uterus or submucosal/intramural fibroids and recurrent implantation or pregnancy failure.

Polycystic ovarian syndrome

Polycystic ovarian syndrome (PCOS) is the leading cause of anovulatory subfertility and has been linked to increased rates of pregnancy loss in women undergoing ART. However, it is unclear whether this effect is due to increased body mass index (BMI), insulin resistance, hyperinsulinemia, hyperandrogenemia, type of ART treatment offered, or altered response to ovarian stimulation. A multivariate logistic regression analysis in a cohort of over 1000 PCOS patients undergoing ART has suggested that the increased rates of pregnancy failure are more likely to be related to the increased prevalence of obesity in this population [20].

Other diagnoses

Thrombophilia

Thrombophilia, and in particular antiphospholipid syndrome (APS), has been associated with both early and later recurrent miscarriages and later pregnancy complications. The theoretical mechanisms for pregnancy failure in APS range from early impairment of endometrial decidualization and trophoblastic invasion to thrombosis of uteroplacental vasculature [21]. In theory, the same mechanism for early pregnancy failure could apply for women undergoing ART. However, a large systematic review and meta-analysis concluded that although case-control studies have reported a higher prevalence of antiphospholipid antibodies (aPL) and Factor V-Leiden (FVL) in women undergoing ART, this finding is not supported by the majority of cohort studies [22]. Accordingly, the American Society for Reproductive Medicine (ASRM) and the Royal College of Obstetricians and Gynaecologists Scientific Advisory Committee currently advise against routine screening for aPL in women undergoing ART [23,24].

Antispermatozoon antibodies

Antispermatozoon antibodies (ASAs) have been considered a possible cause for subfertility, as their incidence is higher in subfertile versus fertile men. However, the presence of ASA does not appear to reduce the chance of achieving a pregnancy following ART, and there are no data suggesting that they increase early pregnancy failure rates [25].

Thyroid antibodies

Thyroid antibodies have been associated with spontaneous pregnancy loss although the exact mechanism is not understood. The pathophysiology may be related to associated autoimmune syndromes, adverse autoantibody reactions on the placenta, cross reactivity with β-hCG, impaired metabolic activity during pregnancy, and confounders such as older age in women with thyroid autoimmune disease.

A meta-analysis of studies has concluded that the pregnancy loss rate in euthyroid women with thyroid antibodies undergoing IVF is twice as high compared to equivalent women without thyroid antibodies. However, there is still a lack of data to justify routine screening for thyroid antibodies or treatment with levothyroxine in euthyroid women [26].

Increased natural killer cells

Immunological mechanisms during the maternal adaptation to the semi-allogenic fetus have been implicated in various types of reproductive failure ranging from subfertility and implantation failure to recurrent miscarriage. The uterine natural killer (NK) cells in particular have been of primary interest in the last couple of decades, as they constitute the majority of endometrial leukocytes and are capable of producing cytokines that may be involved in regulating trophoblast invasion and angiogenesis. Despite the theoretical links, there is to date insufficient evidence to support the measurement of peripheral and uterine NK cells for prognostic purposes. Equally, the administration of immunotherapy in any group of women undergoing ART is currently unsubstantiated and carries a significant financial burden along with a small risk of serious complications [27].

General risk factors

Ethnicity/race

There are marked differences in reproductive outcomes of various racial and ethnic groups, with higher adverse effects occurring most commonly in the ethnic minorities. Data from the SART CORS in the U.S. has recently shown the pregnancy loss rate following ART to be significantly increased by 4%–8% among Asian, Hispanic, and black women compared to white women, although the analysis included later pregnancy losses as well. Several interesting theories to explain these differences have been proposed, such as an increased rate of ovarian aging in Asian women and an increased rate of tubal disease and fibroids in black women [28]. However, conclusions are very difficult to draw as such analyses cannot account for relevant genetic, social, nutritional, and environmental factors.

Weight

Weight is known to adversely affect female reproduction, possibly through abnormal oocyte development, impaired endometrial receptivity, and the metabolic disturbances associated with polycystic ovary syndrome. Current evidence suggests that the extremes of the BMI scale may be associated with increased pregnancy losses in fresh and frozen IVF and ICSI cycles [29]. As a result, all women planning to undergo ART should be strongly advised to optimize their BMI, in order to increase their chances of a successful pregnancy following ART.

Smoking

There is compelling evidence to suggest that smoking significantly lowers the chance of clinical pregnancy and live birth while increasing the chance of pregnancy loss and ectopic pregnancy in women undergoing ART (OR for pregnancy loss: 2.65; 95% CI: 1.33–5.30). The potential mechanisms are varied, ranging from impaired angiogenesis and mutagen damage of oocytes to corpus luteal activity inhibition and reduced endometrial receptivity [30]. In fact, the adverse effects of smoking are not just limited to early development, as they also affect neonatal growth after birth. This highlights the importance of promoting smoking cessation in all women planning to undergo ART.

Anxiety

Subfertility is stressful and anecdotal evidence supports the fact that both stress and anxiety reduce the chances of a successful pregnancy following ART. This may be related to cases where couples relieved from stress (for example, after adopting a child) have conceived naturally, or may be to some extent supported by medical practice, which promotes psychological supportive care (also known as "tender loving care") in certain groups of women with reproductive failure, such as women with unexplained recurrent miscarriage. Interestingly, evidence suggests that emotional distress does not affect the chances of successful outcomes with ART, although the specific outcome of early pregnancy failure has not been separately analyzed [31].

Early pregnancy failure: assisted reproductive technology-dependent factors (Table 5.2)

Ovarian stimulation/ovulation induction

As downregulation and ovarian stimulation protocols become more individualized, it is difficult to ascertain whether a particular method of ovarian stimulation is directly responsible for an increase in early pregnancy failure. The heterogeneity of different ovulation

Table 5.2. The effect of assisted reproductive technology dependent factors on early pregnancy failure rates of women undergoing assisted reproduction

Factor	Effect on early pregnancy failure	Comment
1. Ovarian stimulation		
Stimulation agents	None	No difference between rFSH, HMG, HMG-HP, uFSH-P, and uFSH-HP
GnRH analogues	None	No difference between GnRH agonists and antagonists
Clomiphene	↑	Likely secondary to PCOS
2. Luteal phase support	↑	Optimum regime remains unknown
3. In vitro techniques		
IVF	None	Pregnancy failures similar to natural conceptions
GIFT	None	GIFT/ZIFT are now uncommon
ZIFT	↑	Due to early embryo selection
ICSI	↓	Fewer oocyte abnormalities in male factor infertility
In vitro maturation	?	Limited data
Assisted hatching	?	Limited data
4. Embryonic factors		
Embryo freezing	?	Depends on method of freezing
Low embryo quality	↑	Classifications for embryo quality may vary
Cleavage versus blastocyst transfer	?	Natural selection may help reduce early pregnancy failure rates
Number of oocyte retrievals	None	Quality is more important than number
Number of embryo transfers	↑	Increases after transfer of four or more embryos

GnRH, gonadotrophin releasing hormone; IVF, in vitro fertilization; GIFT, gamete intra-Fallopian transfer; ZIFT, zygote intra-Fallopian transfer; ICSI, intracytoplasmic spermatozoon injection; rFSH, recombinant follicle-stimulating hormone; HMG, human menopausal gonadotrophin; HMG-HP, highly purified human menopausal gonadotrophin; uFSH-P, purified urinary follicle-stimulating hormone; uFSH-HP, highly purified urinary follicle-stimulating hormone; PCOS, polycystic ovarian syndrome.

induction regimes make comparison difficult as the pregnancy failure rates may reflect patient characteristics rather than the treatment itself. Nevertheless, no particular differences in the risk of early pregnancy failure have been attributed to specific downregulation or ovulation induction regimes.

Because the majority of pregnancy failures are the result of aneuploidy, it seems prudent to consider whether ovarian stimulation adversely affects the maternal oocytes. Although the first studies on the human model have been conflicting, a recent analysis of 229 karyotypes of products of conception from women with a history of subfertility found the aneuploidy rate to be 63% versus 70% (nonsignificant) in women who had undergone ovarian stimulation with follicle-stimulating hormone (FSH) versus women who managed to conceive naturally [32].

Stimulation agents

A comprehensive Cochrane review of 30 studies has concluded that the choice of ovarian stimulation agent (recombinant FSH, human menopausal gonadotrophin (HMG), highly purified HMG, purified urinary FSH (FSH-P), and highly purified urinary FSH (FSH-HP)) does not affect the pregnancy failure rates significantly [33]. Conversely, clomiphene citrate has been shown to be linked to an increased risk of pregnancy failure (OR: 1.37; 95% CI: 1.06–1.77) [7], although this may reflect the underlying characteristics of the patients receiving the treatment rather than the treatment itself.

Gonadotrophin releasing hormone analogues

Much controversy arose following the introduction of gonadotrophin releasing hormone (GnRH) antagonists. The theoretical advantages of these agents included: (i) the avoidance of an acute stimulation of endogenous gonadotrophins, (ii) a dramatic reduction in the length of analogue treatment because of their ability to directly inhibit the premature luteinizing hormone (LH) surge, and (iii) a reduction in the gonadotrophin requirement used for ovarian stimulation [34]. However, initial reports suggested that although the risk of ovarian hyperstimulation syndrome (OHSS) was significantly reduced, the clinical pregnancy rate was also reduced by 5% in women receiving GnRH antagonist versus GnRH agonist therapy. However, a further review and meta-analysis of 45 randomized controlled trials refuted the initial findings and reassured clinicians by confirming that pregnancy failure rates are not increased with GnRH antagonist use [35].

Luteal phase support

Although it is accepted that the luteal phase of ART stimulated cycles is abnormal, there is no consensus on the optimum luteal phase support (LPS) regime. Progesterone was traditionally the first agent used for this purpose. Its importance in the first weeks of pregnancy has been known since the early 1970s when Csapo and colleagues reported that removal of the corpus luteum prior to seven weeks led to pregnancy loss, but that this could be avoided if progesterone were administered exogenously [36]. Since then, LPS has been routinely used in ART stimulated cycles, with an occasional study reporting outcomes from patients who did not receive LPS, some of which were terminated prematurely due to unacceptably low pregnancy rates.

Current evidence [37,38] suggests that:

(i) Vaginal and intramural progesterone have similar pregnancy and delivery rates, while oral natural micronized progesterone is not efficient if taken orally.
(ii) hCG is at least as effective as progesterone in achieving pregnancy and preventing pregnancy failure but is associated with higher rates of OHSS.
(iii) GnRH agonist (versus progesterone) use or estrogen supplementation may increase pregnancy and live birth rates further (preliminary evidence).
(iv) LPS beyond 14 days from oocyte retrieval or after the first positive pregnancy test is unlikely to reduce early pregnancy failure rates.
(v) Combinations with ascorbic acid, aspirin, naloxone, and prednisolone are unlikely to reduce early pregnancy failure rates.

In vitro techniques

As mentioned earlier, the question of whether the method of ART or the underlying patient characteristics are responsible for any differences observed in the rates of pregnancy failures is a difficult one. It is important to remember that fresh embryo transfer IVF itself has not generally been associated with higher rates of pregnancy loss compared to spontaneous conception [39]. As a result, different conception modes can be compared to fresh embryo transfer IVF in order to establish whether they are associated with a higher risk of early pregnancy failure.

Gamete and zygote intra-Fallopian transfer

Gamete and zygote intra-Fallopian transfer (GIFT and ZIFT) were traditionally thought to convey high pregnancy and live birth rates before transcervical intrauterine transfer IVF became established. However, since the less invasive conventional IVF method has been adopted, the rates of GIFT and ZIFT have decreased drastically. Evidence suggests that GIFT does not affect the early pregnancy failure rate although ZIFT has been shown to be associated with slightly higher rates of pregnancy loss (OR: 1.22; 95% CI: 1.01–1.47) [7,14]. This may be because embryos used for ZIFT are selected at an earlier stage, and therefore embryo quality can be more difficult to judge.

Intracytoplasmic spermatozoon injection

Only limited trials comparing ICSI versus conventional IVF techniques, in terms of early pregnancy failure, are available. Several large series have failed to show any significant difference in terms of pregnancy loss rates between ICSI and IVF [7,14,39,40], although some centers have reported an improvement in pregnancy rates and a reduction in pregnancy losses with ICSI [15]. Again, it is important to consider that this finding may reflect the underlying diagnosis of the patients rather than the ART method; for instance, if the couple's subfertility is due to a severe male factor, then the oocytes are more likely to be of good quality compared to a couple with female factor subfertility. This viewpoint is supported by a randomized controlled trial that showed that ICSI did not offer any clinical advantages over IVF in couples with non-male factor subfertility [41]. Interestingly, preliminary data regarding a modified form of ICSI, called intracytoplasmic morphologically selected spermatozoon injection (IMSI), suggest that careful morphological selection of spermatozoa may also reduce pregnancy failure rates, although this requires further investigation [42].

In vitro maturation

New developments of in vitro maturation (IVM) of immature oocytes to enable avoidance of ovarian hyperstimulation appear promising. Very limited data are available regarding its effect on early pregnancy failure. One group have reported a higher rate of clinical but not biochemical pregnancy losses using this method. However, they attributed this difference to the underlying PCOS of the patients undergoing treatment rather than the technique itself [40]. More studies will be required before we can draw valid conclusions regarding this technique.

Assisted hatching

Assisted hatching, which involves the artificial rupture of the zona pellucida of the developing embryo, has been used to improve implantation and clinical pregnancy rates in patients undergoing ART. Although assisted hatching is thought to widen the embryonic implantation window by allowing early exchange of metabolites and growth factors [43], there is little evidence to support its routine use. A recent meta-analysis has shown a tendency for increased live birth rates in a subgroup of women with repeated implantation failure, although further studies will be required to establish whether it can reduce the rates of early pregnancy failure in other groups of women undergoing ART [43].

Embryonic factors

Freshly fertilized embryos versus frozen and thawed embryos

Whether there is a difference in clinical outcomes following the use of fresh versus frozen-thawed embryos remains unclear. Traditionally, fresh embryos were thought to perform better than frozen embryos, and this was reflected in national and large published cohort averages, where pregnancy loss rates were reported to be higher for frozen versus fresh embryos [7,39]. However, the questions remained: was this failure rate increased because of embryonic cellular damage from the freezing-thawing process? Was there a selection bias of patients having already failed fresh embryo transfer cycles? Or, were the embryos selected for freezing of "second quality" because the best had been used for the fresh cycles?

More recently, the introduction of the vitrification process, which allows ultra-rapid freezing of the embryo from 37°C to -196°C in less than one second, has meant that the damage at cellular level from ice crystal formation has been drastically reduced [44]. Reports have suggested that implantation and pregnancy rates are increased following vitrification frozen embryo transfer, as the delay of transferring the frozen embryo allows improved endometrial receptivity to develop, which may have been compromised during the dynamic process of controlled ovarian hyperstimulation [44]. However, this has not translated into decreased rates of early pregnancy failure; in fact, preliminary trials have reported increased miscarriage rates in women receiving vitrified frozen embryos [45]. As a result, further large well-designed trials will be required before conclusions can be drawn about this technique.

Quality of embryos

Homogeneity in assessing the quality of embryos is difficult to achieve as laboratories throughout the world may grade embryos at different stages according to different characteristics and standards. Common grading standards include factors such as number of blastomeres, percentage of fragmentation, and degree of multinucleation.

Meta-analyses have shown that high-quality embryos are associated with increased pregnancy rates and overall favorable cumulative outcomes in ART [46]. Retrospective cohort studies have also shown that poor-quality embryos may increase the pregnancy failure rate by approximately 20% compared to good-quality embryos [14]. Interestingly, although good-quality embryos may be thought to have a smaller chance of chromosomal abnormalities, thus allowing for higher pregnancy rates and fewer pregnancy failures, approximately one in three morphologically normal embryos may carry abnormal chromosomes and nearly all of them may display some degree of mosaicism [2,9].

Cleavage stage versus blastocyst stage embryos

Advances in culture media have allowed embryo transfers to shift from the early cleavage stage to the blastocyst stage. Although this carries the risk that there will be no embryos to transfer at days 5 or 6 (or equally that there will be limited embryos to freeze), emerging evidence suggests that allowing a natural selection to occur in this early stage means that pregnancy and live birth rates are increased in women undergoing blastocyst versus cleavage stage embryo transfer. This implies that it improves embryo–endometrial synchronicity facilitating implantation [47], although a reduction in pregnancy failure rates has yet to be reported.

Number of oocytes retrieved

Following conventional ovarian stimulation, a low number of oocytes retrieved after follicle aspiration was thought to be associated with a poor clinical outcome, reflecting poor ovarian reserve. However, it is currently considered to be the quality and not the number of oocytes retrieved that is of importance. A recent meta-analysis has shown that in cycles of mild ovarian stimulation where small numbers of oocytes are retrieved, the implantation rates are not reduced compared to cycles where higher numbers of oocytes are retrieved. Similarly, we may speculate that the rates of early pregnancy failure would not be increased, although the evidence has not yet emerged to clarify this [48].

Number of embryo transfers

There has been a general move to decrease the rates of multiple pregnancies associated with ART, in order to reduce maternal, fetal, and neonatal morbidity and mortality but also to control health costs. Correspondingly, authorities such as the Human Embryology and Fertilisation Authority (HEFA) now advocate the use of elective single embryo transfer in order to reduce the rates of twin births. Recent data suggest that elective single embryo transfer is associated with a lower pregnancy rate compared to double embryo transfer in fresh ART cycles, but this disadvantage can be counteracted by performing an additional frozen single embryo transfer if required. Overall, this gives a higher chance of a singleton live birth when compared to double embryo transfers. In terms of pregnancy loss, it is unclear whether more embryo transfers cause higher rates of pregnancy loss [49], although a multivariate analysis of the SART CORS in the U.S. suggests that the early pregnancy failure rate may increase after four or more embryo transfers [50], which would reflect the increased pregnancy loss rate in higher-order pregnancies.

Interventions and therapies (Table 5.3)

Preimplantation genetic screening and diagnosis

Preimplantation genetic screening and diagnosis (PGS and PGD) commonly involve the chromosomal

Table 5.3. The effect of various treatments on early pregnancy failure rates of women undergoing assisted reproduction

Treatment	Effect on early pregnancy failure	Comment
PGS	↑	Proven adverse effect
Aspirin	None	
Heparin	?	May have role in specific groups or in combination with aspirin
Metformin	None	Reduces rates of OHSS
Endometrioma surgery	?	Conflicting evidence
Myomectomy	↓	Favorable evidence for submucosal myomectomy
Metroplasty	↓	Favorable evidence for septum resection
Acupuncture	?	Conflicting evidence
Glucocorticoids	None	May also be associated with complications

PGS, preimplantation genetic screening; OHSS, ovarian hyperstimulation syndrome.

analysis of one or two biopsied cells of a three-day-old embryo. Preimplantation genetic diagnosis was developed to prevent the birth of children with serious genetic diseases, while PGS is predominantly used to increase pregnancy and live birth rates by diagnosing and excluding chromosomally abnormal embryos prior to performing embryo transfer.

Given that the majority of pregnancy failures following ART may occur due to aneuploidy of the embryos (particularly secondary to increased maternal age and oocyte aging), the introduction of PGS was originally thought to be the panacea for all ART pregnancy failures. However, well-designed randomized controlled trials have shown that PGS in women without genetic disorders undergoing IVF or ICSI lead to significantly reduced ongoing pregnancy rates [51]. The reason behind this seems to lie in the fact that during preimplantation development, human embryos have been shown to have 29%–100% rates of chromosomal mosaicism [2,9]. Therefore, the analyzed cells may not reflect the true chromosomal characteristics of the remaining embryonic cells. Furthermore, PGS does not commonly screen for all chromosomes, and therefore some abnormalities may be missed. Finally, biopsies of embryonic cells may adversely affect the subsequent development of the embryo itself, which may explain the lower ongoing pregnancy rates in the studies performed to date.

Aspirin and heparin

Aspirin has been proposed to potentially improve implantation and ongoing pregnancy rates by increasing uterine blood flow and reducing adverse prostaglandin effects. Aspirin and low molecular weight heparin (LMWH) together have been shown to significantly reduce miscarriage rates in women with APS and recurrent miscarriage, and have become mainstay treatment in this group of patients. As a result, several studies have assessed the effect of aspirin on women undergoing ART. The collective results to date suggest that aspirin versus placebo has no benefit with regards to clinical pregnancy rates and prevention of pregnancy failure [52]. However, recent preliminary studies have suggested that heparin may increase implantation, pregnancy, and live birth rates in women with and without thrombophilia undergoing ART [53]. Ideally, aspirin and heparin alone or in combination should be examined in future randomized controlled trials in women with and without thrombophilia undergoing ART, to establish whether this intervention increases implantation and pregnancy rates and reduces early pregnancy failure rates in specific groups of women.

Metformin

Polycystic ovarian syndrome has been associated with increased rates of pregnancy failure in women undergoing ART. The use of insulin reducing agents such as metformin to counteract the adverse hyperinsulinemic and hyperadrogenemic effects on ovarian response seem a reasonable proposition. Interestingly, the latest Cochrane review has found that metformin does not improve pregnancy or live birth rates in ART cycles of women with PCOS, but significantly reduces the risk of OHSS [54].

Endometrioma surgery

The role of endometriosis in pregnancy failure remains controversial, and there is also a lack of data examining the effect of surgery on pregnancy loss rates. A recent meta-analysis has failed to show any improvements in pregnancy rates or response to ovarian stimulation (i.e., number of oocyte retrievals, amount of gonadotrophins used, estradiol levels) in women with endometriomas undergoing surgery prior to ART treatment [55], suggesting that these interventions are not necessary prior to ART.

Others

Acupuncture has created some interesting controversy with regards to its effect on ART outcomes. An initial review and meta-analysis suggested that it may increase pregnancy and live birth rates when performed at the time of embryo transfer, whereas a more recent meta-analysis including data concerning acupuncture performed during the period of egg retrieval concluded that it does not convey any benefit [56].

Although glucocorticoid treatment in women with autoantibodies undergoing ART cycles or those undergoing assisted hatching has been proposed to be of benefit, there is currently insufficient evidence to support the use of glucocorticoids in any group of women undergoing ART [57].

Monitoring and predicting (Table 5.4)

Paradoxically, a history of early pregnancy failure is a positive predictor for future success from ART treatment. This probably reflects the fact that achieving

Table 5.4. The usefulness of various tests as predictors of early pregnancy failure in women undergoing assisted reproduction

Predictor	Usefulness
Basal FSH, AFC, oocyte number	May reflect ovarian function/ reserve/age and therefore predict early pregnancy failure
Endometrial thickness	Thickness <7 mm and absence of the triple line pattern upon ovulation induction may predict a poor outcome
Spermatozoon DNA damage	May predict poor outcome (preliminary evidence)
Antenatal US monitoring	Absence of a yolk sac 32 days after fertilization is associated with high pregnancy failure rates. Fetal heart-beats are associated with low pregnancy failure rates
β-hCG	Level of >80 mIU/mL 12 days post-embryo transfer is associated with lower pregnancy failure rates

FSH, follicle-stimulating hormone; AFC, antral follicle count; US, ultrasound; β-hCG, beta human chorionic gonadotrophin.

implantation signifies a certain reproductive competence [2]. As a result, although distressing, early pregnancy failure should also reassure couples undergoing ART that they are likely to have a positive future outcome.

Duration of subfertility, antral follicle count (AFC), basal FSH, and number of oocytes retrieved all reflect ovarian function and reserve, and therefore may predict ART success. However, their exact relation to early pregnancy failure remains unknown [46]. In addition, these parameters may also reflect other factors such as maternal age and ovarian stimulation protocols, and therefore should always be interpreted within the clinical context of each patient [48].

Endometrial thickness and pattern have also been implicated as a predictor for ART success, as they may reflect the ability of the receptive endometrium to host the embryo in the early stages of development. The current belief is that an endometrial thickness of <7 mm and the absence of an endometrial triple-line pattern on ultrasound scanning on the day of ovulation induction are associated with reduced clinical pregnancy rates but not miscarriage. On the other hand, a thick endometrium (>14 mm) does not appear to adversely affect pregnancy or miscarriage rates, as hypothesized in the past. Future studies using 3D Doppler ultrasound to assess endometrial and subendometrial blood flow may provide further indices for predicting pregnancy outcomes in women undergoing ART.

Although subfertile men generally have lower counts of conventional spermatozoon parameters, such as concentration, motility, and morphology, these have not been shown to be good predictors of reproductive outcomes. More recent evidence suggests that markers of spermatozoon DNA integrity also differ between subfertile and fertile men, and much interest has risen with regards to their predictive potential. Preliminary data have suggested that higher spermatozoon DNA damage is associated with lower pregnancy rates in IVF, and is associated with higher rates of pregnancy failure in both IVF and ICSI. However, although intriguing, more well-designed randomized controlled trials will be required before such testing can become part of routine ART management [58].

Ultrasound monitoring during early pregnancy may also help predict subsequent failure. Studies on an ART population suggest that measuring variables such as mean sac diameter, crown–rump length, and gestational age at which embryonic life and fetal heartbeats are detected can help predict the risk of miscarriage. Generally, a smaller and slower-developing embryo reflects compromised development and is associated with pregnancy failure. Accordingly, it has been suggested that the absence of a yolk sac after 32 days from fertilization is almost always associated with pregnancy failure, while the detection of fetal heartbeats is associated with very low miscarriage rates [59]. For the ART population, evidence suggests that combining several variables in a multivariate model provides the highest prognostic strength, although there is currently no universally accepted model in use [60].

With regards to β-hCG monitoring in the ART population, it has been suggested that a level of more than 80 mIU/mL at 12 days post-embryo transfer is associated with a subsequent achievement of fetal heartbeats in 95% of the cases, and a live birth rate of 80%. This association appears to hold for fresh, frozen, donor, and non-donor cycles and may prove to be a simple and useful prediction tool to use [61].

Conclusion

The controlled nature of ART, which allows the precise timing of fertilization and embryo transfer to be known, may allow for the development of pregnancy prediction tools that are far more accurate for the ART population than for the general population conceiving naturally.

References

1. Roberts CJ, Lowe CR. Where have all conceptions gone? *Lancet* 1975; **1**: 498–499.
2. Macklon NS, Geraedts JP, Fauser BC. Conception to ongoing pregnancy: the 'black box' of early pregnancy loss. *Hum Reprod Update* 2002; **8**: 333–343.
3. Teklenburg G, Salker M, Molokhia M, et al. Natural selection of human embryos: decidualizing endometrial stromal cells serve as sensors of embryo quality upon implantation. *Plos One* 2010; **5**: e10258.
4. Nybo Andersen AM, Wohlfahrt J, Christens P, Olsen J, Melbye M. Maternal age and fetal loss: population based register linkage study. *BMJ* 2000; **320**: 1708–1712.
5. Wang JX, Norman RJ, Wilcox AJ. Incidence of spontaneous abortion among pregnancies produced by assisted reproductive technology. *Hum Reprod* 2004; **19**: 272–277.
6. Ford JH, MacCormac L, Hiller J. PALS (pregnancy and lifestyle study): association between occupational and environmental exposure to chemicals and reproductive outcome. *Mutat Res* 1994; **313**: 153–164.
7. Schieve LA, Tatham L, Peterson HB, Toner J, Jeng G. Spontaneous abortion among pregnancies conceived using assisted reproductive technology in the United States. *Obstet Gynecol* 2003; **101**: 959–967.
8. Pezeshki K, Feldman J, Stein DE, Lobel SM, Grazi RV. Bleeding and spontaneous abortion after therapy for infertility. *Fertil Steril* 2000; **74**: 504–508.
9. Vanneste E, Voet T, La Caignec C, et al. Chromosome instability is common in human cleavage-stage embryos. *Nat Med* 2009; **15**: 577–583.
10. Collins J, Diedrich K, Franks S, et al. Genetic aspects of female reproduction. *Hum Reprod Update* 2008; **14**: 293–307.
11. Kuliev A, Zlatopolsky Z, Kirillova I, Spivakova J, Cieslak Janzen J. Meiosis errors in over 20,000 oocytes studied in the practice of preimplantation aneuploidy testing. *Reprod Biomed Online* 2011; **22**: 2–8.
12. Luetjens CM, Rolf C, Gassner P, Werny JE, Nieschlag E. Sperm aneuploidy rates in younger and older men. *Hum Reprod* 2002; **17**: 1826–1832.
13. Dain L, Auslander R, Dirnfeld M. The effect of paternal age on assisted reproduction outcome. *Fertil Steril* 2011; **95**: 1–8.
14. Winter E, Wang J, Davies MJ, Norman R. Early pregnancy loss following assisted reproductive technology treatment. *Hum Reprod* 2002; **17**: 3220–3223.
15. Lintsen AM, Eijkemans MJ, Hunault CC, et al. Predicting ongoing pregnancy chances after IVF and ICSI: a national prospective study. *Hum Reprod* 2007; **22**: 2455–2462.
16. Reinblatt SL, Ishai L, Shehata F, et al. Effects of ovarian endometrioma on embryo quality. *Fertil Steril* 2011; **95**: 2700–2702.
17. Barnhart K, Dunsmoor-Su R, Coutifaris C. Effect of endometriosis on in vitro fertilization. *Fertil Steril* 2002; **77**: 1148–1155.
18. Saravelos SH, Cocksedge KA, Li TC. Prevalence and diagnosis of congenital uterine anomalies in women with reproductive failure: a critical appraisal. *Hum Reprod Update* 2008; **14**: 415–429.
19. Pritts EA, Parker WH, Olive DL. Fibroids and infertility: an updated systematic review of the evidence. *Fertil Steril* 2009; **91**: 1215–1223.
20. Wang JX, Davies MJ, Norman RJ. Polycystic ovarian syndrome and the risk of spontaneous abortion following assisted reproductive technology treatment. *Hum Reprod* 2001; **16**: 2606–2609.
21. Rai R, Regan L. Recurrent miscarriage. *Lancet* 2006; **368**: 601–611.
22. Di Nisio M, Rutjes AW, Ferrante N, et al. Thrombophilia and outcomes of assisted reproduction technologies: a systematic review and meta-analysis. *Blood* 2011; **118**: 2670–2678.
23. Practice Committee of American Society for Reproductive Medicine. Anti-phospholipid antibodies do not affect IVF success. *Fertil Steril* 2008; **90**: S172–S173.
24. Scientific Advisory Committee opinion paper 5. Immunological testing and interventions for reproductive failure. RCOG, 2008. (Available at: http://www.rcog.co.uk)
25. Zini A, Fahmy N, Belzile E, et al. Antisperm antibodies are not associated with pregnancy rates after IVF and ICSI: systematic review and meta-analysis. *Hum Reprod* 2011; **26**: 1288–1295.
26. Toulis KA, Goulis DG, Venetis CA, et al. Risk of spontaneous miscarriage in euthyroid women with thyroid autoimmunity undergoing IVF: a meta-analysis. *Eur J Endocrinol* 2010; **162**: 643–652.

27. Tang AW, Alfirevic Z, Quenby S. Natural killer cells and pregnancy outcomes in women with recurrent miscarriage and infertility: a systematic review. *Hum Reprod* 2011; **26**: 1971–1980.

28. Luke B, Brown MB, Stern JE, et al. Racial and ethnic disparities in assisted reproductive technology pregnancy and live birth rates within body mass index categories. *Fertil Steril* 2011; **95**: 1661–1666.

29. Veleva Z, Tiitinen A, Vilska S, et al. High and low BMI increase the risk of miscarriage after IVF/ICSI and FET. *Hum Reprod* 2008; **23**: 878–884.

30. Waylen AL, Metwally M, Jones GL, Wilkinson AJ, Ledger WL. Effects of cigarette smoking upon clinical outcomes of assisted reproduction: a meta-analysis. *Hum Reprod Update* 2009; **15**: 31–44.

31. Boivin J, Griffiths E, Venetis CA. Emotional distress in infertile women and failure of assisted reproductive technologies: meta-analysis of prospective psychosocial studies. *BMJ* 2011; **342**: d223.

32. Massie JA, Shahine LK, Milki AA, Westphal LM, Lathi RB. Ovarian stimulation and the risk of aneuploid conceptions. *Fertil Steril* 2011; **95**: 970–972.

33. van Wely M, Kwan I, Burt AL, et al. Recombinant versus urinary gonadotrophin for ovarian stimulation in assisted reproductive technology cycles. *Cochrane Database Syst Rev* 2011; **16**: CD005354.

34. Kolibianakis EM, Collins J, Tarlatzis BC, et al. Among patients treated for IVF with gonadotrophins and GnRH analogues, is the probability of live birth dependent on the type of analogue used? A systematic review and meta-analysis. *Hum Reprod Update* 2006; **12**: 651–671.

35. Al-Inany HG, Youssef MA, Aboulghar M, et al. Gonadotrophin-releasing hormone antagonists for assisted reproductive technology. *Cochrane Database Syst Rev* 2011; **5**: CD001750.

36. Csapo AI, Pulkkinen MO, Wiest WG. Effects of luteectomy and progesterone replacement therapy in early pregnant patients. *Am J Obstet Gynecol* 1973; **115**: 759–765.

37. Hubayter ZR, Muasher SJ. Luteal supplementation in in vitro fertilization: more questions than answers. *Fertil Steril* 2008; **89**: 749–758.

38. Fatemi HM, Popovic-Todorovic B, Papanikolaou E, Donoso P, Devroey P. An update of luteal phase support in stimulated IVF cycles. *Hum Reprod Update* 2007; **13**: 581–590.

39. Brandes M, Verzijden JC, Hamilton CJ, et al. Is the fertility treatment itself a risk factor for early pregnancy loss? *Reprod Biomed Online* 2011; **22**: 192–199.

40. Buckett WM, Chian RC, Dean NL, et al. Pregnancy loss in pregnancies conceived after in vitro oocyte maturation, conventional in vitro fertilization, and intracytoplasmic sperm injection. *Fertil Steril* 2008; **90**: 546–550.

41. Bhattacharya S, Hamilton MP, Shaaban M, et al. Conventional in-vitro fertilisation versus intracytoplasmic sperm injection for the treatment of non-male-factor infertility: a randomised controlled trial. *Lancet* 2001; **357**: 2075–2079.

42. Souza Setti A, Ferreira RC, Paes de Almeida Ferreira Braga D, et al. Intracytoplasmic sperm injection outcome versus intracytoplasmic morphologically selected sperm injection outcome: a meta-analysis. *Reprod Biomed Online* 2010; **21**: 450–455.

43. Martins WP, Rocha IA, Ferriani RA, Nastri CO. Assisted hatching of human embryos: a systematic review and meta-analysis of randomized controlled trials. *Hum Reprod Update* 2011; **17**: 438–453.

44. Aflatoonian A, Oskouian H, Ahmadi S, Oskouian L. Can fresh embryo transfers be replaced by cryopreserved-thawed embryo transfers in assisted reproductive cycles? A randomized controlled trial. *J Assist Reprod Genet* 2010; **27**: 357–363.

45. Aflatoonian A, Mansoori Moghaddam F, Mashayekhy M, Mohamadian F. Comparison of early pregnancy and neonatal outcomes after frozen and fresh embryo transfer in ART cycles. *J Assist Reprod Genet* 2010; **27**: 695–700.

46. Cai QF, Wan F, Huang R, Zhang HW. Factors predicting the cumulative outcome of IVF/ICSI treatment: a multivariable analysis of 2450 patients. *Hum Reprod* 2011; **26**: 2532–2540.

47. Blake DA, Farquhar CM, Johnson N, Proctor M. Cleavage stage versus blastocyst stage embryo transfer in assisted conception. *Cochrane Database Syst Rev* 2007; **4**: CD002118.

48. Verberg MF, Eijkemans MJ, Macklon NS, et al. The clinical significance of the retrieval of a low number of oocytes following mild ovarian stimulation for IVF: a meta-analysis. *Hum Reprod Update* 2009; **15**: 5–12.

49. McLernon DJ, Harrild K, Bergh C, et al. Clinical effectiveness of elective single versus double embryo transfer: meta-analysis of individual patient data from randomised trials. *BMJ* 2010; **341**: c6945.

50. Baker VL, Luke B, Brown MB, et al. Multivariate analysis of factors affecting probability of pregnancy and live birth with in vitro fertilization: an analysis of the Society for Assisted Reproductive Technology Clinic Outcomes Reporting System. *Fertil Steril* 2010; **94**: 1410–1416.

51. Checa MA, Alonso-Coello P, Sola I, et al. IVF/ICSI with or without preimplantation genetic screening for aneuploidy in couples without genetic disorders: a systematic review and meta-analysis. *J Assist Reprod Genet* 2009; **26**: 273–283.

52. Groeneveld E, Broeze KA, Lambers MJ, et al. Is aspirin effective in women undergoing in vitro fertilization (IVF)? Results from an individual patient data meta-analysis (IPD MA). *Hum Reprod Update* 2011; **17**: 501–509.

53. Urman B, Ata B, Yakin K, et al. Luteal phase empirical low molecular weight heparin administration in patients with failed ICSI embryo transfer cycles: a randomized open-labeled pilot trial. *Hum Reprod* 2009; **24**: 1640–1647.

54. Tso LO, Costello MF, Albuquerque LE, Andriolo RB, Freitas V. Metformin treatment before and during IVF or ICSI in women with polycystic ovary syndrome. *Cochrane Database Syst Rev* 2009; **2**: CD006105.

55. Tsoumpou I, Kyrgiou M, Gelbaya TA, Nardo LG. The effect of surgical treatment for endometrioma on in vitro fertilization outcomes: a systematic review and meta-analysis. *Fertil Steril* 2009; **92**: 75–87.

56. El-Toukhy T, Sunkara SK, Khairy M, et al. A systematic review and meta-analysis of acupuncture in in vitro fertilisation. *BJOG* 2008; **115**: 1203–1213.

57. Boomsma CM, Macklon NS. Does glucocorticoid therapy in the peri-implantation period have an impact on IVF outcomes? *Curr Opin Obstet Gynecol* 2008; **20**: 249–256.

58. Zini A, Sigman M. Are tests of sperm DNA damage clinically useful? Pros and cons. *J Androl* 2009; **30**: 219–229.

59. Deaton JL, Honore GM, Huffman CS, Bauguess P. Early transvaginal ultrasound following an accurately dated pregnancy: the importance of finding a yolk sac or fetal heart motion. *Hum Reprod* 1997; **12**: 2820–2823.

60. Choong S, Rombauts L, Ugoni A, Meagher S. Ultrasound prediction of risk of spontaneous miscarriage in live embryos from assisted conceptions. *Ultrasound Obstet Gynecol* 2003; **22**: 571–577.

61. Lawler CC, Budrys NM, Rodgers AK, et al. Serum beta human chorionic gonadotropin levels can inform outcome counseling after in vitro fertilization. *Fertil Steril* 2011; **96**: 505–507.

Chapter 6

Singleton pregnancy after assisted reproductive technology – the obstetric perspective

Annika K. Ludwig, Michael Ludwig, and Eric R. M. Jauniaux

Introduction

Singleton pregnancies achieved by assisted reproductive technology (ART) are at higher risk than spontaneous pregnancies for adverse perinatal outcomes, including perinatal mortality, preterm birth (PTB), and low birth weight (LBW) [1–3]. Interestingly, spontaneous pregnancies in untreated infertile women are also at higher risk for obstetrical complications and perinatal mortality than spontaneous pregnancies in fertile women [4]. In both groups of women these risks are mainly linked to advanced maternal age. Many women who need ART because of infertility problems are older than the average pregnant woman. Risks for chronic diseases such as obesity, diabetes mellitus, chronic hypertension, cardiovascular disease (CVD), and cancer are known to increase with age and these preexisting medical conditions have a direct impact on both spontaneous and ART pregnancies.

Multiple gestation pregnancies (MGPs) are without any doubt the main complication of ART. All MGP, starting with twin pregnancies, are associated with a higher obstetric risk for both the mother and her fetuses, and the corresponding literature is discussed in Chapter 8. In addition, ART pregnancies may be exposed to additional chronic diseases unrelated to maternal age such as polycystic ovarian syndrome (PCOS) or thyroid disorders, which may increase the risk of an abnormal perinatal outcome. Women requiring ART are also more likely to have had previous pelvic surgery, and in vitro fertilization (IVF) or ART procedures can damage the uterine endometrium, leading to a higher risk of placenta accreta [5].

The presence of a chronic illness increases the risk of the IVF procedure and is also associated with increased obstetric risks and even death (Figure 6.1). The objective of this chapter is to outline the potential obstetric risks for women who undergo ART procedures. We hope that these evaluated risks will lead to guidelines for adequate patient assessment before enrollment in ART programs and a multidisciplinary approach for those women at high risk of obstetric complications.

Perinatal outcome of singleton pregnancies after assisted reproductive technology

A Norwegian population-based study [6] found that ART conceptions are associated with LBW (difference: 25 g, 95% CI: 14–35), shorter duration of gestation (2.0 days, 95% CI: 1.6–2.3), and increased risks of a small for gestational age (SGA) (OR 1.26, 95% CI: 1.10–1.44), and perinatal death (1.31, 95% CI: 1.05–1.65) than were spontaneous conceptions. In the sibling–relationship comparisons, the spontaneous versus the ART conceptions show a difference of only 9 g (95% CI: −18–36) in birth weight and 0.6 days (95% CI: −0.5–1.7) in gestational age. For assisted fertilization versus spontaneous conception in the sibling–relationship comparisons, the odds ratio (OR) for a small for gestational age is 0.99 and that for perinatal mortality is 0.36.

In their systematic review of controlled studies published between 1985 and 2002, Helmerhorst et al. [1] found that for singletons studies with matched controls indicated a relative risk (RR) of 3.27 for very PTB (<32 weeks) and 2.04 for PTB (<37 weeks) in pregnancies after ART (Table 6.1). Relative risks were 3.00 for very LBW (<1500 g), 1.70 for LBW (<2500 g), 1.40 for SGA, 1.54 for Cesarean section, 1.27 for admission to a neonatal intensive care unit, and 1.68 for perinatal mortality. The meta-analysis by Jackson et al. [2] included 15 studies comprising 12 283 IVF and 1.9 million spontaneously conceived

Pregnancy After Assisted Reproductive Technology, ed. Eric R. M. Jauniaux and Botros R. M. B. Rizk. Published by Cambridge University Press.

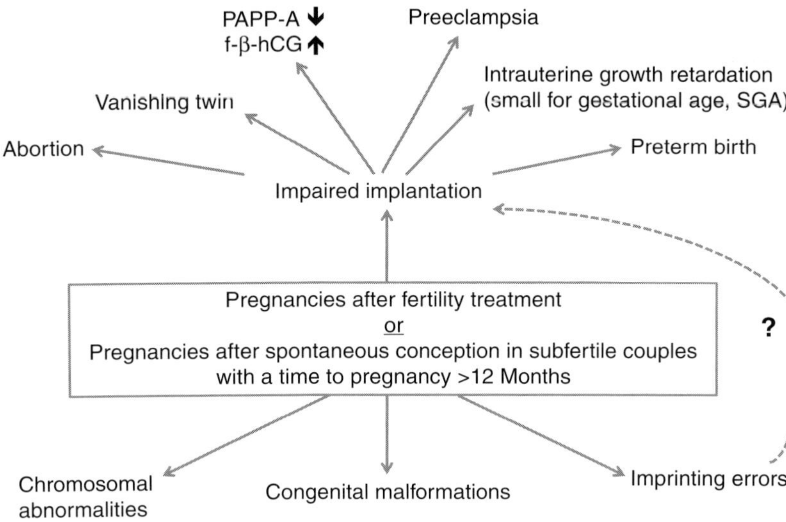

Figure 6.1. The different aspects of pregnancy course and obstetric complications that have been described in patients with subfertility or after assisted reproductive technology. The diagram shows that most complications may be a direct consequence of impaired implantation, which might also be a cause of subfertility in the couples.

Table 6.1. Comparison of the perinatal outcomes in singleton pregnancies following in vitro fertilization in a systematic review (1) and a meta-analysis (2)

Outcome	Helmerhorst et al. [1] RR (95% CI)	Jackson et al. [2] OR (95% CI)
Preeclampsia	NA	1.55 (1.23–1.95)
Placenta previa	NA	2.87 (1.54–5.37)
Stillbirth	NA	2.55 (1.78–3.64)
Premature birth (<37 wks)	2.04 (1.80–2.32)	1.95 (1.73–2.20)
Very premature birth (<32 wks)	3.27 (2.03–5.28)	NA
Low birth weight (<2.500 g)	1.70 (1.50–1.92)	1.77 (1.40–2.22)
Very low birth weight (<1.500 g)	3.00 (2.07–4.36)	2.70 (2.31–3.14)
Small for gestational age (SGA)	1.40 (1.15–1.71)	1.60 (1.25–2.04)
Cesarean section	1.54 (1.44–1.66)	2.13 (1.72–2.63)
Perinatal mortality	1.68 (1.11–2.55)	2.19 (1.61–2.98)
Neonatal intensive care	1.27 (1.16–1.40)	1.60 (1.30–1.96)

Data are presented as relative risks (RR) or odds ratios (OR) with 95% confidence intervals (CI). NA, not available.

singletons, adjusted for age and parity. They found that compared with spontaneous conceptions (Table 6.1), IVF singleton pregnancies are associated with significantly higher ORs of perinatal mortality (OR 2.2), PTB (OR 2.0), LBW (OR 1.8), very LBW (OR 2.7), and SGA (OR 1.6). Early PTB, spontaneous PTB, placenta previa, gestational diabetes, preeclampsia, and neonatal intensive care admission are also significantly more prevalent in the IVF group.

More recently, in their systematic review and meta-analyses, McDonald et al. [3] confirmed that after matching or controlling for maternal age and often other factors, compared to spontaneously conceived singletons, IVF singletons present with increased risks of the two primary outcomes, preterm delivery (RR: 1.84, 95% CI: 1.54, 2.21) and LBW (<2500 g, RR: 1.60, 95% CI: 1.29, 1.98). Singletons conceived through IVF or IVF/ICSI (intracytoplasmic spermatozoon injection) are at increased risk for late PTB (32–36 weeks, RR: 1.52, 95% CI: 1.01, 2.30), moderate PTB (<32–33 weeks, RR: 2.27, 95% CI: 1.73, 2.97), very LBW (<1500 g, RR: 2.65, 95% CI: 1.83, 3.84), and intrauterine growth restriction (IUGR) (RR: 1.45, 95% CI: 1.04, 2.00), LBW (−97 g, 95% CI: −161 g, −33 g), and shorter mean gestations (−0.6 weeks, 95% CI: −0.9 weeks, −0.4 weeks).

There are limited data about the perinatal outcome of non-IVF ART pregnancies. A small Belgian matched-case control study [7] found no differences between pregnancy outcomes after IVF and intrauterine insemination (IUI). The authors concluded that as there is no reason to believe that the IUI technique leads to an increased obstetric or neonatal risk, their data suggest that the worse pregnancy outcome after IVF as compared with spontaneous conceptions is due to the specific patient characteristics rather than to the use of IVF. These data also confirmed previous studies using large registries and showing that IUI treatment does not appear to increase obstetric or perinatal risks compared with matched spontaneous or IVF pregnancies [8,9].

A recent study [10] on the outcome of pregnancies resulting from ovulation induction (OI) found that after stratifying for multiplicity and adjusting for the available confounding factors (region, smoking, maternal age, socioeconomic position, and parity for perinatal health and mother's socioeconomic position for other indicators), most indicators showed worse health among OI children compared with control children. The OI children have poorer perinatal health and more episodes of long hospitalization than the control children. Singleton OI children also have more long-term illnesses in childhood, as measured by child disability allowance, long-term medication use, and hospital care episodes.

Women with unexplained infertility are older and more likely to be primiparous, but after adjusting for age and parity they have a higher incidence of preeclampsia, abruptio placentae, PTD, emergency Cesarean section, and induction of labor in comparison with the general population [11,12]. Subfertility as opposed to infertility also seems to increase perinatal risks, and available data uniformly indicate that it is not the treatments that increase the risks but the underlying causes of subfertility. Similar results have been observed in couples who conceived spontaneously but after a longer waiting time; that is, time to pregnancy (TTP) of >12 months. Perinatal outcome did not differ between women with unexplained infertility and in the general population. Women with unexplained infertility are at higher risk of obstetric complications that persist even after adjusting for age, parity, and fertility treatment. The same group of authors subsequently analyzed the maternity records of 1437 subfertile women and 21 688 controls. They found that after adjusting for age and parity, subfertile women were at increased risk of preeclampsia (OR 1.9), placenta previa (OR 3.9), placental abruption (OR 1.8), PTD (OR 1.7), and delivering LBW (OR 1.4). They were also more likely to undergo induction of labor (OR 1.5), Cesarean section (OR 2.1), and instrumental delivery (OR 2.2). The authors found no differences between treatment-related and treatment-independent pregnancies.

It has been known for more than two decades that women with spontaneous pregnancies have a higher risk of preeclampsia and delivering LBW after a TTP of >12 months compared to women with a TTP of <12 months [13]. By using interview data collected during the second trimester of pregnancy between 1998 and 2001 from women participating in the Danish National Birth Cohort, Basso et al. [14] identified 20 034 and 24 698 singleton live births to primiparous and multiparous women, respectively, for whom preeclampsia information was available from hospital birth records. Among women with no known hypertension, they confirmed a higher risk of preeclampsia in those with longer TTPs, after adjustment for maternal age, prepregnancy body mass index (BMI), and smoking. Compared with primiparas who became pregnant right away, the risk of preeclampsia increased with TTP and then stabilized for women taking six months or longer to conceive, and whose risk of preeclampsia increased by 50%. Multiparas also had an increased risk, but only those reporting a TTP of longer than 12 months (OR 2.47). Using data from the Danish National Birth Cohort, they also analyzed the outcome of 55 906 singleton live births from women who reported their waiting TTP and other covariates in an interview during the second trimester of pregnancy [15]. They found that a TTP of >1 year is associated with an increased risk of PTB among primiparous and multiparous women (OR 1.5 and 1.9, respectively) and that among couples with a TTP of >1 year, infertility treatment is associated with added risk only among multiparas.

Previous uterine surgery, assisted reproductive technology, and placentation disorders

In a nationwide population-based study, Romundstad et al. [16] reviewed the record of 845 384 pregnancies reported to the Medical Birth Registry of Norway between 1988 and 2002. They found a six-fold higher risk of placenta previa in singleton pregnancies conceived by ART compared with naturally conceived pregnancies (OR 5.6). Among mothers who had conceived both naturally and after ART, the risk of placenta previa is nearly three-fold higher in the pregnancy following assisted fertilization (OR 2.9) compared with that in the naturally conceived pregnancy. The use of ART is associated with an increased risk of placenta previa. Their findings suggest that the increased risk of placenta previa may be caused by factors related to the reproductive technology.

Women undergoing ART are known to be at increased risk of obstetrical interventions such as induced labor and elective Cesarean delivery, in particular women aged 40 years and above [4,17] There has been a substantial increase in the occurrence of placenta accreta over the last 50 years with as much as a 10-fold rise in the prevalence to around 1 in 2500 deliveries in many Western countries [18]. Placenta accreta complicates about 5% of pregnancies with placenta previa, and large epidemiological studies have shown that the strongest risk factor for placenta previa is a prior Cesarean section [18]. A single prior Cesarean section is associated with an increase in the prevalence of placenta previa from 0.5% to 5% at term. Thus, it is not surprising that as Cesarean section rates rise, the rate of placenta previa rises, and the rate of placenta accreta follows this trend. Many other factors, which are associated with infertility and ART, such as endometritis, myomectomy, hysteroscopic surgery, IVF procedure, endometrial resection, and the presence of a bicornuate uterus, adenomyosis or submucous fibroids have also been reported as risk factors of placenta accreta [5,18–20]. Where placenta accreta is present, the failure of the placenta to separate normally from the uterus after delivery is always accompanied by severe postpartum hemorrhage. Attempts to remove the adherent tissue may provoke further bleeding and a cascade of ongoing hemorrhage, shock, and coagulation disorders requiring a multidisciplinary approach [18].

Preexisting medical disorders, infertility, and the outcome of assisted reproductive technology pregnancies

Maternal age, primiparity, smoking, BMI, and years of infertility have all been associated with an increased risk of abnormal pregnancy outcome [21]. A recent analysis of the data collected through the national Maternity Experiences Survey (MES) of the Canadian Perinatal Surveillance System [22] has evaluated the outcome of 301 primiparous women aged 35 years or over and 1564 primiparous women aged 20 to 29 years. They found that women of advanced maternal age (AMA) are significantly more likely to have had a miscarriage or infertility treatment, to request or be offered a Cesarean section, and to have a higher rate of Cesarean section, but who are not at higher risks of PTB, LBW, and SGA infants.

Older patient age is naturally associated with an increased incidence of chronic diseases like arthritis, hypertension, and diabetes. However, as for ART singleton pregnancies, most studies have demonstrated similar age- and parity-adjusted risk of pregnancy-induced hypertension and gestational diabetes in IVF and controls. Overall, maternal age seems to have little impact on the rate of obstetric complications in women in their fourth decade of life; however, women aged 50 years or more are at increased risk of preeclampsia and gestational diabetes, and the vast majority of them can expect to deliver via Cesarean section [23–27]. However, independently of maternal age, ART such as oocyte donation could increase the risks of preeclampsia and premature labor. A recent meta-analysis [28] has found that the overall rate of preeclampsia in a total of 2308 deliveries after oocyte donation was 22.6%. Using the data from 11 studies, including a total of 644 oocyte recipients compared to 2320 controls, the authors found that the OR for preeclampsia after oocyte donation is 2.57 compared to conventional ART and 6.60 compared to the control group.

Obesity contributes to worse outcomes following treatment using ART, including lower pregnancy and live birth rates and a higher miscarriage rate [29]. A recent study of the Swedish patient register [30], including 3787 births in women with PCOS compared to 1 191 336 controls, has found that women with PCOS are more often obese and more commonly used ART than women without such a diagnosis

(60.6% versus 34.8% and 13.7% versus 1.5%). Polycystic ovarian syndrome is strongly associated with preeclampsia (OR 1.45) and very PTB (OR 2.21), and has a risk of gestational diabetes that is more than double that of controls. Infants born to mothers with PCOS are more prone to be large for gestational age (OR 1.39), at increased risk of meconium aspiration (OR 2.02) and having a low Apgar score (<7) at five minutes post delivery (1.41). The authors concluded that women with PCOS are at increased risk of adverse pregnancy and birth outcomes that cannot be explained by ART.

A recent prospective study [31] has shown that compared with fertile women, women who conceived by IVF/ICSI have an increased risk of stillbirth that is not explained by confounding factors. The results of this prospective study indicate that the increased risk of stillbirth seen after fertility treatment is a result of the fertility treatment or unknown factors pertaining to couples who undergo IVF/ICSI.

In addition, ART pregnancies seem to be at higher risk of fetal mal-presentation. In particular, breech presentation occurs nearly 50% more often in ART singleton pregnancies than in spontaneously conceived singletons [32]. In general, Cesarean sections and induced deliveries are more likely in ART pregnancies, but over the study period, Romundstad et al. [32] found that the proportion of Cesarean sections in ART pregnancies gradually approached that of spontaneously conceived pregnancies. Increased risk of breech presentation in pregnancies after ART is mediated by lower parity and shorter gestational time. In general, the obstetric management of women with ART pregnancies is gradually approaching the ordinary surveillance of pregnant women.

Overall, these findings confirm that the perinatal outcome of ART gestations depends on mutiple factors and that preexisting medical conditions may play a pivotal role in the risks of obstetric complications in ART pregnancies.

Conclusion

In vitro fertilization singletons have significantly increased risks of PTB, LBW, and other adverse perinatal outcomes compared to spontaneously conceived singletons after matching or controlling for maternal age at least. It remains unclear if these increased risks are attributable to the underlying infertility, characteristics of the infertile couple, or use of ART. Further research is required to clarify the contribution of infertility itself to adverse obstetrical and perinatal outcomes. We recommend a pre-ART medical assessment, which should include a thorough medical questionnaire and medical examination. Further evaluation and treatment should follow to ensure the safety of ART procedures and of ensuing pregnancies.

References

1. Helmerhorst FM, Perquin DA, Donker D, Keirse MJ. Perinatal outcome of singletons and twins after assisted conception: a systematic review of controlled studies. *BMJ* 2004; **328**: 261.
2. Jackson RA, Gibson KA, Wu YW, Croughan MS. Perinatal outcomes in singletons following in vitro fertilization: a meta-analysis. *Obstet Gynecol* 2004; **103**, 551–563.
3. McDonald SD, Han Z, Mulla S, et al. Preterm birth and low birth weight among in vitro fertilization singletons: a systematic review and meta-analyses. *Eur J Obstet Gynecol Reprod Biol* 2009; **146**: 138–148.
4. Allen VM, Wilson RD, Cheung A. Pregnancy outcomes after assisted reproductive technology. *J Obstet Gynaecol Can* 2006; **28**: 220–250.
5. Esh-Broder E, Ariel I, Abas-Bashir N, Bdolah Y, Celnikier DH. Placenta accreta is associated with IVF pregnancies: a retrospective chart review. *BJOG* 2011; **118**: 1084–1089.
6. Romundstad LB, Romundstad PR, Sunde A, et al. Effects of technology or maternal factors on perinatal outcome after assisted fertilisation: a population-based cohort study. *Lancet* 2008; **372**: 737–743.
7. De Sutter P, Veldeman L, Kok P, et al. Comparison of outcome of pregnancy after intra-uterine insemination (IUI) and IVF. *Hum Reprod* 2005; **20**: 1642–1646.
8. Nuojua-Huttunen S, Gissler M, Martikainen H, Tuomivaara L. Obstetric and perinatal outcome of pregnancies after intrauterine insemination. *Hum Reprod* 1999; **14**: 2110–2115.
9. Lansac J, Thepot F, Mayaux MJ, et al. Pregnancy outcome after artificial insemination or IVF with frozen semen donor: a collaborative study of the French CECOS Federation on 21,597 pregnancies. *Eur J Obstet Gynecol Reprod Biol* 1997; **74**: 223–228.
10. Klemetti R, Sevon T, Gissler M, Hemminki E. Health of children born after ovulation induction. *Fertil Steril* 2010; **93**: 1157–1168.
11. Pandian Z, Bhattacharya S, Templeton A. Review of unexplained infertility and obstetric outcome: a 10 year review. *Hum Reprod* 2001; **16**: 2593–2597.

12. Thomson F, Shanbhag S, Templeton A, Bhattacharya S. Obstetric outcome in women with subfertility. *BJOG* 2005; **112**: 632–637.

13. Williams MA, Goldman MB, Mittendorf R, Monson RR. Subfertility and the risk of low birth weight. *Fertil Steril* 1991; **56**: 668–671.

14. Basso O, Weinberg CR, Baird DD, Wilcox AJ, Olsen J. Subfecundity as a correlate of preeclampsia: a study within the Danish National Birth Cohort. *Am J Epidemiol* 2003; **157**: 195–202.

15. Basso O, Baird DD. Infertility and preterm delivery, birthweight, and Caesarean section: a study within the Danish National Birth Cohort. *Hum Reprod* 2003; **18**: 2478–2484.

16. Romundstad LB, Romundstad PR, Sunde A, et al. Increased risk of placenta previa in pregnancies following IVF/ICSI; a comparison of ART and non-ART pregnancies in the same mother. *Hum Reprod* 2006; **21**: 2353–2358.

17. Sheiner E, Shoham-Vardi I, Hershkovitz R, Katz M, Mazor M. Infertility treatment is an independent risk factor for cesarean section among nulliparous women aged 40 and above. *Am J Obstet Gynecol* 2001; **185**: 888–892.

18. Jauniaux E, Jurkovic D. Placenta accreta: pathogenesis of a 20th century iatrogenic uterine disease. *Placenta* 2012; Jan 25. [Epub ahead of print.]

19. Beuker JM, Erwich JJ, Khong TY. Is endomyometrial injury during termination of pregnancy or curettage following miscarriage the precursor to placenta accreta? *J Clin Pathol* 2005; **58**: 273–275.

20. Wood C, Rogers P.A pregnancy after planned partial endometrial resection. *Aust N Z J Obstet Gynyaecol* 1993; **33**: 316–318.

21. Sazonova A, Källen K, Thurin-Kjellberg A, Wennerholm UB, Bergh C. Factors affecting obstetric outcome of singletons born after IVF. *Hum Reprod* 2011; **26**: 2878–2886.

22. Bayrampour H, Heaman M. Comparison of demographic and obstetric characteristics of Canadian primiparous women of advanced maternal age and younger age. *J Obstet Gynaecol Can* 2011; **33**: 820–829.

23. Usta IM, Nassar AH. Advanced maternal age. Part I: obstetric complications. *Am J Perinatol* 2008; **25**: 521–534.

24. Paulson RJ, Boostanfar R, Saadat P, et al. Pregnancy in the sixth decade of life: obstetric outcomes in women of advanced reproductive age. *JAMA* 2002; **288**: 2320–2323.

25. Chibber R. Child-bearing beyond age 50: pregnancy outcome in 59 cases "a concern"? *Arch Gynecol Obstet* 2005; **271**: 189–194.

26. Montan S. Increased risk in the elderly parturient. *Curr Opin Obstet Gynecol* 2007; **19**: 110–112.

27. Franz MB, Husslein PW. Obstetrical management of the older gravida. *Womens Health (Lond Engl)* 2010; **6**: 463–468.

28. Pecks U, Maass N, Neulen J. Oocyte donation: a risk factor for pregnancy-induced hypertension: a meta-analysis and case series. *Dtsch Arztebl Int* 2011; **108**: 23–31.

29. Sobaleva S, El-Toukhy T. The impact of raised BMI on the outcome of assisted reproduction: current concepts. *J Obstet Gynaecol* 2011; **31**: 561–565.

30. Roos N, Kieler H, Sahlin L, et al. Risk of adverse pregnancy outcomes in women with polycystic ovary syndrome: population based cohort study. *BMJ* 2011; **343**: d6309.

31. Wisborg K, Ingerslev HJ, Henriksen TB. IVF and stillbirth: a prospective follow-up study. *Hum Reprod* 2010; **25**: 1312–1316.

32. Romundstad LB, Romundstad PR, Sunde A, et al. Assisted fertilization and breech delivery: risks and obstetric management. *Hum Reprod* 2009; **24**: 3205–3210.

Chapter 7

Early and late pregnancy and psychological complications after assisted reproductive technology

Gamal I. Serour

Introduction

The advent of assisted reproductive technology (ART) has given hope to infertile couples who, a mere 33 years ago, would have had little or no chance of bearing a child.

Assisted reproductive technology has made great strides since the birth of Louise Brown. Today, ART has become a well-established and accepted method for the treatment of female and male infertility and is practiced widely in almost every country in the world. However, debate continues regarding its safety and risks. In countries in Europe with complete reporting, the percentage of babies conceived through ART varied from 1.0% of the national births in Italy to 4.1% in Denmark, and the percentage of ART babies was above 3% [1]. However, not all ART pregnancies are without complications or result in the birth of healthy babies (see Chapters 6 and 8). From patients' perspectives, the birth of a healthy baby is the real measure of success of any infertility treatment.

Assisted reproductive technology pregnancies, like spontaneous pregnancies, may develop complications that threaten such a desired outcome [2]. As couples at the initiation of ART treatment are more anxious than their comparative norms [3], the impact of pregnancy complications is likely to be more seriously perceived by the ART-pregnant patients compared with their comparative norms.

As many aspects of ART pregnancy complications are dealt with in other chapters of this textbook, this chapter is limited to an overview of early and late pregnancy complications with particular emphasis on the psychological complications.

Early pregnancy complications

Miscarriage

Several authors reported a higher incidence of miscarriage in pregnancies resulting from ART than in spontaneous pregnancies [2,4–8]. Serour et al., in a study of 702 ART pregnancies resulting from 3500 ART cycles, reported a miscarriage rate of 20.6% [4], similar to miscarriage rates reported by several other authors [6–8].

Whether the increased miscarriage rate in ART is a direct result of the procedure or simply reflects the population concerned presents some difficulties (see Chapter 5). This is because of several reasons including the use of different definitions of miscarriage, use of highly sensitive assays for beta-human chorionic gonadotrophin (β-hCG) for the diagnosis of pregnancy, the close monitoring of women pregnant after ART, and the exact knowledge of the dates of embryo transfer in ART pregnancies. Other potential factors may lead to this high miscarriage rate in ART pregnancies, including a luteal phase defect following the use of human menstrual gonadotropin (HMG) for ovulation induction, fertilization of postmature ova, and possible adverse effects from handling the oocytes [2].

The importance of increasing maternal age as a confounding factor was illustrated in the 1994 ART Registry results for the U.S. and Canada, with an overall miscarriage rate of 19% compared to a miscarriage rate of 13.2% in women younger than 40 years of age with no male factor, increasing to 30.1% in women over 40 years of age with no male factor [9]. In an analysis of 318 pregnancies resulting from 2386 consecutive ART cycles using autologous oocytes in

Pregnancy After Assisted Reproductive Technology, ed. Eric R. M. Jauniaux and Botros R. M. B. Rizk. Published by Cambridge University Press.

women aged 40 years and above, Serour et al. reported a miscarriage rate of 44.8%. The miscarriage rate increased with one-year age increments for women aged 40 years or older, being 39%, 44.4%, 51.3%, 64.3%, 75%, and 67% for women at ages 40, 41, 42, 43, 44, and >45 years, respectively [10].

The early loss rates of the entire pregnancies are lower in twin than singleton pregnancies resulting from ART [10–15]. The total early loss rate in twin compared with singleton pregnancies was reported to be 20% versus 49%, 5.1% versus 21.8%, 3.7% versus 19.8%, and 11.6% versus 24.6% by Serour et al [10], Tummers et al. [12], Zegers-Hochschild et al. [13], and La Sala et al. [14], respectively. A Portuguese study showed a distinct advantage for twins in the subgroup of younger patients who underwent the intracytoplasmic spermatozoon injection (ICSI) procedure [15].

The much lower figures of early loss rate of entire pregnancies in twin than in singleton pregnancies implies that the uterine milieu during an early twin pregnancy is more supportive compared with that for a singleton pregnancy. It was suggested that the aneuploid twin in dizygotic pairs is frequently protected by the presence of a normal co-twin whereas singletons affected by the same aneuploidy are frequently miscarried [16].

The experience of miscarriage after ART pregnancy is an area of research that is not yet fully explored. Infertility and spontaneous pregnancy loss on their own are associated with considerable grief, loss, and intra- and interpersonal distress.

In ART, the prolonged medical treatment, monitoring, and procedures of oocyte harvesting, embryo transfer, post-transfer treatment, and the post-transfer two-week period of expectations disrupt women's daily lives and routines and they become very focused on their bodies and on securing a satisfactory pregnancy outcome. Their desire to become mothers often increases with repeated treatment failures, further intensifying their investment in having a child [17]. Harris and Daniluki [18] investigated the impact of pregnancy loss for infertile women following conception through ART in a qualitative phenomenological study of women who lost their pregnancy at 2–16 weeks' gestation. Participants' experiences of pregnancy loss were embedded with their experiences of infertility and medical treatment, and shaped by their significant investment in having a child. A particular feature was their marked ambivalence regarding future reproductive options after their pregnancy loss, reflecting a unique overlay of prominent anxiety in their grief experience [18]. They identified nine common themes in the participants' experiences of miscarriage such as the sense of profound loss and grief, shared loss with their partners, injustice and lack of fairness, ongoing reminders of their loss, feelings of social awkwardness, fear of investing in the treatment process of the pregnancy, need to make sense of their experience, and sense of responsibility [18]. As the miscarriage rate increases with maternal age, particularly for women aged 40 years and above, women aged 43 years and above should be discouraged from undergoing ART using their autologous oocytes in favor of egg donation [10]. However, this alternative is not ethically and culturally acceptable in some societies. Couples will have to make their own informed decisions based on the detailed evidence-based information provided to them by the treating physician. If the physician has a conscientious objection to this alternative treatment of egg donations, it is his or her ethical obligation to refer the couple to other clinics where they may obtain this evidence-based treatment [19]. Use of the women's own vitrified oocytes or transplantation of cryopreserved-thawed ovarian cortical tissue are promising future alternatives.

Ectopic pregnancies

In the U.S. during the period 1981–1991, the incidence of ectopic pregnancy (EP) was approximately 1.3%–2% of all reported pregnancies [20]. In the previous decades, the incidence had increased because of the greater prevalence of sexually transmitted diseases, more frequent tubal sterilization and reversal procedures, delayed childbearing, and the wider use of ART [21].

It is worth mentioning that the first ART pregnancy reported by Steptoe and Edwards in 1976 was an EP [22]. Since then, the rate of EP after ART has been quoted as varying widely between 2% and 11% [23,24]. Serour et al. reported a rate of 1.9% in 702 ART pregnancies resulting from 3500 initiated ART cycles [4]. In a relatively recent Finish study of 9175 ART cycles, the rate of EPs per 100 ART births was 5%, which is twice that of earlier studies in Finland [25].

The link between ovulation induction drugs and EP has been contested [2,5]. The most significant risk factor for EP in ART is tubal pathology. Dubuisson et al., in a study of 556 pregnancies resulting from ART, reported an EP rate of 11.1% in patients with a tubal factor, decreasing to 3.4% in unexplained infertility cases, and 2.1% in women with endometriosis

[24]. The pathology examination of the specimens from all three groups showed preexisting tubal lesions. The stimulation protocol, E_2 level, number of embryos transferred, and type of luteal phase support did not significantly affect the EP rate. Asung et al. analyzed 765 cases of EP resulting from 156 454 ART cycles in the U.K. during the period 1991–1999. The EP incidence was significantly higher ($P<0.001$) following in vitro fertilization (IVF) (2.8%) than ICSI (1.3 %) [26]. Within the IVF groups, the EP incidence was inversely correlated with maternal age. The EP rate was 6.1%, 4.1%, 3.9%, 3.0%, and 2% for women in the age groups of <25, 25–29, 30–34, 35–39, and >40 years, respectively, which represented a significant trend ($P<0.004$). There was a small significantly higher incidence of EP when three compared with two embryos were transferred ($P < 0.036$). The strong association of tubal disease with the high incidence of EP supports the practice of prophylactic salpingectomy of unhealthy tubes before ART (see Chapter 3). However, such practice solely for prevention of EP would overtreat 89% of patients by removing their tubes and abolishing any chance of future normal spontaneous pregnancy. In addition, it does not prevent interstitial pregnancy [27]. Ruptured EPs after corneal or tubal stump implantation in ART after salpingectomy have been reported [28,29]. Ko et al. reported a series of six cases of tubal stump pregnancy as a complication of ART. All patients had had unilateral or bilateral laparoscopic salpingectomy owing to tubal pregnancy or hydrosalpinx [30]. In view of the risk of early rupture in tubal stump pregnancy, early diagnosis is warranted to avoid maternal mortality and morbidity.

Ectopic pregnancy following ART may also occur in other sites such as a simultaneous bilateral tubal pregnancy, bilateral simultaneous interstitial EP after salpingectomy, and intramural, ovarian, abdominal, or cervical EP. Cervical EP is associated with reflux of embryos into the cervix after embryo transfer or trauma to the cervix during embryo transfer [2,5]. Early diagnosis of cervical EP is important to avoid severe hemorrhage with advancing gestational age [2].

An empty uterine cavity with a positive β-hCG test four weeks after embryo transfer should be taken seriously. These patients should be followed up very carefully for early diagnosis of EP. Early detection of EP will allow the physician and the patient the choice of minimal access surgery, other minimal interventions, or expectant management of the ectopic pregnancy with decreased maternal morbidity and mortality.

Mol et al. suggested that a single β-hCG measurement nine days after embryo transfer of over 18 IU/L can be used as a cutoff value, justifying expectant management in an asymptomatic patient because the probability of EP is only 1% in these women. Early monitoring is recommended if the value is less than 18 IU/L because the probability of EP in these cases is 38% [31].

Marcus et al. found that three β-hCG levels and a day-13 progesterone measurement combined with a history of pelvic inflammatory disease achieved a predictive value of up to 90% for EP after ART [32]. On a review of the literature, all cases of stump EP were managed with surgery except those reported by Bernardini et al. [33]. They successfully treated interstitial tubal stump pregnancy after unilateral adnectomy with systemic single-dose methotrexate therapy followed by transvaginal colour Doppler ultrasound [33]. Systemic methotrexate is a valid option when laparoscopy is not required for making the diagnosis and the EP is smaller than 4 cm, when the gestational sac is no longer viable, and when EP cannot be safely and easily punctured under echogenic guidance [34].

Heterotopic pregnancies

Coexistent intrauterine and ectopic gestation, or heterotopic pregnancy, is more common after ART. The incidence of heterotopic pregnancy in spontaneous conception varies from 1 in 2600 to 1 in 30 000 pregnancies [35,36].

The rate following ovulation induction and ART is quoted in a review of 139 case reports during the period 1971 to 1993 as approximately 1 in 100 pregnancies [37]. Serour et al., in a series of 702 pregnancies resulting from 3500 consecutive ART cycles, reported two cases of heterotopic pregnancy; an incidence of 0.3% [4].

The increased risk of heterotopic pregnancy in ART is the result of multiple ovulations and embryo transfers in patients with tubal or pelvic disease. Half of the cases studied by Tal et al. had one or more previous EPs and 45% of the women had previous pelvic surgery [37]. The technique of embryo transfer including the volume and viscosity of the medium, deep or superficial insertion of the embryo transfer catheter, and degree of difficulty of the procedure has been proposed as etiological factors for heterotopic pregnancy, but the data are not adequate enough to draw firm conclusions [2,5].

Because of the increasing frequency of this complication, case reports concerned with the management of heterotopic pregnancy are becoming important. Recently Okamura et al. reported on a heterotopic triplet pregnancy after a frozen-thawed embryo transfer in a patient with a remnant tubal ectopic and intrauterine twin pregnancy [38]. The patient had previously undergone a laparoscopic left salpingectomy due to pysosalpinx. A diagnostic emergency laparoscopy based on the suspicion of hemoperitoneum demonstrated an ectopic pregnancy in the remnant isthmic portion of the left tube. Laparoscopic excision of the remnant Fallopian tube was performed [38].

The risk of a tubal pregnancy in addition to an existing intrauterine pregnancy should be thought of after transferring two or more embryos, even in patients who have had a salpingectomy before the ART cycle. Heterotopic pregnancy involving the cervix is even more unusual. A recent case of heterotopic cervical pregnancy was reported by Faschingbauer et al. [39]. They were able to terminate the cervical pregnancy selectively by suction curettage of the cervically located fetus, performed under abdominal ultrasound guidance without complications, with readiness for hysterectomy. A high cervical circulage was positioned and firmly tied to prevent possible massive cervical bleeding from the site of the heterotopic pregnancy. Simultaneous heterotopic intrauterine and cervical pregnancy is a very rare event; 26 cases were reported in the literature of which only two cases followed natural spontaneous conception [39].

Early diagnosis of heterotopic pregnancy by vaginal ultrasonography and/or laparoscopy is important. Once the diagnosis is made, the heterotopic sac is either removed surgically or treated with transvaginal ultrasonographically guided installation of hyperosmolar glucose into the ectopic sac, or potassium chloride injection with aspiration of the pregnancy sac. Clayton et al. compared the heterotopic and intrauterine only pregnancy outcomes after ART in the U.S. during the period 1999–2002. Heterotopic pregnancies were more likely to result in spontaneous or induced abortions than were intrauterine only pregnancies. The RR was 2.05 (95% CI: 1.67–2.51) for spontaneous abortion and 10.28 (95% CI: 6.76–15.65) for induced abortion [40].

Molar pregnancies

Assessment of any potential increased risk of molar pregnancy associated with ART is difficult. Theoretically, the use of immature ova after ovulation induction or the disruption of meiosis and loss of maternal chromosomes as a result of oocyte handling or degeneration could increase the risk of a complete mole. Alternatively, post-mature oocytes are more prone to polyspermy with a resultant heterozygous complete or partial molar pregnancy [41,42]. The literature search, not limited to English language journals in this subject, revealed reports of 38 women with molar pregnancies subsequent to infertility treatment. Cases occurring following ovulation induction used the following drugs: chlomiphene citrate (CC), seventeen cases; hMG/hCG, six cases (one with donor spermatozoa); CC/hMG, three cases; bromocriptine, one case. Additional techniques used were hMG/IVF in seven women, hMG with gamete intra-Fallopian transfer (GIFT) in two women, and CC/hMG/IVF in two cases. The pregnancies were complete moles in 32 women and partial moles in two women. Four cases of choriocarcinoma have been described. In three women, molar pregnancy recurred up to four times. At least six women received chemotherapy. In eight women there was a single coexisting fetus, in eight there were two other fetuses, and in one case there were three coexisting fetuses. In several cases there were live-born babies [2].

Further assessment of this complication is impossible without the collation of data from many centers. In particular, limited information is available about women receiving ovulation induction as their sole treatment; the relatively large number of case reports warrants vigilance for molar pregnancy in patients receiving fertility treatment. The use of modern molecular biology techniques, preimplantation diagnosis, and ICSI will provide further insights into this disease, with possible strategies for prevention in women with recurrent molar pregnancies [43–45].

Late pregnancy complications

It is often reported that women who become pregnant following ART have a higher risk of adverse effects than women who conceive spontaneously. They have a higher risk of preeclampsia and their babies have a higher risk of preterm birth, low birth weight, small size for gestational age, stillbirth, and major malformations [46–49]. A substantial set of data is now available that clearly shows that women who become pregnant after trying to conceive for 12 months or longer have similar adverse effects to those women who undergo ART [48,50]. Infertility per se leads to similar problems to those seen with ART. A background risk seems to exist in subfertile couples that leads to an increased risk of adverse events if a pregnancy occurs. Knowledge of the specific genetic factors that define these risks is not available [51].

Vaginal bleeding

In singleton pregnancies resulting from ART, first-trimester bleeding is associated with increased second-trimester (OR 4.56, 95% C1: 2.76–7.56) and third-trimester bleeding rates (OR 2.85, 95% C1: 1.42–5.73) [52]. In a nation-wide population study of 845 384 pregnancies reported to the Medical Birth Registry of Norway between 1988 and 2002, the risk of placenta previa in 7568 pregnancies conceived after ART was found to be six-fold higher in singleton pregnancies conceived by ART compared with naturally conceived pregnancies (adjusted OR 5.6, 95% C1: 4.4–7) [53]. Among mothers who have conceived both naturally and after ART, the risk of placenta previa was nearly three-fold higher in the pregnancy following ART (adjusted OR 2.9, 95% C1: 1.4–6.1) compared with that in the naturally conceived pregnancy [53].

In a study by Allen et al. of 1182 pregnancies conceived after ART, they reported the incidence of placenta previa to be 2.8% compared with 0.5% in the general population [54].

Pregnancy-induced hypertension and other adverse obstetric and perinatal outcomes

In a study of 702 pregnancies following ART, Serour et al. reported pregnancy-induced hypertension, preterm labor, low birth weight, intrauterine fetal death, and congenital malformations in 10%, 21.5%, 30.5%, 2%, and 2.1% of cases, respectively [4]. It has been suggested that ART pregnancies incur a high risk for hypertension and bleeding, which can in turn lead to reduced birth weight and gestation period.

In order to assess the effects of ART and subfertility during and after pregnancy, Romundstad et al. used the data from the Medical Birth Registry of Norway from January 1984 to June 2006 and conducted a population-based cohort study of women who had conceived singleton babies spontaneously or via ART [55]. They also analyzed the data on pairs of siblings where one baby had been conceived by ART and the other by spontaneous conception, thus allowing the maternal factor to be as constant as possible. A total of 1 209 151 singleton births were recorded; 1 200 992 births (99%) were spontaneously conceived and 8229 births (1%) were conceived after ART. In addition, 2546 women gave birth to both a singleton infant via spontaneous conception, and a singleton infant via ART. In the whole population, babies conceived via ART had more adverse events such as low birth weight, premature delivery, perinatal mortality, and were smaller for their age than babies conceived via spontaneous conception. Among the sibling pairs, ART was not associated with increased risk of low birth weight, premature delivery, small size for gestational age, or perinatal mortality when compared with those spontaneously conceived. These results indicated that the adverse outcomes associated with ART could be attributed to the factors that lead to infertility rather than the factors associated with ART [56].

In a retrospective cohort study of national population data of infants conceived through ART in Australia between 1996 and 2000, preterm birth and low birth weight were more common among singletons and twins conceived with ART and born to nulliparous women. Preterm birth and low birth weight were respectively 1.3- and 1.5-times more likely to occur among singletons conceived by transfer of fresh embryos compared with transfer of frozen embryos. Preterm birth and low birth weight were more common among couples who had female factor infertility compared with male factor infertility [57].

Ludwig recommends follow-up studies are performed to identify possible genes or other factors that lead to high risk of adverse events during and after pregnancy among women in subfertile couples [56]. In women with normal fertility once male factors are overcome, their uterine environment is healthy and so more normal growth can be expected. Whether the ART procedures associated with the infertility contribute to the adverse outcomes has been investigated by many workers, with conflicting results. Some suggest that they are specific adverse effects of ART [58–60]; others conclude that they are related to the health of the infertile women [55,61].

Jacques et al., in a study to compare the prevalence of adverse obstetric and singleton birth outcomes between subfertile women and women from the general population (controls), after adjusting for confounders, reported that women with subfertility compared with controls had increased odds of hypertension or preeclampsia (adjusted OR 1.29, 95 % CI:1.02–1.6), prepartum hemorrhage (adjusted OR 1.41, 95% CI: 1.05–1.89), perinatal death (adjusted OR 2.19, 95% CI: 1.10–4.36), low birth weight (adjusted OR 1.44, 95% CI: 1.11–1.85), preterm birth <37 weeks (adjusted OR 1.32, 95% CI: 1.05–1.67) or <31 weeks (adjusted OR 2.37, 95% CI: 1.35–4.13), and Cesarean delivery (adjusted OR 1.56, 95% CI: 1.37–1.77). There was weak evidence of increased birth defects (adjusted OR 1.3, 95% CI: 0.98–1.72) and gestational diabetes (OR 1.25, 95% CI: 0.96–1.63). No increased risk was found for prelabor rupture of membranes, small for gestational ages, or postpartum hemorrhage [62].

Psychological complications

The findings of increased psychological distress in couples undergoing infertility treatment necessitate providing information and counseling as an essential part of an ART program. Fertility problems are accompanied by a lot of emotional distress, resulting in a considerable proportion of female patients showing severe maladjustment after ART. Although this interferes with their daily life, emotional distress has also been shown to be related to dropout of treatment and deterioration of health behavior. Counseling compared to information alone does not lead to any enhanced reduction in levels of anxiety or depression. The challenge is to identify those individuals who may benefit from specific intervention at an early stage and before pregnancy [2,5].

Assisted reproductive technology may potentially cause psychological problems that are seldom or never encountered during spontaneous conceptions. Moreover, ART may suppress the symptoms of infertility but it does not eliminate them in the sense that it provides a solution to infertility but does not remove the stigmatization of being infertile. Assisted reproductive technology may fulfill the wish of infertile couples via an entirely somatic answer to a subjective problem; it creates risks for a divide between the physiological and psychological aspects of procreation [63].

Methodological and conceptual difficulties exist in researching this area including difficulty in matching controls, small sample sizes, debate on the validity of the various questionnaires used, and a tendency to positive self-reporting in couples undergoing ART [2]. In retrospective studies, perception of the stress of treatment may be influenced by the impact of treatment failure.

A prospective longitudinal study of 144 couples found that at intake for ART treatment, women were more anxious than their partners and comparative norms, but those who conceived were less depressed and more positive about their relationships [3]. A study of forty-five couples during ART treatment, pregnancy, and delivery reported that the psychological burden of the treatment exceeded the physical burden, and pregnancy was more stressful than in controls with spontaneous conceptions [64]. However, mothers experienced the delivery, and fathers the pregnancy, as more exceptional than controls, and fathers enjoyed the pregnancy more than their control equivalents. The positive aspects of ART also were recorded by Boivin and Takefman, with higher levels of optimism (as well as more stress and changes to marital and social relationships) in women during a treatment cycle compared to a non-treatment cycle [65].

In a study by Colpin and Soenen, parenting and the children's psychological development do not differ significantly between ART families and control families [66]. Pinborg et al., in a Danish National cohort study of 472 ART twins and 634 ART singletons, reported the implications for families are stronger in ART twins compared with ART singletons.Both ART and non-ART twin parents experienced more marital stress (OR 2.9, 95% CI: 2.2–3.8) and twins had more impact on the mother's life (OR 1.7, 95% CI: 1.2–2.4) compared with singletons [67].

The impact of high-order multiple pregnancy has been reported in a series of articles assessing the psychological consequences of having triplets, up to four years after delivery [68]. Only one of twelve pregnancies was spontaneous. At one year, the majority of mothers reported difficulties related to home help, social isolation, marital relationship, and relationships with the children. Eight of the twelve mothers expressed psychological difficulties, and three were treated for depression. By four years after birth, all mothers reported emotional distress (mainly fatigue and stress), four women had a high depression score and were on psychotropic medication, and four mothers spontaneously expressed regrets about having triplets [68].

Monti et al. studied depressive symptoms during late pregnancy and early parenthood following ART in a case-control longitudinal study. Women who conceived by ART were compared with men and with women following spontaneous conceptions. The sample included 87 subjects, 48 ART (25 mothers, 23 fathers, response rate of 30%), and 39 non-ART mothers evaluated by the Edinburgh Postnatal Depression Scale (EPDS) at 30–32 weeks of gestation and at one week and three months after delivery [63]. The EPDS score was higher in ART women compared with non-ART women during all assessments, and higher during the third trimester of pregnancy and at one week postpartum compared with ART men. The prevalence of depressed subjects was significantly higher in ART women compared with non-ART women during the antenatal assessment. The authors concluded that ART pregnancies are more frequently associated with symptoms that may persist after delivery, suggesting a greater emotional vulnerability of these women. The risk of depression during and following ART pregnancies needs monitoring to avoid adverse effects of postpartum depression on the mother–infant relationship and the infant's psychological development.

Men are also at risk of depression during ART. Although psychological distress scores are significantly higher among women than men for symptoms of depression, state anxiety, infertility specific distress, and general perceived stress, the partners of women undergoing ART are at risk of similar psychological problems [69]. Finally, a large number of life events perceived as having a negative impact on the quality of life may indicate chronic stress, and the results of a recent study indicate that stress may reduce the chances of a successful outcome following IVF, possibly through psychobiological mechanisms affecting medical end-points such as oocyte retrieval outcome [70].

Conclusion

Assisted reproductive technology pregnancies are associated with slightly increased risks of physical and psychological complications. These risks are most probably related to the genetic or other factors of subfertility of these patients rather than the technology of ART. However more research is needed in this area. Meanwhile, physicians providing ART services should carefully select, counsel, and monitor their ART patients all through the procedure until the time of delivery and in the postpartum period to ensure the safest possible outcome for both the mother and the baby to be born. Such a continuum of care, although ideal, may not be available in all settings. Physicians must make all the necessary arrangements to ensure follow-up of ART pregnancy women and their newborns. Early identification of women at risk of psychological complications enables the provision of timely psychosocial support and the focusing of psychosocial resources on those who need it most.

References

1. De Mouzon J, Goossens V, Bhattacharya S, et al. Assisted reproductive technology in Europe, 2006: results generated from European registers by ESHRE. *Hum Reprod* 2010; **25**: 1851–1862.
2. Serour GI. Complications of assisted reproductive techniques: a review. *Assist Reprod* 1999; **9**: 214–232.
3. Slade P, Emery J, Lieberman BA. A prospective, longitudinal study of emotions and relationships in in vitro fertilization treatment. *Hum Reprod* 1997; **12**: 183–190.
4. Serour GI, Aboulghar M, Mansour R, et al. Complications of medically assisted conceptions in 3, 500 cycles. *Fertil Steril* 1998; **70**: 638–642.
5. Serour GI. Complications of Assisted Reproductive Technology. In: Botros R, Juan A, Garcia-Velasco, Hassan Sallam, Antonis Makrigiannakis, eds. *Infertility and Assisted Reproduction*. 1st edn. Cambridge, UK: Cambridge University Press, 2008; 604–618.
6. Kupka MS, Dorn C, Richter O, Felberbaum R, van der Ven H. Impact of reproductive history on in vitro fertilization and intracytoplasmic sperm injection outcome; evidence from the German IVF Registry. *Fertil Steril* 2003; **80**: 508–516.
7. Schieve LA, Tatham L, Peterson HB, Toner J, Jeng G. Spontaneous abortion among pregnancies conceived using assisted reproductive technology in the United States. *Obstet Gynecol* 2003; **101**: 959–967.
8. Wang JX, Norman RJ, Wilcox AJ. Incidence of spontaneous abortion among pregnancies produced by assisted reproductive technology. *Hum Reprod* 2004; **19**: 272–277.
9. Society for Assisted Reproductive Technology and American Society for Reproductive Medicine. Assisted reproductive technology in the United States and Canada: 1994 results generated from the American Society for Reproductive Medicine/Society for Assisted Reproductive Technology registry. *Fertil Steril* 1996; **66**: 697–705.
10. Serour GI, Mansour R, Serour A, et al. Analysis of 2,386 consecutive cycles of in vitro fertilization or intracytoplasmic sperm injection using autologous oocytes in women aged 40 years and above. *Fertil Steril* 2010; **94**: 1707–1712.

11. Matias A, La Sala GB, Blickstein I. Early loss rates of entire pregnancies after assisted reproduction are lower in twin than in singleton pregnancies. *Fertil Steril* 2007; **88**: 1452–1454.

12. Tummers P, De Sutter P, Dhont M. Risk of spontaneous abortion in singleton and twin pregnancies after IVF/ICSI. *Hum Reprod* 2003; **18**: 1720–1723.

13. Zegers-Hochschild F, Bravo M, Fernandex, et al., Multiple gestation as a marker of reproductive efficacy: learning from assisted reproductive technologies. *Reprod Biomed Online* 2003; **8**: 125–129.

14. La Sala GB, Nucera G, Gallinelli A, et al. Spontaneous embryonic loss following in-vitro fertilization with and without intracytoplasmic sperm injection. *Fertil Steril* 2004: **82**: 1536–1539.

15. Matias A, Oliveria C. da Silva JT. et al. The effect of ICSI. Maternal age and embryonic stage on early clinical loss rate of twin versus singleton pregnancies. *Eur J Obstet Gynecol Reprod Biol* 2007: **130**: 212–215.

16. Hall JG. Pediatricians beware: the age of ART is upon us. *J Pediatr* 2005; **146**: 450–452.

17. Daniluki JC. Gender and infertility In: Lieblum SR. ed. *Infertility: Psychological Issues and Counseling Strategies*. New York, NY: Wiley, 1997; 103–125.

18. Harris DL, Daniluki JC. The experience of spontaneous pregnancy loss for infertile women who have conceived through assisted reproduction technology. *Hum Reprod* 2010; **25**: 714–720.

19. Serour GI. Islamic perspectives in human reproduction: ethical issues in ART. *Reprod Biomed Online* 2008; **17**: S34–S38.

20. Sariya M, Berg CJ, Shulman H, Green CA, Atrash HK. Estimates of the annual number of clinically recognized pregnancies in the United States, 1981–1991. *Am J Epidemiol* 1999; **149**: 1025–1029.

21. Takeda A, Manabe S, Mitsui T, Nakamura H. Spontaneous ectopic pregnancy occurring in the isthmic portion of the remnant tube after ipsilateral adnexectomy: report of two cases. *J Obstet Gynaecol Res* 2006; **32**: 190–194.

22. Steptoe PC, Edwards RG. Reimplantation of a human embryo with subsequent tubal pregnancy. *Lancet* 1976; **1**: 880–882.

23. Bryant J, Sullivan EA, Dean JH. Supplement to assisted reproductive technology in Australia and New Zealand. *Assist Reproductive Technology Series*. Number 8. Publication of AIHW National Prenatal Statistics Unit, no. PER 26. Sydney, Australia, 2004.

24. Dubuisson JB, Aubriot FX, Mathieu L, et al. Risk factors for ectopic pregnancy in 556 pregnancies after in vitro fertilization: implications for preventive management. *Fertil Steril* 1991; **56**: 686–690.

25. Klemetti R, Sevon T, Gissler M, Hemminiki E. Complication of IVF and ovulation induction. *Hum Reprod* 2005; **20**: 3293–3300.

26. Asung E, Cuckle HS, Dirnfeld M, Grudzinskas GJ. Ectopic pregnancy following IVF/ICSI-ET in the United Kingdom, HFEA Register (1991–1999). Abstracts of the 19th annual meeting of ESHRE, Madrid, Spain 2003; xviii34–xviii35.

27. Rebic-Pucelj M, Tomazevic T, Vogler A, Meden-Vrtovec H. Risk factors for ectopic pregnancy after in vitro fertilization and embryo transfer. *J Assist Reprod Genet* 1995; **12**: 594–598.

28. Agarwal SK, Wisot AL, Garzo G, Meldrum DR. Corneal pregnancies in patients with prior salpingectomy undergoing in vitro fertilization and embryo transfer. *Fertil Steril* 1996; **65**: 659–660.

29. Arbab F, Boulieu D, Bied V, et al. Uterine rupture in first or second trimester of pregnancy after in vitro fertilization and embryo transfer. *Hum Reprod* 1996; **11**: 1120–1122.

30. Ko PC, Liang CC, Lo TS, Huang HY. Six cases of tubal stump pregnancy: complication of assisted reproductive technology. *Fertil Steril* 2011; **95**: 2432.el–e4.

31. Mol BWJ, Van der Venn F, Hajenius PJ, et al. Diagnosis of ectopic pregnancy after in vitro fertilization and embryo transfer. *Fertil Steril* 1997; **68**: 1027–1032.

32. Marcus SF, Macnamee M, Brinsden P. The prediction of ectopic pregnancy after in vitro fertilization and embryo transfer. *Hum Reprod* 1995; **10**: 2165–2168.

33. Bernardini L, Valenzano M, Foglia G. Spontaneous interstitial pregnancy on a tubal stump after unilateral adnectomy followed by transvaginal colour Doppler ultrasound. *Hum Reprod* 1998; **13**: 1723–1726.

34. Carson SA, Buster JE. Ectopic pregnancy. *N Engl J Med* 1993; **329**: 1174–1181.

35. Dicken D, Goldman G, Feldberg D, Ashkenazi J, Goldman JA. Heterotopic pregnancy after IVF-ET: report of a case and a review of the literature. *Hum Reprod* 1989; **4**: 335–336.

36. De Vroe RW, Pratt JH. Simultaneous intrauterine and extrauterine pregnancy. *Am J Obstet Gynecol* 1948; **56**: 1119–1123.

37. Tal J, Haddad S, Gordon N, Timor-Tritsch I. Heterotopic pregnancy after ovulation induction and assisted reproductive technologies: a literature review from 1971 to 1993. *Fertil Steril* 1996; **66**: 1–12.

38. Okamura Y, Arakane F, Nagayoshi-Taura Y, et al. Heterotopic triplet pregnancy: report of a patient with

remnant tubal ectopic and intrauterine twin pregnancy after frozen-thawed embryo transfer. *Reprod Med Biol* 2011; **10**: 283–286.

39. Faschingbauer F, Mueller A, Voigt F, Beckmann MW, Goecke TW. Treatment of heterotopic cervical pregnancies. *Fertile and Steril* 2011; **95**: 1787.e9–e13.

40. Clayton HB, Shieve LA, Peterson HB, et al. A comparison of heterotopic and intrauterine-only pregnancy outcomes after assisted reproductive technologies in the United States from 1999 to 2002. *Fertil Steril* 2007; **87**: 303–309.

41. Johannes CB, Caro JJ, Hartz SC, Marrs R. Adverse effects of ovulatory stimulants: a review. *Assist Reprod Rev* 1993; **3**: 68–74.

42. Van de Geijn EJ, Yedema CA, Hemrika DJ, Schutte MF, ten Velden JJ. Hydatidiform mole with coexisting twin pregnancy after gamete intra-fallopian transfer. *Hum Reprod* 1992; **7**: 568–572.

43. Edwards R, Crow J, Dale S, et al. Preimplantation diagnosis and recurrent hydatidiform mole. *Lancet* 1990: **335**: 1030–1031.

44. Reubinoff BE, Lewin A, Verner M, et al. Intracytoplasmic sperm injection combined with preimplantation genetic diagnosis for the prevention of recurrent gestational trophoblastic disease. *Hum Reprod* 1997; **12**: 805–808.

45. Shozu M, Akimoto K, Kasai T, Inoue M, Michikura Y. Hydatidiform mole associated with multiple gestations after assisted reproduction: diagnosis by analysis of DNA fingerprint. *Mol Hum Reprod* 1998; **4**: 877–880.

46. Helmerhorst FM, Perquin DA, Donker D, Keirse MJ. Perinatal outcome of singletons and twins after assisted conception: a systematic review of controlled studies. *BMJ* 2004; **328**: 261–264.

47. Jackson RA, Gibson KA, Wu YW, Croughan MS. Perinatal outcomes in singletons following in vitro fertilization: a meta-analysis. *Obstet Gynecol* 2004; **103**: 551–563.

48. Sutcliffe AG, Ludwig M. Outcome of assisted reproduction. *Lancet* 2007; **370**: 351–359.

49. Hansen M, Bower C, Milne E, de Klerk N, Kurinczuk JJ. Assisted reproductive technologies and the risk of birth defects – a systematic review. *Hum Reprod* 2005; **20**: 328–338.

50. Horsthemke B, Ludwig M. Assisted reproduction: the epigenetic perspective. *Hum Reprod Update* 2005; **11**: 473–482.

51. Ludwig M, Katalinic A, Gross S, et al. Increased prevalence of imprinting defects in patients with Angelman syndrome born to subfertile couples. *J Med Genet* 2005; **42**: 289–291.

52. Sutter PD, Bontinck J, Schutysers V, et al. First-trimester bleeding and pregnancy outcome in singletons after assisted reproduction. *Hum Reprod* 2006; **21**: 1907–1911.

53. Romundstad LB, Romundstad PR, Sunde A, et al. Increased risk of placenta previa in pregnancies following IVF/ICSI; a comparison of ART and non-ART pregnancies in the same mother. *Hum Reprod* 2006; **21**; 2353–2358.

54. Allen C, Bowdin S, Harrison RF, et al. Pregnancy and perinatal outcomes after assisted reproduction: a comparative study. *Ir J Med Sci* 2008; **177**: 233–241.

55. Romundstad LB, Romundstad PR, Sunde A, et al. Effects of technology or maternal factors on perinatal outcome after assisted fertilisation: a population-based cohort study. *Lancet* 2008; **372**: 737–743.

56. Ludwig M. Are adverse outcomes associated with assisted reproduction related to the technology or couples subfertility. *Nat Clin Pract Urol* 2009; **6**: 8–9.

57. Wang YA, Sullivan EA, Black D, et al. Preterm birth and low birth weight after assisted reproductive technology-related pregnancy in Australia between 1996 and 2000. *Fertil Steril* 2005; **83**: 1650–1658.

58. De Geyter C, De Geyter M, Steimann S, Zhang H, Holzgreve W. Comparative birth weights of singletons born after assisted reproduction and natural conception in previously infertile women. *Hum Reprod* 2006; **21**: 705–712.

59. Shih W, Rushford DD, Bourne H, et al. Factors affecting low birth weight after assisted reproduction technology: difference between transfer of fresh and cryopreserved embryos suggests an adverse effect of oocyte collection. *Hum Reprod* 2008; **23**: 1644–1653.

60. Wang JX, Norman RJ, Kristiansson P. The effect of various infertility treatments on the risk of preterm birth. *Hum Reprod* 2002; **17**: 945–949.

61. Lambert RD. Safety issues in assisted reproductive technology: aetiology of health problems in singleton ART babies. *Hum Reprod* 2003; **18**: 1987–1991.

62. Jacques AM, Amor DJ, Baker HWG, et al. Adverse obstetric and perinatal outcomes in subfertile women conceiving without assisted reproductive technologies. *Fertil Steril* 2010; **94**: 2674–2679.

63. Monti F, Agostini F, Fagandini P, La Scala GB, Blickstein I. Depressive symptoms during late pregnancy and early parenthood following assisted reproductive technology. *Fertil Steril* 2009; **91**: 851–857.

64. Van Balen F, Naaktgeboren N, Trimbos-Kemper TCM. In-vitro fertilization: the experience of treatment, pregnancy and delivery. *Hum Reprod* 1996; **11**: 95–98.

65. Boivin J, Takefman JE. Impact of the in-vitro fertilization process on emotional, physical and relational variables. *Hum Reprod* 1996; **11**: 903–907.

66. Colpin H, Soenen S. Parenting and psychological development of IVF children: a follow up study. *Hum Reprod* 2002; **17**: 1116–1123.

67. Pinborg A, Loft A, Schmidt L, Andersen AN. Morbidity in a Danish National cohort of 472 IVF/ICSI twins, 1132 non-IVF/ICSI twins and 634 IVF/ICSI singletons: health-related and social implications for the children and their families. *Hum Reprod* 2003; **18**: 1234–1243.

68. Garel M, Salobir C, Blondel B. Psychological consequences of having triplets: a 4 year follow-up study. *Fertil Steril* 1997; **67**: 1162–1165.

69. Wichman CL, Ehlers SL, Wichman SE, Weaver AL, Coddington C. Comparison of multiple psychological distress measures between men and women preparing for in vitro fertilization. *Fertil Steril* 2011; **95**: 717–721.

70. Ebbesen SM, Zachariae R, Mehlsen MY, et al. Stressful life events are associated with a poor in-vitro fertilization (IVF) outcome: a prospective study. *Hum Reprod* 2009; **24**: 2173–2182.

Chapter 8

Multiple gestation pregnancy after assisted reproductive technology

Eric R. M. Jauniaux

Introduction

With the development of new assisted reproductive techniques (ARTs) in the late 1970s, multiple gestation pregnancy (MGP) rates have increased markedly around the world. If differences in perinatal outcome between spontaneous and ART pregnancies remain the matter of constant debate (see Chapters 6 and 7), all MGPs are associated with a significant increase in perinatal complication rates for both the fetuses and their mothers. Twins are born with an average gestational age three weeks lower than that for spontaneous and ART singletons and with a mean birth weight ranging between 800 and 1000 g lower [1]. These perinatal risks are directly linked to the number of fetuses developing in utero and, overall, perinatal mortality rates are reported to be four-fold higher for twins and six-fold higher for triplets than for singletons [1].

The social, economic, and human costs of MGPs following ART have led to numerous clinical, legal, and political debates, and there is no doubt that MGPs remain the single biggest risk associated with ART. The problems associated with ART twins and higher-order MGPs are mainly due to the perceived need to stimulate excess follicles and transfer excess embryos in order to achieve higher pregnancy rates [1]. In particular, the most frequent measure of success of any one in vitro fertilization (IVF) center has been the number of pregnancies or live births, irrespective of outcomes. The initial data seemed to support the practice of transferring as many embryos as available, with lower pregnancy rates when only one or two embryos were transferred compared to three or more. As a result, in many ART clinics between 35% and 50% of IVF conceptions have been and still are twins, triplets, or higher-order MGPs.

The increase in the number of MGPs is related not only to these historical clinical incentives but also to increasing child-bearing age and the desire from older couples to achieve a pregnancy at all costs [2]. Most IVF patients tend to be aware of the risks associated with triplet and higher-order MGPs; however, many are unaware of twin-associated perinatal risks, particularly cerebral palsy and infant mortality [2]. Furthermore many patients, who recognized the risks of twin pregnancies, remained unconcerned and older patient age remains associated with an increased desire for a twin pregnancy [3]. Knowledge of risks tend to prompt partners toward a preference for a single embryo transfer (SET), but there is less impact on women themselves who tend to want a pregnancy at whatever cost, even if the resulting children had health problems [4]. Responses differ in the U.S. and Europe, which in the U.S. are linked to a more competitive and costly IVF market associated with a desire for higher pregnancy rates. In turn, educational interventions have a greater effect in the U.S., suggesting that knowledge of the risks for both mothers and babies of twin pregnancies was lower than in Europe [3].

As IVF techniques have improved and the risks and consequences of higher-order MGPs are well documented, rules and regulations regarding the number of embryos that can be transferred have progressively been restricted to two in many Europeans countries. However, many IVF centers, in particular in less-regulated countries, continue to promote the transfer of more than two embryos in older women who are often are at higher obstetric risks than younger ones. The evidence has shown that for most infertile couples, costs of treatment are secondary to the overwhelming desire for a child, and that they are also prepared to travel to private ART clinics in less-regulated or unregulated countries if it increases their chances of a pregnancy [5]. In the U.K. where access to public-funded IVF continues to be limited, many

Pregnancy After Assisted Reproductive Technology, ed. Eric R. M. Jauniaux and Botros R. M. B. Rizk. Published by Cambridge University Press.

infertile couples travel abroad [5]. Additional reasons for fertility tourism include cheaper treatments abroad than in the private sector in the U.K., better success rates due to the higher number of embryo transfers overseas, faster speed of treatment, and the availability of an acceptable ethnic oocyte donor. Within this context, fertility tourism often results in higher-order MGPs which, when the couple return to the U.K. for obstetric care, will essentially be managed by the National Health Service.

A decade ago, clinicians in Scandinavian countries began to carry out trials of replacing one rather than two embryos. Finland was the first country to implement this with more than 30% single embryo transfers (SETs) [6]. This has resulted in a twin birth rate reduction from 17.1 in 1998 to 14.9 per 1000 births in 2004. A recent meta-analysis has shown that compared with a double embryo transfer (DET), an elective single transfer increases the chances of delivering a full-term singleton live birth and reduces the risk of MGP and low birth weight (LBW) [7]. Furthermore, this study also confirms that an additional frozen cycle results in live birth rates similar to those with double embryo transfers. As shown in Belgium, when public-funded IVF is offering freezing of good-quality embryos as part of the treatment, this results in more couples accepting SET [8]. This depends on existing funding arrangements, which differ from country to country, but reducing the MGP rates should continue to be a high priority for ART strategies at national and international levels. League tables of ART success should now provide the true measure of success of IVF, which is the number of "births emphasizing a successful singleton at term" or BESST [9] rather than pregnancy rates or any other misleading statistics.

This chapter reviews the consequences of MGPs following ART and the factors that may influence the perinatal risk associated with multiple pregnancies.

Multiple gestation pregnancy outcome: spontaneous versus assisted reproductive techniques

Multiple gestation pregnancies are associated with greater risks for both mothers and their babies than singleton pregnancies, including higher rates of early and late miscarriages, pregnancy-induced hypertension (PIH), prepartum bleeding, postpartum hemorrhage (PPH), and operative delivery for mothers; and of prematurity, intrauterine growth restriction (IUGR), and small for gestational age (SGA), intrauterine death (IUD), and LBW for the babies [1,10]. Overall, MGPs increase the risks for preterm delivery (PTD) by 50%, admission to a neonatal intensive care unit two-fold, and Cesarean delivery by 30% [10,11].

Mothers carrying a MGP are also more likely to present with pregnancy-associated nausea and vomiting, gestational hypertension, PIH, and gestational diabetes than those carrying singletons [1,10,11]. The most serious maternal complication is hypertension, with or without proteinuria. The prognosis is fairly good for PIH with an accompanying substantial rise in plasma volume. Hypertension associated with hemoconcentration and proteinuria has a much worse prognosis. In addition, multiple gestation appears to neutralize the protective effect of parity against the risk of PIH generally found in successive singleton pregnancies [1]. The dilutional anemia associated with pregnancy is often aggravated by the iron deficiency generally accentuated in multiple gestations. The incidence of anemia is doubled in twin pregnancies, increasing the risk of premature labor and the severity of a PPH. Other obstetrical problems include increased operative delivery, uterine rupture, and placenta abruptio, all with consequent prolonged hospitalization. Finally, depression is more common in mothers of multiple births than with singletons [1].

Multiple gestations require more intensive clinical and ultrasonographic monitoring. The frequency of these investigations is largely determined by the number of fetuses and the chorionicity (Figure 8.1). Thus, MGPs impose higher costs on health services from conception to many years after delivery and there are also psychological, medical, social, and financial implications for parents [1,12,13]. Higher-order MGPs resulting from fertility tourism in countries with no regulation regarding ET are an additional and unpredictable burden on the National Health Service [5]. The financial concerns arise mainly from the direct costs of prematurity, neonatal intensive care, drug therapy, imaging, and other diagnostic procedures [1]. Higher costs are also incurred after discharge, due to chronic health problems and developmental disabilities. The hospital costs for each twin or triplet ranges between two and 10 times that of a singleton depending on the type of healthcare available, that is, public versus private, and in particular, the access to private neonatal intensive care for very premature babies [12,13]. The lifetime costs to the healthcare system and community of higher MGPs could be

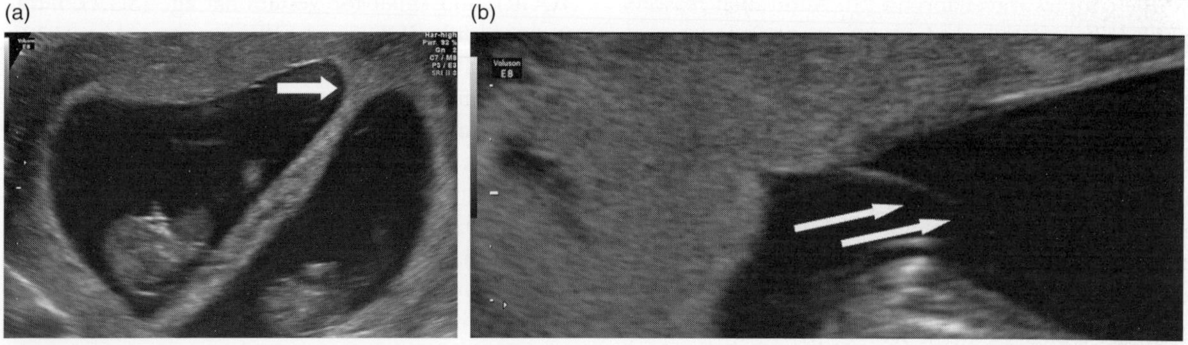

Figure 8.1. Ultrasound images of the inter-twin membrane at 11 weeks of gestation (arrows) showing (a): a dichorionic pregnancy, and (b): a monochorionic pregnancy.

100–200 times that of a singleton. Allowing for inflation of healthcare costs (at 5% per year), the 2000 ESHRE (European Society of Human Reproduction and Embryology) workshop group on MGPs projected costs of delivering MGPs for twins, triplets, and quadruplets of U.S.$ 58 865 USD, 170 282 USD, and 281 698 USD, respectively [1]. These costs emphasize the desire of medical professionals and healthcare providers to reduce MGPs [13].

Many early comparative studies have suggested that there is an increased rate of obstetric complications, PTB, LBW, perinatal mortality, Cesarean delivery, and birth defects for twins conceived by IVF (and IVF/ICSI (intracytoplasmic spermatozoon injection)) compared with spontaneously conceived twins and twins conceived by other ART. However, more recent series showed no significant differences for gestational age at delivery, fetal birth weight, perinatal morbidity and mortality, and rate of malformations [11,14,15]. A recent systematic review and meta-analyses of perinatal outcomes of IVF twins identified 12 case-control studies, including 4385 twins conceived after IVF or IVF/ICSI and 11 793 spontaneous twins, published between 1978 and 2008 [16]. Selecting only those with an appropriate control group of spontaneously conceived twins that matched for maternal age and often other factors, this review has confirmed an increased risk of PTB, LBW (<2500 g), lower mean birth weight, and admission to a neonatal intensive care unit (NICU) in IVF twin pregnancies, but the risks of very LBW (VLBW), extremely LBW, and IUGR are similar. It is likely that the slightly higher incidence of Cesarean sections and NICU admittance in IVF twins is due to more precautions being taken in the highly valued ART twin pregnancies. More recent population-based studies comparing spontaneous with ART twins from different parts of the world have also all concluded that maternal and perinatal outcomes were similar in both groups [14,17]. Overall, IVF/ICSI twins may have a significant but small increased risk of prematurity and LBW than spontaneous twins even after exclusion of monozygotic (MZ) twins. However, in comparison with IVF singletons, they do noticeably worse. This human cost is without any doubt the main argument for single ET, particularly in low-income countries and other countries with limited access to specialist neonatal care.

A number of systematic reviews have shown that birth defects are increased after IVF/ICSI and there has been a particular interest in imprinting syndromes (Chapter 10). Multiple gestation pregnancies are obviously at higher risk of birth defects than singleton ones due to a natural increase in the risk of structural defects and/or aneuploidies associated with the higher number of fetuses present. The vast majority of studies on malformations in IVF twins are based on a limited number of cases with varying definitions of malformations and different or no matching criteria, resulting in a wide range of malformation rates from 25 to 115 per 1000 in IVF twin infants [10]. Taken together, some types of malformations are known to appear at a higher rate in spontaneous twins than in singletons, such as anomalies of the central nervous system and of the gastrointestinal tract. Some of these excess risks have also been found in IVF twins, but the risk increase is moderate and requires a large database to be demonstrated.

A very large registry-based study has produced strong evidence for an increased risk of placenta previa in both singleton and twin IVF pregnancies (18). Similarly, there is an increased incidence of abnormal cord insertion including vasa previa in IVF

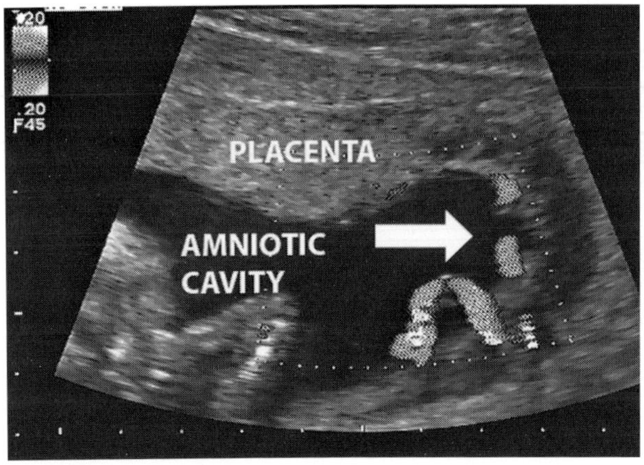

Figure 8.2. Ultrasound view of a singleton in vitro fertilization pregnancy at 15 weeks of gestation showing the velamentous insertion of the umbilical cord into the placental membranes (arrow).

(Figure 8.2) compared to spontaneous twins (19). The mechanical placement of the embryo with interference of the natural rotation of the blastocyst is thought to be related to these findings. The actual incidence of placenta previa is low, approximately 0.2% for spontaneously conceived singleton and twin pregnancies, 1.6% in singleton IVF pregnancies, and 0.8% in twin IVF pregnancies [11]. These numbers are even lower for vasa previa and thus the vast majority of IVF pregnancies will not be affected by placenta previa or vasa previa (Figure 8.2).

There are limited data on the impact of non-IVF-related ART on the outcome of MGPs. The use of gonadotrophins for ovarian induction (OI) is the most important cause of multiple pregnancies in ART patients in the U.S., with one-third of multiple pregnancies being caused by non-IVF ovarian stimulation [20]. Several authors have suggested that LBW in IVF singletons is associated with ovarian stimulation but a more recent study has shown no correlation between OI parameters and birth weight [21]. Overall, studies of twins following IVF and twins after OI have shown no significant difference in outcomes between the two groups [11].

Interpretation of most published reports on long-term outcome in ART twins is constrained by numerous methodological limitations, especially small sample size, ensuring limited statistical power. Many data collections are corrupted by selection bias, in particular by the fact that only a small proportion of the total number of ART births from the selected population appears to have been enrolled at the start of the studies. Additionally, in some studies no or an inadequate comparison group is included, loss to follow-up is high, and the follow-up period is often too short to identify neurodevelopmental sequelae. One of the most important parameters concerning the evaluation of the data on long-term outcome in IVF twins is that the three- to four-fold increased risk of cerebral palsy in spontaneously conceived twins versus singletons is not found when IVF twins are compared with IVF singletons [10]. However, as suggested by Pinborg [10] in her exhaustive review, this may in turn be due to a higher risk of cerebral palsy in IVF singletons.

Vanishing twin after assisted reproductive technology

The disappearance of an entire gestational sac or one of the fetuses after documented fetal heart activity in multiple pregnancies is referred to as the vanishing twin (VT) phenomenon [22]. The incidence of VT is slightly higher than that of clinical miscarriage (30% versus 20%) in first-trimester singleton pregnancies but a VT is likely to have the same pathophysiology and similar etiology; for instance, the association with a chromosomal abnormality [23]. This could explain why the rate of VT after IVF/ICSI is lower, at around 9% [24], as the IVF procedure of embryo selection decreases the risk of transferring morphologically abnormal conceptions. Early implantation crowding, resulting in an unfavorable placentation of one of the gestational sacs, or the consequence of major intra-uterine bleeding with the formation of a large hematoma involving the definitive placenta of one of the gestational sacs have also been proposed as possible etiologies for a VT [25].

The main differential diagnosis of a VT phenomenon if the pregnancy has not be diagnosed as a twin pregnancy earlier in gestation is with a threatened miscarriage presenting with a subchorionic hematoma. This pregnancy complication affects around 10%–15% of early pregnancies and a recent hematoma will appear as a sonolucent space in the free membranes next to the placenta, sometimes mimicking a second sac. A twin pregnancy combining a normal fetus and placenta with a complete hydatidiform mole will also present with vaginal bleeding starting in the first trimester of pregnancy. However, in the case of the VT, the abnormal sac is clearly defined (Figure 8.3) and may contain embryonic remnants, whereas in the subchorionic hematoma it appears as

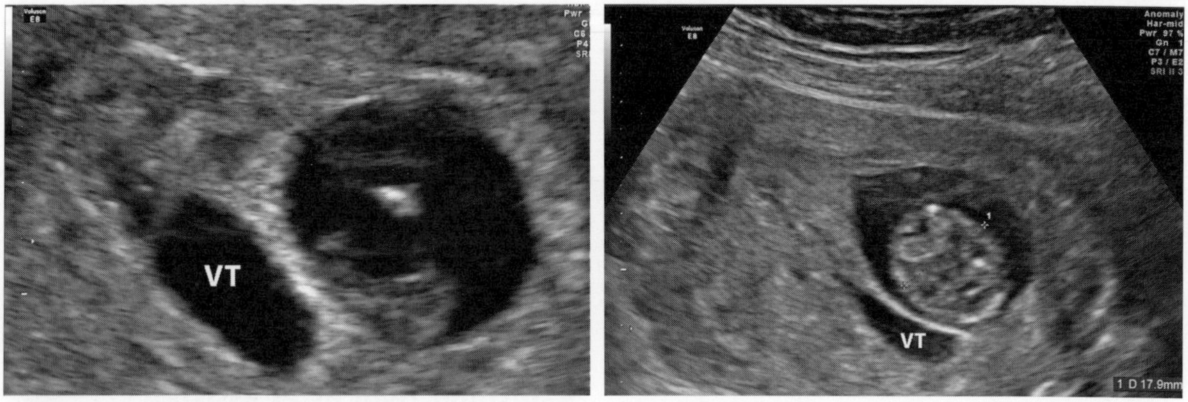

Figure 8.3. Ultrasound views of a vanishing twin (VT) at (a): 11 and (b): 12 weeks of gestation. Note the small gestational sac on the lower left of the normal sac containing a live fetus.

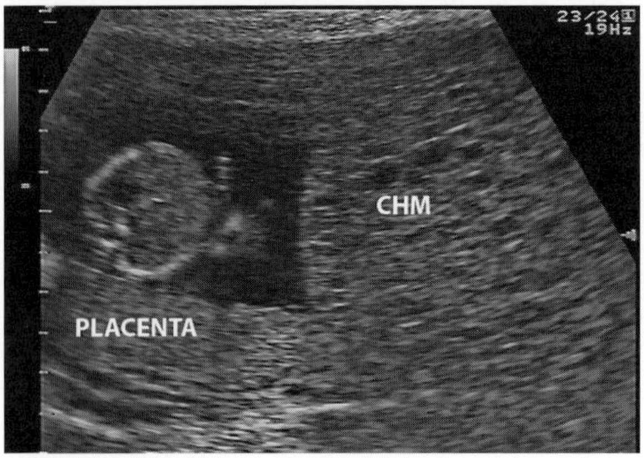

Figure 8.4. Ultrasound view at 14 weeks of a normal gestational sac with a live fetus and normal placenta (left), coexisting with a complete hydatidiform mole (CHM) (right).

a clot displacing the free placental membranes, and a complete mole is a heterogeneous mass often presenting with the typical "snowstorm appearance" (Figure 8.4). By contrast to VT gestational sacs or threatened miscarriages, molar pregnancies are rare findings and even rarer within a MGP. Their association with ART remains difficult to prove due to their extremely rare incidence.

Although the VT phenomenon occurs with a similar incidence in both spontaneous pregnancy and pregnancies conceived using ART, most available data are from ART populations [24,25]. This is due to the fact that ART pregnancies are generally monitored with ultrasound throughout the first trimester when the incidence of VT is at its highest whereas spontaneous MGPs would only be diagnosed during the first trimester in the case of complications such as maternal bleeding.

Compared with uncomplicated control ART pregnancies with the same number of viable fetuses, there is an increase in adverse obstetrical outcomes after the vanishing twin/triplet phenomenon, including PTD, SGA, LBW, and VLBW (<1500 g). The increased risk of PTD and very PTD and of LBW and VLBW has been found comparing VT survivors with uncomplicated singletons [26,27]. This risk seems to be almost entirely due to a VT occurring after eight weeks of gestation, and a large U.S. register study found that the risk of LBW was higher, the higher the number of fetal hearts shown on early ultrasonography for both singletons and twins [28]. By contrast, the VT phenomenon in triplet pregnancies increases the live birth rate and decreases the risk of preterm delivery [24,29].

In recent large studies, no association has been found between a VT phenomenon and an increased risk of preeclampsia (PE), placenta previa, and placental abruption, but an increased risk of SGA has been observed in comparison with singletons from a single gestation [30], and the risk increases with increasing gestational age at the time of the start of the VT. No difference has been found in the incidence of congenital malformations and perinatal death [25].

The knowledge about the risk of long-term consequences for the singleton survivor of a vanished co-twin is limited. The Danish multicenter [10] survey revealed a nearly two-fold increased risk of cerebral palsy in singleton survivors of a vanished co-twin, but because of the limited sample size, it did not reach statistical significance. However, a significant correlation between the gestational age at onset of VT and the risk of development of neurological sequelae has been reported. One of the major causes for the slightly adverse obstetric outcome in IVF/ICSI singletons is the higher rate of singletons from VT gestations, which is another argument for single ET [10].

Multiple gestation pregnancy and advanced maternal age

Advanced maternal age has traditionally been defined as an age of more than 35 years at delivery and it has been associated with increased obstetric morbidity and interventions. The average age at delivery increased between the late 1970s and mid-1990s: from 26 to 29 years old in Denmark, France, Finland, and Sweden and to 30 years in the Netherlands [10]. This trend has resulted in a progressive shift of deliveries to the 30–39 year age group and around a quarter of twin birth rates is now attributable to the reproductively aging women.

As a result of ART using oocyte donation, menopausal women are now able to become pregnant in their 50s and 60s. Between 1977 and 1998, the number of women giving birth at 35–39, 40–44, and >45 years increased by around 10, 9, and 50 times, respectively [31]. Independently of maternal age, oocyte donation could increase the risks of PE and premature labor (see Chapters 6 and 11). Older patient age is naturally associated with an increased incidence of chronic diseases like arthritis, hypertension, and diabetes. However, as for ART singleton pregnancies, most studies have demonstrated similar age- and parity-adjusted risk of PIH and gestational diabetes in IVF and control twin pregnancies [10]. Overall, maternal age seems to have little impact on the rate of obstetric complications in women in their fourth decade of life; however, women aged 50 years or more, are at increased risk of PE and gestational diabetes, and the vast majority of them can expect to deliver via Cesarean section [31–35].

As a result of ART, the twin birth rate to women aged 40–44 years old nearly doubled between 1990 and 2001 and that of triplets increased four-fold in women aged ≥35 years old between 1975 and 1998 [36,37]. The epidemiological study of the obstetric outcome of twin pregnancy in older mothers has generated conflicting results. Some authors have found no difference in the rate of PE, premature delivery, LBW, and neonatal asphyxia rates in nulliparas of ≥35 years of age with a dichorionic twin pregnancy compared to younger women [38–40]. By contrast, others have reported a higher rate of VLBW [41] and PE [42] in women aged ≥35 years old. Some authors have reported that the mean gestational age at delivery, mean individual birth weight, mean total birth weight, and neonatal death rates were more favorable in older mothers carrying twins [43] and that women >40 years of age carrying triplets had a lower incidence of PTD [44].There is also no universally accepted explanation for the better outcome of triplet pregnancy in the older gravida. One possible explanation is that prior pregnancies with organ growth, cell proliferation, hypertrophy, apoptosis, differentiation, matrix synthesis, and remodeling influence later outcomes [37]. Better socioeconomical status and thus financial resources available may also provide an explanation for the more favorable outcome of higher-order MGPs in older women.

However, these epidemiological studies rarely provide information on confounders such as socioeconomical status and type of ART used. Furthermore, there is limited information on the long-term impact of coping with a multiple pregnancy and young children in older versus younger women.

Zygocity and chorionicity after assisted reproductive technology

Multiple gestation pregnancies arise more frequently from the fertilization of two (dizygotic) or more separate oocytes than from a single fertilized oocyte that subsequently divides before day 8 of gestation into two embryonic structures forming a monozygotic (MZ) twin pregnancy. Dizygotic (DZ) twins are always dichorionic (DC)/diamniotic (DA), whereas MZ twins are mainly (>75%) monochorionic (MC)/DA, sometimes DC/DA, and rarely (<1%) MC/monoamniotic (MA). Apart from exceptionally rare cases, MC twins are MZ. Overall, MZ twin pregnancies in Caucasians account for 30% of all naturally conceived twins or 0.3%–05% of all pregnancies. This universally low incidence of MZ twinning is constant worldwide and independent of environmental factors, suggesting a genetic contribution [45].

Monozygotic twin pregnancies are of concern due to a higher rate of associated perinatal complications compared to DC twins. In particular, MC twins have a 15%–20% risk of twin–twin transfusion syndrome (TTTS) and MA/MC twins are at additional risk of cord accident due to cord entanglement. Almost all MC twins have vascular anastomoses and these are the

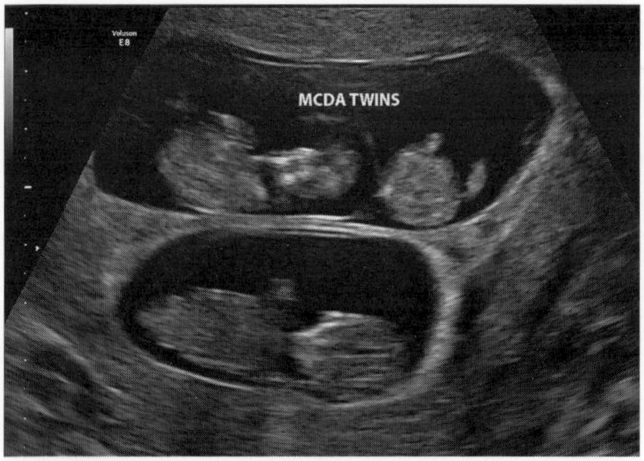

Figure 8.5. In vitro fertilization/intracytoplasmic spermatozoon injection triplet pregnancy resulting from two embryo transfers at 11 weeks of gestation, showing a monochorionic, diamniotic (MCDA) twin pair (above) and a singleton fetus (below).

pathophysiological basis of the TTTS, which if untreated is associated with a 90% fetal mortality [46]. Apart from some defects that may result from intrauterine crowding including foot deformities, dislocation of the hip, and skull asymmetry, MC twins also have a two- to three-fold higher incidence of structural anomalies such as congenital heart defects compared to spontaneously conceived DZ twins. Overall, MC twin pregnancies are associated with a three-fold increase in perinatal mortality and a 10-fold increase in prenatally acquired neurological lesions. In the case of an MC twin pair included in a triplet pregnancy (Figure 8.5), the incidence of neurological sequelae could be as high as 40–100 times those found in a singleton pregnancy population.

Although the great majority of ART twinning result in a DZ twin pregnancy, the rate of MZ twinning after ART has been the topic of a lot of debate. Monozygotic twin pregnancies were first reported to occur at a significantly higher rate following ART and in particular after ICSI [45,47]. All three configurations of MZ placentation have been observed following ART, suggesting that MZ twinning occurs at various times during embryo development and by a variety of mechanisms [45]. Ovarian stimulation, zona pelucida manipulation including intracytoplasmic spermatozoon injection (ICSI), and assisted hatching (AH), maternal age, and factors associated with in vitro embryo culture may contribute to the division of the fertilized oocyte.

Studies from the 1970s and 1980s have reported MZ twinning rates following ART procedures between two and 12 times higher than the natural occurrence of around 0.4% [10,45]. In the more recent Danish twin birth cohort between 1995 and 2000, the rate of MZ twinning was estimated to be 1.6% in IVF twins versus 31% in controls by using Weinberg's differential method based on the number of opposite-gender twin-sets [48]. This low rate of MZ after IVF compared to older studies may be due to the fact that assisted hatching and blastocyst culture are rarely performed in Denmark [10]. By dividing the MZ rate with the mean number of embryos transferred, Sills and co-workers [49] reached a result very close to the background MZ rate and they found no increased MZ rate by AH and ICSI, suggesting that the higher MZ rate in IVF can primarily be explained by the increased number of implantations due to multiple ET. Thus, the lower average number of ET in Scandinavia compared to most other European countries and North America can also explain the lower MZ rate found in the Danish study compared with previous reports.

Studies published in the last decade have confirmed that women undergoing ovarian stimulation delivered MZ twins at nearly twice the rate of controls [50] and that a higher proportion of twins conceived following ovarian stimulation with clomiphene citrate were MZ compared with iatrogenic cases where no clomiphene citrate was used [51]. Finally, maternal age may contribute to an increased incidence of MZ twins, but the contribution is likely to be minimal in ART cases [10].

Elective multiple pregnancy reduction after assisted reproductive technology

Elective reduction or "multifetal pregnancy reduction" (MFPR) is the invasive procedure performed because of an excess number of fetuses in utero to maximize the chances of a delivery of at least one healthy child. Selective termination is the reduction of a fetus in a multiple gestation due to an abnormality detected in that fetus [5,10]. The procedure is now performed under continuous ultrasound control at around 11 weeks of gestation by injecting into the chest of each fetus 1–2 mL of potassium chloride (KCl) [52–54]. The fetuses selected for reduction are preferably those located in the upper part of the uterus for technical reasons or those presenting with an increased nuchal translucency or any other ultrasonographic markers of risk of aneuploidy. Some authors advocate karyotyping by chorionic villous sampling (CVS) prior to MFPR [52], but this requires an additional procedure and thus increases the risk of post-procedure loss. As most IVF couples opt against an invasive procedure for fetal karyotyping [55] and the screening for fetal aneuploidy using the 11–14 week scan is efficient in MGPs [56], many fetal medicine units propose a nuchal translucency scan at 11–14 weeks and amniocentesis at 15–17 weeks or later based on the results of a mid-pregnancy detailed fetal anatomy ultrasound examination.

Multifetal pregnancy reduction and selective termination for an abnormal fetus in a DC twin pregnancy have been used for about 30 years, and in experienced hands appears to be safe and effective. The spontaneous pregnancy loss rate in twin pregnancies is 7% but exceeds 12% when the pregnancy started with three or more fetuses [10]. Overall, the post-procedure loss rate after first-trimester reduction by means of intracardiac/thoracic KCl injection ranges between 4% and 7% [52–54]. The risk of miscarriage seems to be associated with the final number of fetuses (4.5% for triplets, 8% for quadruplets, and 11% for quintuplets), but for triplets the decrease in pregnancy loss risk for 3 to 1 reduction is not as much as 3 to 2 [52]. The lowest pregnancy loss rates are for those cases reduced from triplets, or more, to twins. The data from the most recent collaborative series indicate substantial improvement of reduced twins as compared to triplets and suggest that for cases starting as triplets or quadruplets reduced to twins do as well as pregnancies starting as twins [52–54]

The demographics of multiple pregnancy patients having evolved over the past two decades, with increasing proportions resulting from ART, the number of triplets resulting from two ETs, one of which splits, resulting in a pair of MC twins and a singleton has also increased. In particular, in the U.K. the introduction of a limit in the number of ETs to two in IVF/ICSI has increased the relative number of triplet pregnancies, including a singleton and an MZ twin pair referred to a specialist fetal medicine unit offering elective reduction [5]. A recent study has shown that reduction of the monochorionic pair in IVF triplet pregnancies conferred a significantly greater likelihood of delivery at ≥34 weeks and an average gestational length that was 52 days longer compared with triplet pregnancies in which the monochorionic pair was not reduced [57].

Accurate determination of chorionicity (Figure 8.1) is pivotal before performing an MFPR, as the techniques involving percutaneous injections can only be performed safely in DC or trichorionic MGPs. In MC twins any substance given to one twin will enter the circulation of the other via the placental anastomoses. Multiple other methods of interrupting the affected twin's circulation have been attempted with variable success, including cord ligation, cord coagulation, or laser cord occlusion. Recent advances in vascular-occlusive techniques have allowed the possibility of selective termination in monochorionic pregnancies in the presence of discordant anomalies or, indeed, multifetal reduction in non-trichorionic triplets, with radiofrequency ablation appearing to be the most successful [58,59]. However, the techniques vary in complexity and complication rates, which increase with gestation.

Conclusion

Having more than one child per birth, whether resulting from the use of ART or not, increases psychosocial risks for the parents [60]. Iatrogenic twinning and higher-order MGPs have become the main side effect of ART. The considerable higher risk of adverse obstetric outcome in IVF twins than in singletons and the 20-fold higher ART twin birth rate is still one, if not the most serious, adverse effect of ART. A recent U.S. study has shown that the financial burden of ART-associated preterm deliveries is estimated to be approximately US$ 1 billion annually [61]. This figure has remained essentially unchanged between 2001 and 2006, despite the decreasing number of embryos transferred, due to the increasing total number of ART cycles performed. Although the data of the case-control and cohort studies comparing the obstetric outcome of ART with spontaneous MGPs remain controversial, there is no doubt that MGPs are high-risk pregnancies from a clinical, social, and financial point of view. This point is particularly important for low-income countries where there is very limited or no access to specialist obstetrics and neonatal care.

Maternal age at first pregnancy has become a new clinical parameter of modern obstetrics. Maternal age is known to influence perinatal outcomes but to a lesser extent than the number of fetuses and zygosity of the MGPs. Other new parameters have also made their entry in obstetric risk evaluation, such as maternal obesity, making many previous epidemiological studies on ART MGPs obsolete. Maternal age has usually been adjusted for in many studies, as has parity, but it is still difficult in most series of ART pregnancies to find accurate information on other clinically important confounders such as underlying cause of infertility and smoking status. In addition for MGPs, authors still rarely provide details on chorionicity, which is the single most important factor with a direct impact on obstetric outcome and in particular on birth weight, prematurity, and mode of delivery. Less obvious confounders such as previous obstetric outcome, socioeconomic status, incidence of VT or MFPR are also rarely available in most epidemiological studies. It is also unknown whether some IVF technologies or the etiology of the infertility may contribute to specific abnormalities such as conjoined twins [62] or long-term adverse outcomes in childhood (see Chapter 9). Future epidemiological studies will only yield valuable information if they include as many of these new and old confounders as possible in their analyses.

Once the MGP is established and has reached the end of the third month, elective MFPR involves extremely difficult decisions for infertile couples and should only be used as a last resort. For many people, any deliberate termination of a fetus is inherently controversial and abortion laws vary among countries with Ireland and Poland, and the majority of countries outside Europe, and North America having strict laws against any form of abortion except sometimes in the case of life-threatening maternal medical conditions. The clinical evidence in favor of MFPR in pregnancies with more than four fetuses to twins is undisputed. Despite the recent improvements in expectant management of triplets with reasonable perinatal outcomes, the evidence suggests that reduction to twins significantly reduces the risk of preterm delivery without an increase in miscarriage rates. Despite the fact that for all MGPs, including twins, reduction to a lower number of fetuses reduces fetal losses, prematurity, and maternal and infant mortality and morbidity, the ethical debate around MFPR is likely to remain complex for many decades to come (see Chapter 15). What is certain is that MFPR should not continue to be an alternative for single ET.

Assisted reproductive technology centers should include the previously discussed information with the obstetric and neonatal risks, stressing the advantages of having one child per birth. Within this context, public-funded IVF, including single ET and freezing of good-quality embryos as part of the treatment, should be the way forward [3,4,6–9,63,64].

References

1. The ESHRE Capri Workshop Group. Multiple gestation pregnancy. *Hum Reprod* 2000; **15**: 1856–1864.
2. Ryan GL, Zhang SH, Dokras A, Syrop CH, Van Voorhis BJ. The desire of infertile patients for multiple births. *Fertil Steril* 2004; **81**: 500–503.
3. Leese B, Denton J. Attitudes towards single embryo transfer, twin and higher order pregnancies in patients undergoing infertility treatment: a review. *Hum Fertil* 2010; **13**: 28–34.
4. Scotland GS, McNamee P, Peddie VL, Bhattacharya S. Safety versus success in elective single embryo transfer: women's preferences for outcomes of in vitro fertilisation. *BJOG* 2007; **114**: 977–983.
5. McKelvey A, David A, Shenfield F, Jauniaux ER. The impact of cross-border reproductive care or 'fertility tourism' on NHS maternity services. *BJOG* 2009; **116**: 1520–1523.
6. Martikainen H, Titinen A, Thomas C, et al. One versus two embryo transfer after IVF and ICSI: a randomized study. *Hum Reprod* 2001; **16**: 1900–1903.
7. McLemon DJ, Hamid K, Bergh C, et al. Clinical effectiveness of single versus double embryo transfer: meta-analysis of individual patient data from randomised trials. *BMJ* 2011; **345**: c6945.
8. Gerris J. The near elimination of triplets in IVF. *Reprod Biomed Online* 2007; **15**: 40–44.
9. Min JK, Breheny SA, MacLachlan V, Healy DL. What is the most relevant standard of success in assisted reproduction? The singleton, term gestation, live birth rate per cycle initiated: the BESST endpoint for assisted reproduction. *Hum Reprod* 2004; **19**: 3–7.
10. Pinborg A. IVF/ICSI twin pregnancies: risks and prevention. *Hum Reprod Update* 2005; **11**: 575–593.
11. Halliday J. Outcomes of IVF conceptions: are they different? *Best Pract Res Clin Obstet Gynaecol* 2007; **21**: 67–81.
12. Ledger WL, Anumba D, Marlow N, Thomas CM, Wilson EC. The costs to the NHS of multiple births after IVF treatment in the UK. *BJOG* 2006; **113**: 21–25.
13. Chambers GM, Chapman MG, Grayson N, Shanahan M, Sullivan EA. Babies born after ART treatment cost more than non-ART babies: a cost analysis of inpatient birth-admission costs of singleton and multiple gestation pregnancies. *Hum Reprod* 2007; **22**: 3108–3115.
14. Vasario E, Borgarello V, Bossotti C, et al. IVF twins have similar obstetric and neonatal outcome as spontaneously conceived twins: a prospective follow-up study. *Reprod Biomed Online* 2010; **21**: 422–428.

15. Murphy MF, Neale RE, Hey K, et al. Pregnancy outcome among twins conceived after subfertility treatment compared with natural twins: a population-based study. *Twin Res Hum Genet* 2006; **9**: 279–284.

16. McDonald S, Han Z, Mulla S, et al. Preterm birth, and low birth weight among in vitro fertilization twins: a systematic review and meta-analyses. *Eur J Obstet Gynecol Reprod Biol* 2010; **148**: 105–113.

17. Boulet SL, Schieve LA, Nannini A, et al. Perinatal outcomes of twin births conceived using assisted reproduction technology: a population-based study. *Hum Reprod* 2008; **23**: 1941–1948.

18. Romundstad LB, Romundstad PR, Sunde A, et al. Increased risk of placenta previa in pregnancies following IVF/ICSI; a comparison of ART and non-ART pregnancies in the same mother. *Hum Reprod* 2006; **21**: 2353–2358.

19. Gavriil P, Jauniaux E, Leroy F. Pathologic examination of placentas from singleton and twin pregnancies obtained after in vitro fertilization and embryo transfer. *Pediatr Path* 1993; **13**: 453–462.

20. Ombelet W, Martens G, De Sutter P, et al. Perinatal outcome of 12,021 singleton and 3108 twin births after non-IVF-assisted reproduction: a cohort study. *Hum Reprod* 2006; **21**: 1025–1032.

21. Griesinger G, Kolibianakis EM, Diedrich K, Ludwig M. Ovarian stimulation for IVF has no quantitative association with birthweight: a registry study. *Hum Reprod* 2008; **23**: 2549–2554.

22. Jauniaux E, Elkhazen N, Leroy F, et al. Clinical and morphologic aspects of the vanishing twin phenomenon. *Obstet Gynecol* 1988; **72**: 577–581.

23. Greenwold N, Jauniaux E. Collection of villous tissue under ultrasound guidance to improve the cytogenetic study of early pregnancy failure. *Hum Reprod* 2002; **17**: 452–456.

24. Barton SE, Missmer SA, Hornstein MD. Twin pregnancies with a 'vanished' embryo: a higher risk multiple gestation group? *Hum Reprod* 2011; **26**: 2750–2753.

25. Jauniaux E, Van Oppenraaij RH, Burton GJ. Obstetric outcome after early placental complications. *Curr Opin Obstet Gynecol* 2010; **22**: 452–457.

26. Pinborg A, Lidegaard O, Freiesleben NC, Andersen AN. Consequences of vanishing twins in IVF/ICSI pregnancies. *Hum Reprod* 2005; **20**: 2821–2829.

27. Shebl O, Ebner T, Sommergruber M, Sir A, Tews G. Birth weight is lower for survivors of the vanishing twin syndrome: a case-control study. *Fertil Steril* 2008; **90**: 310–314.

28. Schieve LA, Meikle SF, Ferre C, et al. Low and very low birth weight in infants conceived with use of assisted reproductive technology. *N Engl J Med* 2002; **346**: 731–737.

29. Skiadas CC, Missmer SA, Benson CB, Acker D, Racowsky C. Spontaneous reduction before 12 weeks' gestation and selective reduction similarly extend time to delivery in in vitro fertilization of trichorionic-triamniotic triplets. *Fertil Steril* 2010; **95**: 596–599.

30. Pinborg A, Lidegaard O, Freiesleben NC, Andersen AN. Vanishing twins: a predictor of small-for-gestational age in IVF singletons. *Hum Reprod* 2007; **22**: 2707–2714.

31. Usta IM, Nassar AH. Advanced maternal age. Part I: obstetric complications. *Am J Perinatol* 2008; **25**: 521–534.

32. Paulson RJ, Boostanfar R, Saadat P, et al. Pregnancy in the sixth decade of life: obstetric outcomes in women of advanced reproductive age. *JAMA* 2002; **288**: 2320–2323.

33. Chibber R. Child-bearing beyond age 50: pregnancy outcome in 59 cases "a concern"? *Arch Gynecol Obstet* 2005; **271**: 189–194.

34. Montan S. Increased risk in the elderly parturient. *Curr Opin Obstet Gynecol* 2007; **19**: 110–112.

35. Franz MB, Husslein PW. Obstetrical management of the older gravida. *Womens Health (Lond Engl)* 2010; **6**: 463–468.

36. Martin JA, Hamilton BE, Ventura SJ, et al. Births: final data for 2001. *Natl Vital Stat Rep* 2002; **51**: 1–102.

37. Oleszczuk JJ, Keith LG, Oleszczuk AK. The paradox of old maternal age in multiple pregnancies. *Obstet Gynecol Clin North Am* 2005; **32**: 69–80.

38. Suzuki S. Obstetric outcomes in nulliparous women aged 35 and over with dichorionic twin pregnancy. *Arch Gynecol Obstet* 2007; **276**: 573–575.

39. Zhang J, Meikle S, Grainger DA, Trumble A. Multifetal pregnancy in older women and perinatal outcomes. *Fertil Steril* 2002; **78**: 562–568.

40. Suzuki S, Mikaye H. Perinatal outcomes of elderly primiparous dichorionic twin pregnancies conceived by in vitro fertilization compared with those conceived spontaneously. *Arch Gynecol Obstet* 2010; **281**: 87–90.

41. Prapas N, Kalogiannidis I, Prapas I, et al. Twin gestation in older women: antepartum, intrapartum complications, and perinatal outcomes. *Arch Gynecol Obstet* 2006; **273**: 293–297.

42. Haydon M, Gaffaney CL, Saul L, et al. Twin pregnancies in women greater than 40 years of age: could advanced age improve obstetric outcome? *Am J Obstet Gynecol* 2006; **195**: S108.

43. Martin J, Curtin S, Saulnier M, Mousavi J. Development of the matched multiple birth file. In:

1995–1997 Matched Multiple Birth Dataset. NCHS CD-ROM series 21, no. 12. National Center for Health Statistics Hyattsville, MD, 2000.

44. Keith LG, Goldman RD, Breborowicz G, Blickstein I. Triplet pregnancies in the mothers age 40 or older: a matched control study. *J Reprod Med* 2004; **49**: 683–688.
45. Aston KI, Peterson CM, Carrell DT. Monozygotic twinning associated with assisted reproductive technologies: a review. *Reproduction* 2008; **136**: 377–386.
46. Huber A, Hecher K. How can we diagnose and manage twin-twin transfusion syndrome. *Best Pract Res Clin Obstet Gynecol* 2004; **18**: 543–556.
47. Schachter M, Raziel A, Friedler S, et al. Monozygotic twinning after assisted reproductive techniques: a phenomenon independent of micromanipulation. *Hum Reprod* 2001; **16**: 1264–1269.
48. Pinborg A, Loft A, Rasmussen S, et al. Neonatal outcome in a Danish national cohort of 3438 IVF/ICSI and 10362 non-IVF/ICSI twins born in 1995–2000. *Hum Reprod* 2004; **19**: 435–441.
49. Sills ES, Moomjy M, Zaninovic N, et al. Human zona pellucida micromanipulation and monozygotic twinning frequency after IVF. *Hum Reprod* 2000; **15**: 890–895.
50. Kallen B, Olausson PO, Nygren KG. Neonatal outcome in pregnancies from ovarian stimulation. *Obstet Gynecol* 2002; **100**: 414–419.
51. Derom C, Leroy F, Vlietinck R, Fryns JP, Derom R. High frequency of iatrogenic monozygotic twins with administration of clomiphene citrate and a change in chorionicity. *Fertil Steril* 2006; **85**: 755–757.
52. Evans MI, Ciorica D, Britt DW, Fletcher JC. Update on selective reduction. *Prenat Diagn* 2005; **25**: 807–813.
53. Antsaklis A, Anastasakis E. Selective reduction in twins and multiple pregnancies. *J Perinat Med* 2011; **39**: 15–21.
54. Wimalasundera RC. Selective reduction and termination of multiple pregnancies. *Semin Fetal Neonatal Med* 2010; **15**: 327–335.
55. Holmes A, Jauniaux E. Parental choice for aneuploidy screening in assisted conception versus spontaneously conceived twins. *Reprod Biomed Online* 2004; **8**: 243–245.
56. Maymon R, Jauniaux E, Holmes A, et al. Nuchal translucency measurement and pregnancies outcomes after assisted conception versus spontaneously conceived twins. *Hum Reprod* 2001; **16**: 1999–2004.
57. Skiadas CC, Missmer SA, Benson CB, Acker D, Racowsky C. Impact of selective reduction of the monochorionic pair in in vitro fertilization triplet pregnancies on gestational length. *Fertil Steril* 2010; **94**: 2930–2931.
58. Moise KJ Jr, Johnson A, Moise KY, Nickeleit V. Radiofrequency ablation for selective reduction in the complicated monochorionic gestation. *Am J Obstet Gynecol* 2008; **198**: 198.e1–5.
59. Paramasivam G, Wimalasundera R, Wiechec M, et al. Radiofrequency ablation for selective reduction in complex monochorionic pregnancies. *BJOG* 2010; **117**: 1294–1298.
60. Roca-de Bes M, Gutierrez-Maldonado J, Gris-Martínez JM. Comparative study of the psychosocial risks associated with families with multiple births resulting from assisted reproductive technology (ART) and without ART. *Fertil Steril* 2011; **96**: 170–174.
61. Bromer JG, Ata B, Seli M, Lockwood CJ, Seli E. Preterm deliveries that result from multiple pregnancies associated with assisted reproductive technologies in the USA: a cost analysis. *Curr Opin Obstet Gynecol* 2011; **23**: 168–173.
62. Mercan R, Oktem O, Salar Z, et al. Conjoined twins after intracytoplasmic sperm injection and transfer of day-3 embryos. *Fertil Steril* 2011; **96**: e 111–114.
63. Khalaf Y, Bewley S, Braude P. Reducing multiple pregnancies after assisted reproduction treatment: Québec says 'Yes, we can!' *Reprod Biomed Online* 2011; **23**: 407–410.
64. Roberts SA, McGowan L, Mark Hirst W, et al. Reducing the incidence of twins from IVF treatments: predictive modelling from a retrospective cohort. *Hum Reprod* 2011; **26**: 569–575.

Chapter 9

Pregnancy after intracytoplasmic spermatozoon injection

Willem Verpoest and Paul Devroey

Introduction

Intracytoplasmic spermatozoon injection (ICSI) has been the subject of ongoing debate about its indications and safety ever since its introduction in clinical practice nearly 20 years ago [1]. Intracytoplasmic spermatozoon injection is, at this moment, still the most powerful tool available to treat severe male infertility. Its most important advantage is that it offers couples with severe male factor infertility the possibility to produce offspring with their own gametes. This includes cases of severe (1–5 million/mL) and extreme (<1 million/mL) oligospermia and of obstructive azoospermia or non-obstructive azoospermia, in which spermatozoa can be retrieved by microsurgical epididymal spermatozoon aspiration (MESA), percutaneous epididymal spermatozoon aspiration (PESA), testicular epididymal spermatozoon extraction (TESE), or testicular epididymal spermatozoon aspiration (TESA), depending on the indications [2–4].

An additional advantage of ICSI is that fertilization failure only occurs in less than 3% of treatment cycles [5], which allows the clinician to proceed to ICSI in cases of multiple failures of classical in vitro fertilization (IVF) and poor fertilization rate. Many external and often uncontrollable factors such as spermatozoon morphology, spermatozoon motility, or the presence of reactive oxygen species do not seem to have any major impact on the outcome of ICSI. These external factors may interfere with classical IVF and therefore lead to fertilization failure, which can be avoided by applying ICSI.

Other indications for the use of ICSI include the presence of a high concentration of anti-spermatozoon antibodies, cancer patients in remission where spermatozoa were cryopreserved prior to chemo- and radiotherapy, patients with ejaculatory dysfunction, patients with retrograde ejaculation, and patients where semen was banked prior to vasectomy [6]. Intracytoplasmic spermatozoon injection is also indicated when preimplantation genetic diagnosis (PGD) for monogenic diseases is applied, in order to avoid spermatozoon presence on the outside of the zona pellucida of the embryo at the cleavage stage, which may lead to DNA contamination. Intracytoplasmic spermatozoon injection is often applied in PGD with the aim of increasing the fertilization rate, especially in male factor infertility. However, ICSI is not considered necessary for preimplantation aneuploidy screening (PGS), but is sometimes applied because of male factor infertility and/or to maximize fertilization rates [7].

Of all assisted reproductive technology (ART) treatments recorded, 63% is performed by ICSI, and the proportion of ICSI versus standard IVF is continuing to increase [8,9]. A similar development is observed in the U.S. [10] with the proportion of ICSI increasing from 11.0% in 1995 to 57.5% in 2004, despite the fact that male factor infertility as an indication did not increase significantly. Many theoretical concerns related to the use of ICSI have been raised, including issues related to technical, biological, and genetic hazards. Breaching the oocyte membrane by the injection pipette potentially causes damage to the spindle apparatus of the oocyte, while the use of poor-quality spermatozoa is thought to induce developmental and genetic abnormalities in the offspring. Concerns about potential risks of ICSI do not concern only the technique as such, but also the influence on genetic and epigenetic mechanisms, which may lead to a higher prevalence of chromosomal anomalies, congenital abnormalities, developmental abnormalities, and obstetric complications [11].

Pregnancy After Assisted Reproductive Technology, ed. Eric R. M. Jauniaux and Botros R. M. B. Rizk. Published by Cambridge University Press.

This chapter addresses the most important issues concerning pregnancy after ICSI.

Procedure-related risks in pregnancy after intracytoplasmic spermatozoon injection

The piercing of the oocyte membrane by the injection pipette may cause damage to the second meiotic (metaphase II) spindle apparatus [12]. Studies in the hamster [13] and a primate model [14] have demonstrated that despite correct positioning of the first polar body at right angles to the site of injection, spindle damage is possible because the localization of the first polar body does not indicate the exact localization of the spindle. These findings were confirmed in human oocytes. Polarized microscopy should resolve this problem by locating the position of the birefringent spindle [15]. Misalignment between the meiotic spindle and the first polar body has been shown to be associated with an increased risk of fertilization abnormalities, more specifically a high proportion of tripronucleated zygotes and failure to extrude the second polar body, although the cleavage potential of normally fertilized embryos was not impaired [16].

Physical and biochemical disturbances and dislocation of the ooplasm during spermatozoon injection or disturbance of the meiotic spindle may occur secondary to the ICSI procedure. This may lead to aneuploidy and an increased risk of chromosomal anomalies due to mechanical disturbance, or errors in the second meiotic division or in mitosis during early cleavage divisions. There is conflicting evidence on this issue. One study found the chromosome breakage rate in uncleaved oocytes after failed ICSI to be higher than after failed conventional in vitro fertilization [17,18]. Another study comparing chromosome breakage rate after failed ICSI or IVF found a higher breakage rate after conventional IVF than after ICSI [19].

An equally important concern is the introduction of contaminating foreign material into the oocyte's cytoplasm; for example, polyvinylpyrrolidone that may contain endotoxins. Although clear evidence is not available to support this risk, this product has been withdrawn from the market by its manufacturer and replaced by products controlled for endotoxin contamination. Semen may potentially be contaminated with microbiological organisms, which may therefore be introduced into the oocyte. On the basis of the current literature, this hazard is assumed to be minimal or nonexistent for bacteria [20], but the issue is less clear for viruses (e.g., human papilloma virus [21]). Theoretically, prions may be introduced during an ICSI procedure [22]. One experiment proved the possibility of integrating foreign DNA by ICSI in mice, producing transgenic offspring, but the reproducibility of the technique was debatable [23]. More recently, foreign DNA was successfully integrated into non-human primate oocytes during ICSI; however, this did not produce transgenic offspring [24]. Finally, ICSI induces changes in the Ca^{2+}- induced transients, demonstrating clear differences in the synchrony of fertilization events in ICSI compared with IVF [25].

Procedure-unrelated risks in pregnancy after intracytoplasmic spermatozoon injection

Perinatal risks

The miscarriage rate in pregnancies after ICSI (17.6%) does not appear to be increased compared with IVF pregnancies (16.7%) [26]. An analysis of 424 consecutive single ICSI pregnancies showed a prematurity rate of 7.6%, a low birth weight (LBW) rate of 10.3%, and a perinatal mortality rate of 13.5/1000 [27,28]. These rates are similar to a comparable IVF population, and slightly higher than those for spontaneous pregnancies when controlled for multiple pregnancies. A large population-based retrospective analysis in the U.S. estimated the relative risk (RR) of LBW after ICSI at 2.6 (95% CI: 2.4–2.7) for singletons, while the perinatal mortality rate was estimated at 13.2/1000 [29]. This increased risk of LBW, remarkably, was not increased further for multiple births, and did not differ between ICSI and IVF populations. A systematic review by Helmerhorst et al. confirmed these findings, adding that the RR of other outcome factors such as very preterm birth (<32 weeks), preterm birth (<37 weeks), small for gestational age (SGA) rate, Cesarean section rate, and admission to a neonatal care unit were increased significantly in matched studies of ART children. The perinatal outcome is not significantly worse in ART multiple pregnancies when matched with non-ART controls, but morbidity remains higher in multiple pregnancies [30].

The adverse outcome of some pregnancies resulting from ART is largely attributable to a persistently high multiple pregnancy rate, not exclusively as a result of IVF/ICSI, and more likely as a result of ovulation induction. The multiple pregnancy rate after IVF is 29% for twin pregnancies and 3.7% for triplet pregnancies [31]. Perinatal risks associated with multiple pregnancies are significantly higher than those of singleton pregnancies. The preterm delivery rate is reported to be as high as 60% in twin pregnancies, compared to 14% in singleton pregnancies, while the risk for LBW is 50% in twin pregnancies compared to 9% in singletons. However, singleton pregnancies are also reported to be independently associated with an increased risk of adverse pregnancy outcome compared to unassisted singleton conceptions, including preterm birth, LBW, congenital anomalies, and perinatal complications [29,30,32].

Patients pregnant after ICSI request more antenatal care and are having more ultrasound scans performed than women conceiving spontaneously. Despite this intensified follow-up, consumption of supplementary iodine and periconceptional folic acid is found to be below standard in ART patients, and attention ought to be paid to counseling ART patients carefully on the necessity of these supplements [33].

Congenital abnormalities

A major concern is the incidence of inborn abnormalities in children conceived by ICSI. Bonduelle et al. published, in 1999, the results on a follow-up cohort of 1987 children conceived by ICSI, which showed no increased risk of major congenital malformations as compared to the general population, the latter of which was based on information registered in the National Birth Registry [34]. Major malformations were defined as abnormalities causing dysfunction or requiring surgical correction. A Danish study by Loft et al. published in 1999 on 730 ICSI children showed no increase in major malformation rate as compared to the general population [35]. A Swedish study by Wennerholm et al. on 1139 ICSI children showed a higher incidence of congenital malformations compared to those registered in a control group of all newborns in the Swedish Medical Birth Registry. This increase is attributed to a high rate of multiple births in the ICSI group. Hypospadias was more prevalent in ICSI children in this study, potentially related to paternal infertility [36]. These findings were confirmed in the large Swedish study published by Ericson and Kallen in 2001, where 9111 children born after ART were compared to a population-based control group, and where the prevalence of hypospadias again appeared to be increased in the subgroup of ICSI children (RR 2.9; 95% CI: 1.4–5.4). The increased odds ratio (OR) of 1.47 for congenital malformations after IVF and ICSI disappeared when confounding factors (year of birth, maternal age, parity, period of unwanted childlessness, multiple pregnancies) were taken into account (OR 1.10) [37].

An interesting study by Hansen et al. in Western Australia between 1993 and 1997 analyzed the incidence of major birth defects in ART children at their first birthday. This demonstrated an OR for major birth defects (International Classification of Diseases, 9th revision (ICD-9)) of 2.0 (95% CI: 1.5–2.9) for the 837 IVF children and 2.0 (95% CI: 1.3–3.2) for the 301 ICSI children, as compared to a control population of naturally conceived children (n=4000) after correction for maternal age, parity, gender of the infant, and correlation between siblings [38].

Ludwig and Katalinic published results on a large cohort of stillbirths registered as early as 16 weeks' gestational age and live births in a population of ICSI children compared to a prospective population-based birth registry of spontaneously conceived children. The dropout rate for this study was very low at 4.3%, and the findings showed a major malformation rate in ICSI children of 8.6% according to EUROCAT (European Registry of Congenital Anomalies and Twins) criteria, compared to 6.9% in a control population, with a crude RR of 1.25 (95% CI: 1.11–1.40) [39]. These results were refined with a more appropriate control cohort in a more recent publication, showing an RR of major congenital malformations in ICSI children and fetuses beyond a gestational age of 16 weeks of 1.44 (95% CI: 1.25–1.65); when corrected for risk factors that have an effect on malformation rate in univariate analysis, that is, maternal age, parental malformations, and history of a previous stillbirth or fetus or child with a major malformation, the RR for malformation was 1.24 (95% CI: 1.02–1.50) [40]. The significance disappeared in twins and triplets presumably because of the low sample-size.

The Western Australian group of Hansen and colleagues published results of a systematic review of all studies (25) and reviewer-selected studies (7) relating to the prevalence of birth defects in infants conceived after IVF and/or ICSI compared with spontaneously conceived children. Their conclusion is that there is a statistically significant increased risk of birth defects of the order of 30%–40%. The pooled OR for birth defects was 1.40 (95% CI: 1.28–1.53) and 1.29 (95% CI: 1.21–1.37) for both the 7- and the 25-study groups included. The authors do not consider the review appropriate for inferring differences between the two techniques (IVF and ICSI) [41]. The use of an appropriate control group for the study of structural birth defects in an infertile population undergoing ART is essential, and previous reports have highlighted the absence of such control groups in many of the analyses and meta-analyses published [42]. Zhu et al. [43] attempted to compare structural birth defects in children conceived by ART of infertile couples versus those observed in spontaneously conceived children in infertile couples and spontaneously conceived children in fertile couples, and on the basis of an increased hazard ratio for overall birth defects in the two former categories, suggested common causal pathways of some of the determinants of infertility with mechanisms that cause congenital malformations. This study, however, showed a significantly increased incidence of genital organ malformations in children conceived by ART in infertile couples in comparison to children conceived spontaneously by infertile couples, consistent with previous findings by Hansen et al. and Rimm et al. [41,42].

When comparing birth defects following IVF versus ICSI, no significant differences have been reported. Bonduelle and colleagues published data on neonatal outcome of a cohort of 2889 infants born after ICSI (1991–1999) and 2995 children born after IVF (1983–1999) [44], showing no increased risk of malformations following ICSI compared to IVF.

There is concern for the effect of very poor spermatozoon quality on the health of ICSI children, especially when non-ejaculated spermatozoa are used. Studies into the incidence of adverse health outcomes, birth parameters, major anomaly rates, and chromosomal aberrations in ICSI versus spontaneously conceived children have so far not been able to establish a significant effect of the source of spermatozoa used for ICSI [45,46].

The largest multicenter cohort study results on follow-up of five-year-old children conceived after ICSI [47] showed an increased risk of congenital malformations in ICSI singletons (OR 2.77; 95% CI: 1.41–5.46) and IVF singletons (OR 1.80; 95% CI: 0.85–3.81), compared with naturally conceived children. This increased incidence of major congenital malformations in the ICSI group was partially due to a higher incidence of urogenital malformations in ICSI boys. Moreover, ICSI and IVF children were more likely to need medical or surgical intervention in the first years of life than children who were conceived spontaneously. A longer-term outcome study in eight-year-old singleton ICSI children (n=150) born at ≥32 weeks' gestation confirmed a higher rate of major congenital malformations in the ICSI children (10%) compared to spontaneously conceived children (3.3%) [48]. The same authors also reported a higher major malformation rate in children conceived from frozen-thawed ICSI embryos (6.4%) compared to frozen-thawed IVF embryos (3.1%) (OR 2.15; 95% CI: 1.10–4.20). The perinatal outcome was similar in both groups [49].

There also appears to be an increased interest in the risk of neurological sequelae in children conceived by IVF/ICSI. A population-based retrospective cohort study [50] suggests that children born after IVF have an increased risk of developing neurological problems (OR 1.7 overall), especially cerebral palsy (OR 3.7) which, according to the authors, is largely due to the high frequency of twin pregnancies, LBW, and prematurity among IVF babies, both singletons and twins. The study is of value, but the authors were not able to distinguish between different fertilization techniques; that is, IVF and ICSI. The question remains whether fertilization techniques, artificial culture media, ovarian stimulation, or subfertility are the underlying causes of this increased risk. Another study by Pinborg and colleagues [51] did not show a difference in neurological sequelae after IVF, neither in singletons nor in twins, and there was no difference with regard to fertilization techniques (IVF or ICSI). Neurological development was similar in ICSI versus spontaneously conceived children, at ≥32 weeks' gestation, at birth, and at eight years of age [48]. These findings were confirmed in a more recent prospective study into neuromotor development and mental health of ICSI singletons at five and a half years of age and compared to spontaneously conceived children: no significant differences were detected [52]. Vision and hearing develops normally in five and a half-year-old ICSI children compared to spontaneously conceived children [53].

As ICSI is also performed in most cases of PGD, and because embryo biopsy as well as prolonged embryo culture potentially contributes to the risks associated with ICSI, follow-up of children conceived by ICSI and selected by PGD is important. A small study on gestational age and auxiological outcome of 102 neonates born after PGD did not show statistical differences compared to ICSI children [54]. A study on the outcome of 480 PGD children showed comparable term and birth weight data [55]. Preimplantation genetic diagnosis children have been reported to have a lower gestational age at birth as well as a LBW, in comparison to spontaneously conceived children, although the studies so far are small in sample size [56]. The largest series of PGD children studied so far was reported recently, and did not show significant differences between ICSI/PGD and ICSI children in terms of gestational age at birth and birth weight [57]. An even larger study on 995 children confirmed these findings and refuted previous findings of an increased perinatal mortality rate for PGD singletons and multiples in comparison to ICSI offspring [58]. (For an overview, please see Table 9.1.)

Chromosomal abnormalities after intracytoplasmic spermatozoon injection

The first results in 1994 of a small cohort of 43 prenatal tests on 56 consecutive ICSI fetuses did not reveal any chromosomal abnormalities following ICSI conception [59]. However, as more ICSI procedures were being carried out, reports of a high incidence of chromosomal abnormalities started emerging. In't Veld et al. [60] and Van Opstal et al. [61] reported 9/71 chromosomal abnormalities in prenatal tests of ICSI fetuses, noting maternal age. On the contrary, other data did not confirm these risks and failed to show an increased rate of chromosomal abnormalities [35,62–66].

A large systematic prospective follow-up study of ICSI children at our hospital, with prenatal diagnosis and postnatal follow-up, showed a 2.6% rate of abnormal karyotypes [34,67]. Follow-up of the data published by Bonduelle and colleagues in 2002 again demonstrated a significantly higher incidence of chromosomal abnormalities (3.0%) when compared to the general population [68]. In this follow-up program, 85% of ICSI couples were seen and counseled before the start of and in early pregnancy, while 60% of fetuses actually underwent prenatal diagnosis. They reported a three-fold risk of de novo chromosomal anomalies (1.6% versus 0.5% in the general population), mainly related to a higher rate of sex chromosomal anomalies and partly related to a higher number of autosomal structural anomalies. There is a four-fold risk of inherited chromosomal abnormalities (1.4% versus 0.3%–0.4% in the general population; $P<0.001$), related to a higher rate of constitutional chromosomal anomalies, mainly in the fathers. A significantly higher percentage of 2.1% of de novo prenatal chromosomal anomalies was observed for spermatozoon concentrations of $<20.10^6$/mL, as compared to 0.24% when the sperm concentrationatozoon was $\geq 20.10^6$/mL. A statistical difference was found for motility criteria, but not for morphology.

A recent study by Kim et al. analyzed the prevalence of chromosomal abnormalities in spontaneous abortion after ART, and did not find a significant difference of cytogenetic abnormalities between the ICSI group (54.3%), the IVF group (55.3%), and a control group of spontaneous abortion after spontaneous conception (48.8%) [69]. However, the ICSI for the male factor infertility subgroup showed a significantly higher risk of chromosomal abnormalities than the ICSI group having non-male factors (65.8% versus 34.2%, OR 1.529, 95% CI: 1.092–2.141). (For an overview please see Table 9.2.)

The etiology of this higher incidence of chromosomal abnormalities is probably multifactorial. First, there is an atypical decondensation and delayed replication of the male genome in ICSI; current semen preparation techniques do not select against aneuploid spermatozoa [70,71]. The preferential localization of the sex chromosomes in the anterior spermatozoon head may lead (in combination with the delayed replication in the paternal genome) to a higher number of sex chromosome abnormalities in the fetuses [72,73].

Second, DNA damage is increased substantially in infertile men and inversely related to spermatozoon concentration, motility, and morphology [74]. A subgroup of men may therefore have a genetic background to their fertility problem, and could pass this genetic abnormality on to their offspring, if ICSI proves to be successful. The incidence of male karyotype abnormalities with sex-chromosomal or structural aberrations is inversely related to the number of spermatozoa in the ejaculate, hence is higher among ICSI fathers (4.8% of ICSI men, 1.5% of ICSI women, 0.5% in the general population). The incidence of sex chromosome abnormalities in azoospermic men is as high as 14%. Additionally, there is an increased rate of sex-chromosome aneuploidy (2.91%) in the spermatozoa of oligozoospermic men compared to a control population (0.69%) [75].

Table 9.1. Congenital malformations

Country	Authors	Year	Study population	Major ICSI	Minor ICSI	Major IVF	Minor IVF	Major Normal	Minor Normal	Criteria	RR
Belgium	Bonduelle et al. [95]	1996	ICSI (n=423)	3.30%	20.50%	N/A	N/A	N/A	N/A	N/A	
Australia	Kurinczuk et al. [96]	1997	ICSI (n=420) vs. NC (n=100 454)	7.40%	0.70%	N/A	N/A	3.80%	0.50%	ICD-9	
Belgium	Bonduelle et al. [34]	1999	ICSI (n=1987) vs. IVF (n=130)	2.30%	N/A	4.60%	N/A	N/A	N/A	N/A	
Denmark	Loft et al. [35]	1999	ICSI (n=730)	2.20%	1.20%	N/A	N/A	N/A	N/A	N/A	
England	Sutcliffe et al. [97]	1999	ICSI (n=123) vs. NC (n=123)	4.90%	11%	N/A	N/A	4.10%	7.30%	ICD-10	
Sweden	Wennerholm et al. [36]	2000	ICSI (n=1139)	3.20%	3.50%	N/A	N/A	N/A	N/A	ICD-8, ICD-9, ICD-10	OR 1.19 (95% CI: 0.79–1.81) after stratification for confounding factors including multiple pregnancies
Sweden	Ericson et al. [37]	2001	ICSI + IVF (n=9111)	N/A	N/A	N/A	N/A	N/A	N/A	ICD-8, ICD-9, ICD-10	OR 1.10 (95% CI: 0.68–1.81) after stratification for confounding factors
U.S.	Palermo et al. [98]	2000	ICSI (n=3573) vs. IVF (n=3277)	1.10%	0.80%	1.70%	1.30%	N/A	N/A		
Germany	Ludwig et al. [33]	2006	ICSI (n=2809)	9.10%	N/A	N/A	N/A	7.20%	N/A	EUROCAT	

England	Sutcliffe et al. [99]	2001	ICSI (n=208 singletons) vs. NC (n=221 singletons); singletons only	4.80%	N/A	N/A	N/A	4.50%	N/A	ICD-10	OR 1.759 (95% CI: 0.873–3.543)
Australia	Hansen et al. [38]	2002	ICSI (n=301) vs. IVF (n=837) vs. NC (n=4000)	8.60%	0.3% (by one year)	9.00%	0.80%	4.20%	0.60%	ICD-9	
Netherlands	Anthony et al. [100]	2002	ICSI + IVF (n=4224) vs. NC (n=314 605)	0.70%	1.30%	N/A	N/A	0.50%	1.10%		
Germany	Ludwig et al. [39]	2002	ICSI (n=3372) vs. NC (n=30 940)	8.60%	N/A	6.90%	N/A	N/A	N/A	EUROCAT	1.25 (95% CI: 1.11–1.40)
Sweden	Stromberg et al. [101]	2002	IVF (n=5680 singletons; 2060 twins) vs. NC (n=11 360 singletons; 4120 twins)	N/A	N/A	N/A	N/A	N/A	N/A	N/A	OR 1.7 (95% CI: 1.3–2.2) overall for need of rehabilitation services; OR 3.7 (95% CI: 2.0–6.6) overall for cerebral palsy
Holland	Moll et al. [93]	2003	observed vs. expected numbers of retinoblastoma from Nov 2000-Feb 2002							retinoblastoma	7.2 (95% CI: 2.4–17.0; 1% conceived by IVF) or 4.9 (1.6–11.3; 1.5% IVF)
Denmark	Pinborg et al. [51]	2004	ICSI/IVF (twins=3393, singletons=5130) vs. NC (n=10 239)	0.9% (twins)	0.8% (singletons)	IVF and ICSI				1.0% (control twins)	Neurological sequelae OR 1.3 ICSI vs. IVF twins; 0.5% ICSI vs. IVF singletons
Germany	Katalinic et al. [40]	2004	ICSI (n=3372) vs. NC (8016)	8.70%	N/A	N/A	N/A	6.1%	N/A	children and fetuses >16 weeks	1.44 (95% CI: 1.25–1.65)

Table 9.1. (cont.)

Country	Authors	Year	Study population	Major ICSI	Minor ICSI	Major IVF	Minor IVF	Major Normal	Minor Normal	Criteria	RR
Multicenter	Bonduelle et al. [47]	2005	5-year-olds (ICSI (n=540) vs. IVF (n=437) vs. NC (n=538)	4.20%	N/A	N/A	N/A	N/A	N/A		ICSI OR 2.77 (95% CI: 1.41–5.46); IVF OR 1.88 (CI: 0.85–3.81)
Meta-analysis	Hansen et al. [41]	2005	meta-analysis of selected studies								
Belgium	Belva et al. [48]	2007	8-year-olds ICSI (n=150) vs. NC (n=147)	10.00%	N/A	N/A	N/A	3.30%	N/A		RR 2.94 (95% CI: 1.09–7.89)
Belgium	Belva et al. [49]	2008	ICSI cryo children (n=547) vs. IVF cryo children (n=390)	6.40%	N/A	3.10%	N/A	N/A	N/A		OR 2.15 (95% CI: 1.10–4.20)

ICSI, intracytoplasmic spermatozoon injection; IVF, in vitro fertilization; RR, relative risk; NC, natural conception; ICD, International Classification of Diseases; OR, odds ratio; CI, confidence interval.

Table 9.2. Chromosomal abnormalities

Country	Authors	Year	Study Population	Criteria	RR
Belgium	Bonduelle et al. [59]	1994	Prospective ICSI cohort	43 prenatal tests	No chromosomal abnormalities
Netherlands	In 't Veld et al. [60]	1995	Selected population	15 prenatal tests	5 sex-chromosome abnormailities
France	Testart et al. [62]	1996	Selected population	83 prenatal tests	No de novo abnormalities; only inherited from parents
Netherlands	Van Opstal et al. [61]	1997	Selected population	71 prenatal tests	12.7% chromosomal aberrations
Belgium	Govaerts et al. [63]	1998	Retrospective 145 ICSI vs. 145 IVF	101 prenatal tests	1 de novo; no increased risk
U.S.	Munné et al. [102]	1998	79 IVF couples vs. 53 ICSI couples	Preimplantation diagnosis	No difference IVF vs. ICSI
Belgium	Bonduelle et al. [103]	1998	Prospective ICSI cohort	1082 prenatal tests	De novo abnormalities 1.66%; sex chromosome 0.83%; autosomal chromosome 0.83%
Denmark	Loft et al. [35]	1999	National cohort study	209 prenatal karyotypes	3.3% abnormal karyotypes
Sweden	Wennerholm et al. [36]	2000	National cohort	149 prenatal karyotypes	2.7% abnormal karyotypes
Egypt	Aboulghar et al. [104]	2001	ICSI neonates	430 ICSI babies	Non-significantly increased risk abnormal karyotype; autosomal and sex chromosome abnormalities equal
Belgium	Van Steirteghem et al. [66]	2002	Prospective ICSI cohort	1437 prenatal tests	2.9% abnormal karyotypes
Belgium	Bonduelle et al. [68]	2002	Prospective ICSI cohort	1586 prenatal tests	De novo: x2 (1.6%); sex chromosome abnormalities: x3 (0.6%); inherited chromosome abnormalities: x4 (1.4%)
U.S.	Kushnir and Frattarelli [105]	2009	Retrospective ICSI and IVF abortions	355 miscarriage specimens	ICSI 52.6% vs. IVF 47.2% aneuploidy rate (NS)
Korea	Kim et al. [69]	2010	Spontaneous abortion ICSI vs. IVF vs. control	406 miscarriage specimens	ICSI 54.3%, IVF 55.3%, control 48.4% cytogenetic abnormalities (NS)

RR, relative risk; ICSI, intracytoplasmic spermatozoon injection; IVF, in vitro fertilization.

Structural chromosomal anomalies include the presence of microdeletions on the long arm of the Y chromosome (Yq deletions) in some men, which will be passed on to the next male generation by ICSI. This microdeletion of a DNA sequence in the long arm of the Y chromosome (Yq11; azoospermia factor (AZF) region) is associated with extreme oligoasthenoterato-zoospermia (OAT) or azoospermia. The incidence of microdeletions in these patients varies from 1% to 55% with a mean of 8% depending on the inclusion criteria and the applied diagnostic technology [76]. There is a high likelihood of transmission of these deletions, hence infertility to male offspring by applying ICSI [77]; however, infertility is not an absolute finding for all Yq deletions [78]. In a mathematical model, it has been estimated that the incidence of Yq deletions will stabilize rapidly over the next generations, even if ICSI treatment becomes very successful [79]. Autosomal Y homologues or other unknown recessive gene defects may exist, and many genes related to spermatogenesis may be interlinked in gene networks. Mutations in the androgen receptors; for instance, increased CAG repeats in the androgen receptor gene, have been reported to cause male infertility. Globozoospermia and immotile cilia syndrome are now increasingly considered to be hereditary disorders. It has been reported that single-copy gene mutations on the X chromosome may be involved in male infertility as well. Any mutation or deletion, be it inherited or de novo, is potentially related to infertility in men [80].

Third, there are reports that the transmission of paternal mitochondrial DNA (mtDNA) may be increased as a result of ICSI, leading to an increased risk of inheritance of paternal mtDNA diseases. However, to date, there is no evidence of spermatozoon mtDNA being transmitted through the offspring following ICSI. Furthermore, in a report by St. John et al., spermatozoon mtDNA was not detected in abnormal embryos generated to blastocyst by ICSI [81].

Finally, centrosome deficiencies may occur in immature spermatozoa in OAT or azoospermia, ultimately producing mosaicism in embryos [82].

Epigenetic risks after intracytoplasmic spermatozoon injection

Genomic imprinting implies a mechanism of DNA methylation and results in the expression of only one of the parental copies of a gene. The functions of imprinted genes include embryonic and placental growth and development, carcinogenesis, and neurological development alongside a number of other functions. Dysregulation of genomic imprinting, for example, by non-methylation can result in congenital syndromes in humans such as Beckwith–Wiedemann syndrome (BWS), Silver–Russell syndrome, Prader–Willi syndrome, Angelman syndrome, and other neurogenetic diseases. There have been reports of unusually high incidences of BWS in children conceived by ART, and cases of Angelman syndrome after ART have also been reported [83].

The etiology of imprinting defects after ICSI is believed to involve a disruption in the normal process of DNA-methylation of parental genes. Attempts to detect specific abnormalities of known DNA-methylation patterns have not revealed abnormalities in a small sample of 92 children conceived by ICSI [84]. The use of immature haploid germ cells, for example as may happen when epididymal or testicular spermatozoa or even elongated or round spermatids are used, may give rise to genomic imprinting defects due to incomplete imprinting at the gamete level. Manning et al. investigated whether males with abnormal semen parameters may inherently have an abnormal paternal imprint. This study failed to find differences in spermatozoon imprinting status when compared with men with normal semen parameters [85]. A more recent study by Marques and colleagues [86], however, suggests that in relation to normozoospermia, abnormal spermatogenesis, as reflected in oligozoospermia, is associated with a rise in defective genomic imprinting, potentially leading to transmission of paternal imprinting errors. There may therefore be a higher risk of DNA-methylation defects in children born after ICSI. As with any other disorder that occurs with such a low incidence, large-scale cohort studies must be undertaken to see if ICSI is pathogenetic in this group of disorders, whether the origin of genome imprinting defects is maternal or paternal, and whether culture media may contribute to imprinting defects. The absolute risk of imprinting disorders after IVF/ICSI is still small (estimated at 1/20 000 for Angelman syndrome, compared to 1/200 000–400 000 in the general population), and the incidence is too low to explain higher rates of inborn abnormalities in ART [83].

A more recent study [87] revealed an increased incidence of genomic imprinting disorders in oocytes following ovulation induction and in vitro maturation. This may not only be due to maternal background factors such as age, but also to external factors such as suboptimal or abnormal follicular fluid biochemistry and cytoplasmic development. Moreover, aneuploidy rates in human oocytes are known to be substantially higher compared with animal species oocytes which, as far can be assessed, could be due to ovarian stimulation as this is the only setting in which aneuploidy in oocytes was determined. Other factors such as spermatozoon quality [88–90] and embryo culture conditions [91] can affect the chromosomal constitution of an embryo, giving rise to post-zygotic abnormalities such as mosaicism. These abnormalities will not be eliminated by omission of ovarian stimulation. Baart et al. [92], however, were able to demonstrate that the proportion of chromosomal abnormalities can be reduced by reducing the dosage of gonadotrophins for ovarian stimulation.

A study by Moll and colleagues [93] reported the observed incidence of retinoblastoma in children born after IVF to be significantly higher than was to be expected in the same period of time: RR 7.2, 95% CI: 2.4–17.0, assuming 1% of children is born after IVF and RR 4.9, 95% CI: 1.6–11.3 if 1.5% of children is born after IVF. Retinoblastoma may arise as a result of localized hypermethylation, as may other sporadic cancers. Other studies do not confirm these findings, and the findiings need to be interpreted with caution as they are prone to selection bias ("clustering" of cases). A recent report studying 26 692 IVF children showed an increase in risk of developing cancer (OR 1.45; 95% CI: 1.10–1.91), as registered in the Swedish Cancer Registry and compared to a group of spontaneously conceived children and corrected for background characteristics. The prevalence of histiocytosis was remarkably high. None of the registered maternal characteristics was significantly linked with the pathogenesis of cancer in the offspring, whereas high birth weight and preterm birth as neonatal factors were identified as intermediary factors [94].

Conclusion

Intracytoplasmic spermatozoon injection is a well-established technique that provides thousands of couples with the chance to conceive a child of their own. Pregnancy after ICSI carries a small yet increased risk of perinatal complications including LBW, preterm delivery, congenital abnormalities, and chromosomal abnormalities. Although the absolute risk of these complications is still low, the consistency of the findings in progressively larger cohort analyses and the clinical implications of these complications warrant a constant vigilance among health practitioners monitoring ICSI pregnancies and children, as well as correct counseling of the couples undergoing ICSI of the potential hazards involved. In view of the widespread application of ICSI, calls should also be made for establishing follow-up programs of the children conceived by ICSI and affiliated techniques, as is currently only happening in well-organized National Registries and a few local initiatives by large fertility centers.

On balance, the benefits of ICSI in terms of obstetric and perinatal health seem to outweigh the risks involved, and couples should not be withheld the chance of conceiving on condition that they are well informed.

References

1. Palermo GD, Joris H, Devroey P, Van Stierteghem AC. Pregnancies after intracytoplasmic sperm injection of single spermatozoon into an oocyte. *Lancet* 1992; **340**: 17–18.
2. Tournaye H, Devroey P, Liu J, et al. Microsurgical epididymal sperm aspiration and intracytoplasmic sperm injection: a new effective approach to infertility as a result of congenital bilateral absence of the vas deferens. *Fertil Steril* 1994; **61**: 1045–1051.
3. Tournaye H, Liu J, Verheyen G, et al. The use of testicular sperm for intracytoplasmic sperm injection in patients with necrozoospermia. *Fertil Steril* 1996; **66**: 331–334.
4. Tournaye H. Management of male infertility by assisted reproductive technologies. *Baillières Best Pract Res Clin Endocrinol Metab* 2000; **14**: 423–435.
5. Liu J, Nagy Z, Joris H, et al. Analysis of 76 total fertilization failure cycles out of 2732 intracytoplasmic sperm injection cycles. *Hum Reprod* 1995; **10**: 2630–2636.
6. Devroey P, Van Steirteghem. A review of ten years experience of ICSI. *Hum Reprod Update* 2004; **10**: 19–28.
7. Liebaers I, Sermon K, Staessen C, et al. Clinical experience with preimplantation genetic diagnosis and intracytoplasmic sperm injection. *Hum Reprod* 1998; **13**: 186–195.
8. Nyboe Andersen A, Carlsen E, Loft A. Trends in the use of intracytoplasmatic sperm injection marked variability between countries. *Hum Reprod Update* 2008; **14**: 593–604.
9. Nyboe Andersen A, Goossens V, Bhattacharya S, et al. Assisted reproductive technology and intrauterine

inseminations in Europe, 2005: results generated from European registers by ESHRE: ESHRE. The European IVF Monitoring Programme (EIM), for the European Society of Human Reproduction and Embryology (ESHRE). *Hum Reprod* 2009; **24**: 1267–1287.

10. Jain T, Gupta RS. Trends in the use of intracytoplasmic sperm injection in the United States. *N Engl J Med* 2007; **357**: 251–257.
11. Chang PL, Sauer MV, Brown SY. Chromosome microdeletion in a father and his four infertile sons. *Hum Reprod* 1999; **14**: 2689–2694.
12. Dumoulin JCM, Coonen E, Bras M, et al. Embryo development and chromosomal anomalies after ICSI: effect of the injection procedure. *Hum Reprod* 2001; **16**: 306–312.
13. Silva CP, Kommimeni K, Oldenbourg R, Keefe DL. The first polar body does not predict accurately the location of the metaphase II meiotic spindle in mammalian oocytes. *Fertil Steril* 1999; **71**: 719–721.
14. Hewitson L, Dominko T, Takahashi D, et al. Unique checkpoints during the first cell cycle of fertilization after intracytoplasmic sperm injection in rhesus monkeys. *Nat Med* 1999; **5**: 431–433.
15. Keefe D, Liu L, Wang W, Silva C. Imaging meiotic spindles by polarization light microscopy: principles and applications to IVF. *Reprod Biomed Online* 2003; **7**: 24–29.
16. Rienzi L, Ubaldi F, Martinez F, et al. Relationship between meiotic spindle location with regard to polar body position and oocyte developmental potential after ICSI. *Hum Reprod* 2003; **18**: 1289–1293.
17. Bergere M, Selva J, Volante M, et al. Cytogenetic analysis of uncleaved oocytes after intracytoplasmic sperm injection. *J Assist Reprod Genet* 1995; **12**: 322–325.
18. Edirisinghe WR, Murch A, Junk S, Yovich JL. Cytogenetic abnormalities of unfertilized oocytes generated from in-vitro fertilization and intracytoplasmic sperm injection: a double-blind study. *Hum Reprod* 1997; **12**: 2784–2791.
19. Plachot M. Les risques specifiques de l'ICSI. *Contracept Fertil Sex* 1996; **24**: 577–580.
20. Michelmann HW. Influence of bacteria and leukocytes on the outcome of in vitro fertilization (IVF) or intracytoplasmic sperm injection (ICSI). *Andrologia* 1998; **30**: 99–101.
21. Brossfield JE, Chan PJ, Patton WC, King A. Tenacity of exogenous human papillomavirus DNA in sperm washing. *J Assist Reprod Genet* 1999; **16**: 325–328.
22. Lacey RW, Dealler SF. Vertical transfer of prion disease. *Hum Reprod* 1994; **9**: 1792–1800.
23. Perry ACF, Wakayama T, Kishikawa H, et al. Mammalian transgenesis by intracytoplasmic sperm injection. *Science* 1999; **284**: 1180–1183.
24. Chan AW, Luetjens CM, Dominko T, et al. TransgenICSI reviewed: foreign DNA transmission by intracytoplasmic sperm injection in rhesus monkey. *Mol Reprod Dev* 2000; **56**: 325–328.
25. Tesarik J. Oocyte activation after intracytoplasmic sperm injection of mature and immature sperm cells. *Hum Reprod* 1998; **13**: 117–127.
26. American Society for Reproductive Medicine; Society for Assisted Reproductive Technology Registry. Assisted reproductive technology in the United States: 1999 results generated from the American Society for Reproductive Medicine/Society for Assisted Reproductive Technology Registry. *Fertil Steril* 2002; **78**: 918–931.
27. Wisanto A, Magnus M, Bonduelle M, et al. Obstetric outcome of 424 pregnancies after intracytoplasmic sperm injection. *Hum Reprod* 1995; **10**: 2713–2718.
28. Aytoz A, Camus M, Tournaye H, et al. Outcome of pregnancies after intracytoplasmic sperm injection and the effect of sperm origin and quality on this outcome. *Fertil Steril* 1998; **70**: 500–505.
29. Schieve L, Meikle S, Ferre C, et al. Low and very low birthweight in infants conceived with use of assisted reproductive technology. *N Engl J Med* 2002; **346**: 731–737.
30. Helmerhorst FM, Perquin DAM, Donker D, Keirse MJ. Perinatal outcome of singletons and twins after assisted conception: a systematic review of controlled studies. *BMJ* 2004; **328**: 261.
31. Reynolds MA, Schieve LA, Martin JA, Jeng G, Macaluso M. Trends in multiple births conceived using assisted reproductive technology, United States 1997–2000. *Pediatrics* 2003; **111**: 1159–1162.
32. Jackson RA, Gibson KA, Wu YW, Croughan MS. Perinatal outcomes in singletons following in vitro fertilization: a meta-analysis. *Obstet Gynecol* 2004; **103**: 551–563.
33. Ludwig AK, Katalinic A, Steinbicker V, Diedrich K, Ludwig M. Antenatal care in singleton pregnancies after ICSI as compared to spontaneous conception: data from a prospective controlled cohort study in Germany. *Hum Reprod* 2006; **21**: 713–720.
34. Bonduelle M, Camus M, De Vos A, et al. Seven years of intracytoplasmic sperm injection and follow-up of 1987 subsequent children. *Hum Reprod* 1999; **14**: 243–264.
35. Loft A, Petersen K, Erb K, et al. A Danish national cohort of 730 infants born after intracytoplasmic

sperm injection (ICSI) 1994–1997. *Hum Reprod* 1999; **14**: 2143–2148.

36. Wennerholm UB, Bergh C, Hamberger L, et al. Obstetric outcome of pregnancies following ICSI, classified according to sperm origin and quality. *Hum Reprod* 2000; **15**: 1189–1194.

37. Ericson A, Kallen B. Congenital malformations in infants born after IVF: a population based study. *Hum Reprod* 2001; **16**: 504–509.

38. Hansen M, Kurinczuk JJ, Bower C, Webb S. The risk of major birth defects after intracytoplasmic sperm injection and in vitro fertilization. *N Engl J Med* 2002; **346**: 725–730.

39. Ludwig M, Katalinic A. Malformation rate in fetuses and children conceived after ICSI: results of a prospective cohort study. *Reprod Biomed Online* 2002; **5**: 171–178.

40. Katalinic A, Rösch C, Ludwig M. Pregnancy course and outcome after intracytoplasmic sperm injection: a controlled, prospective cohort study. *Fertil Steril* 2004; **81**: 1604–1616.

41. Hansen M, Bower C, Milne E, de Klerk N, Kurinczuk JJ. Assisted reproductive technologies and the risk of birth defects – a systematic review. *Hum Reprod* 2005; **20**: 328–338.

42. Rimm AA, Katayama AC, Diaz M, Katayama KP. A meta-analysis of controlled studies comparing major malformation rates in IVF and ICSI infants with naturally conceived children. *J Assist Reprod Genet* 2004; **21**: 437–443.

43. Zhu JL, Basso O, Obel C, Bille C, Olsen J. Infertility, infertility treatment and congenital malformations: Danish national birth cohort. *BMJ* 2006; **333**: 679.

44. Bonduelle M, Liebaers I, Deketelaere V, et al. Neonatal data on a cohort of 2889 infants born after ICSI (1991–1999) and of 2995 children born after IVF (1983–1999). *Hum Reprod* 2002; **17**: 671–694.

45. Ludwig M, Katalinic A. Pregnancy course and health of children born after ICSI depending of parameters of male factor infertility. *Hum Reprod* 2003; **18**: 351–357.

46. Belva F, De Schrijver F, Tournaye H, et al. Neonatal outcome of 724 children born after ICSI using non-ejaculated sperm. *Hum Reprod* 2011; **26**: 1752–1758.

47. Bonduelle M, Wennerholm U-B, Loft A, Tarlatzis BC, et al. A multi-centre cohort study of the physical health of 5-year-old children conceived after intracytoplasmic sperm injection, in vitro fertilization and natural conception. *Hum Reprod* 2005; **20**: 413–419.

48. Belva F, Henriet S, Liebaers I, et al. Medical outcome of 8-year-old singleton ICSI children (born ≥32 weeks' gestation) and a spontaneously conceived comparison group. *Hum Reprod* 2007; **22**: 506–515.

49. Belva F, Henriet S, Van den Abbeel E, et al. Neonatal outcome of 937 children born after transfer of cryopreserved embryos obtained by ICSI and IVF and comparison with outcome data of fresh ICSI and IVF cycles. *Hum Reprod* 2008; **23**: 2227–2238.

50. Strömberg B, Dahlquist G, Ericson A, et al. Neurological sequelae in children born after in-vitro fertilisation: a population-based study. *Lancet* 2002; **359**: 461–465.

51. Pinborg A, Loft A, Schmidt L, et al. Neurological sequelae in twins born after assisted conception: controlled national cohort. *BMJ* 2004; **329**: 311.

52. Ludwig A, Katalinic A, Thyen U, et al. Neuromotor development and mental health at 5.5 years of age of singletons born at term after intracytoplasmic sperm injection ICSI: results of a prospective controlled single-blinded study in Germany. *Fertil Steril* 2009; **91**: 125–132.

53. Ludwig AK, Hansen A, Katalinic A, et al. Assessment of vision and hearing in children conceived spontaneously and by ICSI: a prospective controlled, single-blinded follow-up study. *Reprod Biomed Online* 2010; **20**: 391–397.

54. Desmyttere S, De Schepper J, Nekkebroeck J, et al. Two-year auxological and medical outcome of singletons born after embryo biopsy applied in preimplantation genetic diagnosis or preimplantation genetic screening. *Hum Reprod* 2009; **24**: 470–476.

55. Tur-Kaspa I, Horwitz A, Ginsberg N, et al. Clinical outcome of PGD. *Fertil Steril* 2005; **84**: 599.

56. Banerjee I, Shevlin M, Taranissi M, et al. Health of children conceived after preimplantation genetic diagnosis: a preliminary outcome study. *Reprod Biomed Online* 2008; **16**: 376–381.

57. Liebaers I, Desmyttere S, Verpoest W, et al. Report on a consecutive series of 581 children born after blastomere biopsy for preimplantation genetic diagnosis. *Hum Reprod* 2010; **25**: 275–282.

58. Desmyttere S, Verpoest W, De Rycke M, et al. Neonatal outcome of 995 children conceived after embryo biopsy compared to children born after intracytoplasmic sperm injection. *Hum Reprod* 2010; **25**: 2945–2950.

59. Bonduelle M, Desmyttere S, Buysse A, et al. Prospective follow-up study of 55 children born after subzonal insemination and intracytoplasmic sperm injection. *Hum Reprod* 1994; **9**: 1765–1769.

60. In't Veld P, Brandenburg H, Verhoeff A, Dhont M, Los F. Sex chromosomal anomalies and intracytoplasmic sperm injection. *Lancet* 1995; **345**: 773.

61. Van Opstal D, Los FJ, Ramlakhan S, et al. Determination of the parent origin in nine cases of

prenatally detected chromosome aberrations found after intracytoplasmic sperm injection. *Hum Reprod* 1997; **12**: 682–686.

62. Testart J, Gautier E, Brami C, et al. Intracytoplasmic sperm injection in infertile patients with structural chromosome abnormalities. *Hum Reprod* 1996; **11**: 2609–2612.

63. Govaerts I, Devreker F, Koenig I, et al. Comparison of pregnancy outcome after intracytoplasmic sperm injection and in vitro fertilization. *Hum Reprod* 1998; **13**: 1514–1518.

64. Van Golde R, Boada M, Veiga A, et al. A retrospective follow-up study on intracytoplasmic sperm injection. *J Assist Reprod Genet* 1999; **16**: 227–232.

65. Antoni K, Hamori M. Distribution of fetal malformations and chromosomal disorders in 1290 ICSI newborns between 1993 and 2000. *Hum Reprod* 2001; **16**: 39.

66. Van Steirteghem A, Bonduelle M, Liebaers I, Devroey P. Children born after assisted reproductive technology. *Am J Perinatol* 2002; **19**: 59–65.

67. Liebaers I, Bonduelle M, Van Assche E, Devroey P, Van Steirteghem A. Sex chromosome abnormalities after intracytoplasmic sperm injection. *Hum Reprod* 1995; **346**: 1095.

68. Bonduelle M, Van Assche E, Joris H, et al. Prenatal testing in ICSI pregnancies: incidence of chromosomal anomalies in 1586 karyotypes and relation to semen parameters. *Hum Reprod* 2002; **17**: 2600–2614.

69. Kim JW, Lee WS, Yoon TK, et al. Chromosomal abnormalities in spontaneous abortion after assisted reproductive treatment. *BMC Med Genet* 2010; **11**: 153.

70. Luetjens CM, Payne C, Schatten G. Non-random chromosome positioning in human sperm and sex chromosome anomalies following intracytoplasmic sperm injection. *Lancet* 1999; **353**: 1240.

71. Sbracia M, Baldi M, Cao D, S et al. Preferential location of sex chromosomes, their aneuploidy in human sperm, and their role in determining sex chromosome aneuploidy in embryos after ICSI. *Hum Reprod* 2002; **17**: 320–324.

72. Bourgain C, Nagy ZP, De Zutter H, et al. Ultrastructure of gametes after intracytoplasmic sperm injection. *Hum Reprod* 1998; **13**: 107–116.

73. Terada Y, Luetjens CM, Sutovsky P, Schatten G. Atypical decondensation of the sperm nucleus, delayed replication of the male genome, and sex chromosome positioning following intracytoplasmic human sperm injection (ICSI) into golden hamster eggs: does ICSI itself introduce chromosomal anomalies? *Fertil Steril* 2000; **74**: 454–460.

74. Sakkas D, Manicardi GC, Bizzaro D. Sperm nuclear damage in the human. *Adv Exp Med Biol* 2003; **518**: 73–84.

75. Van Assche E, Bonduelle M, Tournaye H, et al. Cytogenetics of infertile men. *Hum Reprod* 1996; **11**: 1–24.

76. Van Landuyt L, Lissens W, Stouffs K, et al. Validation of a simple Yq deletion screening programme in an ICSI candidate population. *Mol Hum Reprod* 2000; **6**: 291–297.

77. Page DC, Silber S, Brown LG. Men with infertility caused by AZFc deletion can produce sons by intracytoplasmic sperm injection but are likely to transmit the deletion and infertility. *Hum Reprod* 1999; **14**: 1722–1726.

78. Saut N, Terriou P, Navarro A, Levy N, Mitchell MJ. The human Y chromosome genes BPY2, CDY1 and DAZ are not essential for sustained fertility. *Mol Hum Reprod* 2000; **6**: 789–793.

79. Kremer JA, Tuerlings JH, Borm G, et al. Does intracytoplasmic sperm injection lead to a rise in the frequency of microdeletions in the AZFc region of the Y chromosome in future generations? *Hum Reprod* 2001; **13**: 2808–2811.

80. Stouffs K, Tournaye H, Liebaers I, Lissens W. Male infertility and the involvement of the X chromosome. *Hum Reprod Update* 2009; **15**: 623–637.

81. St John JC, Lloyd R, El Shourbagy S. The potential risks of abnormal transmission of mtDNA through assisted reproductive technologies. *Reprod Biomed Online* 2003; **8**: 34–44.

82. Schatten H, Sun QY. The role of centrosomes in mammalian fertilization and its significance for ICSI. *Mol Hum Reprod* 2009; **15**: 531–538.

83. Gosden R, Trasler J, Lucifero D, Faddy M. Rare congenital disorders, imprinted genes, and assisted reproductive technology. *Lancet* 2003; **361**: 1975–1977.

84. Manning M, Lissens W, Bonduelle M, et al. Study of DNA methylation patterns at chromosome 15q11-q13 in children born after ICSI reveals no imprinting defects. *Mol Hum Reprod* 2000; **6**: 1049–1053.

85. Manning M, Lissens W, Liebaers I, Van Steirteghem A, Weidner W. Imprinting analysis in spermatozoa prepared for intracytoplasmic sperm injection (ICSI). *Int J Androl* 2001; **24**: 87–94.

86. Marques CJ, Carvalho F, Sousa M, Barros A. Genomic imprinting in disruptive spermatogenesis. *Lancet* 2003; **363**: 1700–1702.

87. Sato A, Otsu E, Negishi H, et al. Aberrant DNA methylation of imprinted loci in superovulated oocytes. *Hum Reprod* 2007; **22**: 26–35.

88. Obajasu M, Kadam A, Sultan K, Fateh M, Munne S. Sperm quality may adversely affect the chromosome constitution of embryos that result from intracytoplasmic sperm injection. *Fertil Steril* 1999; **72**: 1113–1115.

89. Pfeffer J, Pang MG, Hoegerman SF, et al. Aneuploidy frequencies in semen fractions from ten oligoasthenoteratozoospermic patients donating sperm for intracytoplasmic sperm injection. *Fertil Steril* 1999; **72**: 472–478.

90. Vegetti W, Van Assche E, Frias A, et al. Correlation between semen parameters and sperm aneuploidy rates investigated by fluorescence in-situ hybridization in infertile men. *Hum Reprod* 2000; **15**: 831–838.

91. Van Blerkom J, Henry G. Oocyte dysmorphism and aneuploidy in meiotically mature human oocytes after ovarian stimulation. *Hum Reprod* 1992; **7**: 379–390.

92. Baart EB, Martini E, Eijkemans MJ, et al. Milder ovarian stimulation for in-vitro fertilization reduces aneuploidy in the human preimplantation embryo: a randomized controlled trial. *Hum Reprod* 2007; **22**: 980–988.

93. Moll AC, Imhof SM, Cruysberg JR, et al. Incidence of retinoblastoma in children born after in-vitro fertilization. *Lancet* 2003; **361**: 309–310.

94. Källen B, Finnström O, Lindam A, et al. Cancer risk in children and young adults conceived by in vitro fertilization. *Pediatrics* 2010; **126**: 270–276.

95. Bonduelle M, Wilikens A, Buysse A, et al. Prospective follow-up study of 877 children born after intracytoplasmic sperm injection (ICSI), with ejaculated epididymal and testicular spermatozoa and after replacement of cryopreserved embryos obtained after ICSI. *Hum Reprod* 1996; **11**: 131–155.

96. Kurinczuk JJ, Bower C. Birth defects in infants conceived by intracytoplasmic sperm injection: an alternative interpretation. *BMJ* 1997; **315**: 1260–1266.

97. Sutcliffe AG, Taylor B, Li Jun, et al. Children born after intracytoplasmic sperm injection: population control study. *BMJ* 1999; **318**: 704–705.

98. Palermo GD, Neri Q, Hariprashad JJ, et al. ICSI and its outcome. *Semin Reprod Med* 2000; **18**: 161–169.

99. Sutcliffe AG, Saunders K, Thornton S, Lieberman BA, Grudzinskas JG. Outcome in the second year of life after in-vitro fertilization by intracytoplasmic sperm injection: a UK case-control study. *Lancet* 2001; **357**: 2080–2084.

100. Anthony S, Buitendijk SE, Dorrepaal CA, et al. Congenital malformations in 4224 children conceived after IVF. *Hum Reprod* 2002; **17**: 2089–2095.

101. Stromberg B, Dahlquist G, Ericson A, et al. Neurological sequelae in children born after in vitro fertilization: a population-based study. *Lancet* 2002; **359**: 461–465.

102. Munné S, Marquez C, Reing A, Garrisi J, Alikani M. Chromosome abnormalities in embryos obtained after conventional in vitro fertiization and intracytoplasmic sperm injection. *Fertil Steril* 1998; **69**: 904–908.

103. Bonduelle M, Legein J, Hofmans K, Liebaers I, Van Steirteghem A. Mental development of 201 ICS children at 2 years of age. *Lancet* 1998; **351**: 1553.

104. Aboulghar H, Aboulghar M, Mansour R, et al. A prospective controlled study of karyotyping for 430 consecutive babies conceived through intracytoplasmic sperm injection. *Fertil Steril* 2001; **76**: 249–253.

105. Kushnir VA, Frattarelli JL. Aneuploidy in abortuses following IVF and ICSI. *J Assist Reprod Genet* 2009; **26**: 93–97.

Chapter 10

Pregnancy outcome after oocyte and embryo cryopreservation

Eleonora Porcu and Antonia Bazzocchi

Cryopreservation is essential for correct and appropriate clinical application of assisted reproductive technologies (ARTs). Reproductive cryopreservation is crucial for ART efficiency and flexibility in infertile patients. In addition, reproductive storage is a precious tool for fertility preservation in cancer patients. However, as in all reproductive methodologies, safety must be focused and short- and long-term children follow-up studies are mandatory. The first children conceived from frozen oocytes and embryos are now adults and a number of subjects are presently adolescents; therefore, information is available on their health and development and some conclusions can be drawn.

Oocyte cryopreservation

While embryo and spermatozoon cryopreservation are well-established techniques among in vitro fertilization (IVF) centers, it is only recently that clinically effective human oocyte cryopreservation has become a reality. Oocyte cryopreservation is an important complement to ART. It represents a major method in preservation of female fertility in prepuberal patients in need of immediate gonadotoxic therapy and in all women who desire to preserve fertility in cases of surgical removal of ovaries, radiotherapy, and chemotherapy. Oocyte freezing can find an application in cycles complicated by ovarian hyperstimulation syndrome or failure to obtain spermatozoa. In addition, oocyte cryopreservation overcomes ethical and legal concerns in contrast with conventional embryo cryopreservation. The technique can also simplify the oocyte donation process for IVF. A potential increasing demand of oocyte cryopreservation could be associated with the desire of the women to preserve their fertility in order to postpone pregnancy.

To maintain long-term viability after long-term storage, living cells must be brought into a state of suspended animation, in which they remain for indefinite periods of time and from which they can be brought back to viability at some point in the future. The temperature of liquid nitrogen (−196°C) appears to be adequate for these purposes. At these low temperatures, water exists only in a solid state and no biological reactions take place. The only possible alteration may be related to DNA damage caused by background radiation that, however, does not seem to compromise the chance of survival. Because human oocytes are viable at 37°C and are almost totally inactive at −196°C, the lapse-time of major danger occurs during the temperature decreasing and rewarming phases.

The human oocyte is one of the largest cells in the body, measuring approximately 130 μm and has a low surface area to volume ratio; the consequence is that the oocyte is more prone to water retention and consequent damage caused by ice crystals. Although the avoidance of chilling injury is the most important goal to improve survival rates, several other parameters have been taken into account in oocyte cryopreservation: cell characteristics, permeability to the cryoprotectants, toxicity, temperature, and time of exposure to the cryoprotectants. Cryoprotectants protect cells by forming hydrogen bonds with water molecules, eliminating ice formation, and preventing damage caused by high salt concentration.

From 1986 when the first pregnancy with frozen oocytes was achieved [1], until 1997 when intracytoplasmic spermatozoon injection (ICSI) was first used to fertilize frozen-thawed oocytes [2], there have only been a few live births from frozen-thawed oocytes. Conventional slow-freezing methods are associated with relatively low success rates, although survival rates seem to be acceptable and vary from 33% to 100 % [3–16]. Several improvements in culture conditions, cryoprotectant use, and oocyte selection have

Pregnancy After Assisted Reproductive Technology, ed. Eric R. M. Jauniaux and Botros R. M. B. Rizk. Published by Cambridge University Press.

led to better clinical results and a more extensive application of the technique worldwide.

The slow-freezing method needs low initial cryoprotectant concentrations, which are associated with lower toxicity; concentration increases only when the cells decrease their metabolism. At a temperature of –6°C, by introducing a seed ice crystals may be induced to grow gradually toward the oocytes. The temperature is then slowly decreased up to −196°C. During thawing, a rapid transition of temperature is preferred to prevent recrystallization of water.

The technical approach most widely attempted is based on a slow-cooling/rapid-thawing method using 1,2-propanediol and sucrose as cryoprotectants. Many modifications in the slow-freezing protocol have been proposed in order to stabilize the plasma membrane and promote the retention of an intact chromosome segregation apparatus. A high concentration of sucrose (0.2–0.3 M) and differential sucrose concentration during dehydration and rehydration have been described [17,18].

In recent years, vitrification has been introduced as an alternative to slow freezing. Vitrification is the process by which water is prevented from forming ice due to the viscosity of a highly concentrated cryoprotectant cooled at an extremely rapid rate. Recent advances in vitrification methods have led to an ovum survival rate over 85% and pregnancy rates comparable to those achieved with fresh ova [19–21].

It has recently been demonstrated that when comparing slow freezing with vitrification, the latter might have a lower impact on the oocyte meiotic spindle [22,23]. However, the clinical efficiency and safety of vitrification is still under investigation.

As regards the efficiency of oocyte cryopreservation, Porcu et al. [14] published data documenting comparable pregnancy rates between thawed oocytes and thawed embryos, confirming the applicability of the technique. Recently, the Italian centers have published data on the clinical outcomes in 940 thawed oocyte cycles [24]. In Italy, oocyte cryopreservation is more widespread than in other countries because the Italian law bans embryo cryopreservation. The eight centers participating in the observational study used the same freezing and thawing protocols to cryopreserve the surplus oocytes (slow-freezing/rapid-thawing protocol with 1,2-propanediol and a high sucrose concentration (0.2 M) as cryoprotectants). On the whole, the survival rate of thawed oocytes was 55.8 % and the fertilization rate was 72.5%. The pregnancy rate per transfer was 17% compared to 27.9% in fresh cycles, and the pregnancy rate per cycle was 13.7% in freezing cycles versus 26.2 % in fresh cycles. It must be underlined that data largely differed among centers; in fact, the survival rate varied from 30.8+/−27.7% to 67.2+/−25.8% and the pregnancy rate per embryo transfer varied from 9.5% to 31%. These data underline the importance of IVF laboratory interventions in the cryopreservation procedure. Moreover, the authors note that patients who had achieved a pregnancy in a fresh cycle have better outcomes in cryopreservation cycles, confirming the strict connection between success rates and gamete quality.

The number of births from thawed oocytes has increased significantly in recent years, although oocyte cryopreservation is still considered an experimental procedure in accordance with its relatively slow start and early lack of reproducibility [25]. Consequently, the interest in the pregnancy outcomes from frozen oocytes and in the health of the children born has been increasing.

Some studies showed a higher incidence of certain disorders of pregnancy such as preeclampsia, gestational diabetes, placenta previa, placental abruption, preterm delivery, and elective Cesarean section in pregnancies achieved through fresh techniques of IVF [26,27]. The risks identified to date do not seem to be associated with the techniques per se, but rather as being attributable to the higher incidence of multiple pregnancies and to intrinsic parental characteristics.

The first report that evaluated the safety of oocyte cryopreservation was published by Porcu et al. [28]. Results regarding 17 pregnancies obtained from oocyte cryopreservation were reported in terms of obstetric and perinatal outcomes and follow-up of children. These preliminary observations gave a first reassurance about the health of babies born. Eleven pregnancies out of seventeen ended with the delivery of thirteen healthy children (nine females and four males). The amniocentesis performed in all but one pregnancy showed a normal karyotype. Obstetric complications registered were: two preterm deliveries, one placenta previa, and one gestational hypertension. Mean gestational age at birth was 260+/−17 days whereas mean birth weight was 2730+/−537 g. The mean Apgar score at five minutes was 7.9+/−0.9. No malformations were detected in the newborns. Cesarean section was performed in nine cases. The follow-up of the children showed a normal physical and cognitive development in all the children. These positive observations were confirmed in a subsequent study conducted on 70 children [29] and on 105 babies

[30]. In the latter, 149 pregnancies resulted in the birth of 105 babies, 73 in singleton pregnancies and 32 in twin pregnancies, with a 23% miscarriage rate. The mean gestational age at birth was 38.9 weeks, whereas the mean birth weight was 3.353 kg in singletons and 2.599 kg in twins.

Recently, data regarding a very large population of 936 babies born after oocyte cryopreservation have been published [31]. Authors built a database including all verified live-born infants between 1986 and 2008; 58 reports, which included 609 live-born babies (308 from slow freezing, 289 from vitrification, and 12 from both methods), were reviewed. An additional 327 live births were documented (Table 10.1).

The rate of birth anomalies that resulted was 1.3 % (12), which is comparable with that in spontaneous pregnancies. The anomalies observed were: ventricular septal defects (3), choanal atresia (1),biliary atresia (1), Rubinstein–Taybi syndrome (1), Arnold–Chiari syndrome (1), cleft palate (1), clubfoot (3), and skin hemangioma (1) (Table 10.2).

Birth weight, gestational age, and prematurity cannot be correctly evaluated in this study because the parameters are not expressed separately for single and multiple births, as the authors underline. However, the multiple gestation rate was 19%. The mean gestational age and weight at birth of the 30 babies reported in case reports were, respectively, 36.9+/−0.6 weeks and 2720+/−116 g in the slow-freezing group and 39+/−1 weeks and 3318+/−201 g in the vitrification group.

These conclusions are comparable with those achieved by Chian et al., [32] who reported the obstetric and perinatal outcomes of 200 infants born in 165 pregnancies from oocyte vitrification. The multiple birth rate was 17% (26 twins and 2 triplets). The Cesarean section rate was 37% in singleton pregnancies and 96% in multiple pregnancies, whereas the mean birth weight was 2920+/−37 g for singletons and 2231+/−55 g for multiples. The incidence of congenital malformations was 2.5 % (two ventricular septal defects, one biliary atresia, one clubfoot, and one skin hemangioma) [32] (Table 10.3).

Another review of published data concerning live births after oocyte cryopreservation has been published by Wennerholm [33], who collected neonatal information about 148 children born from oocyte slow-freezing and 221 children born after vitrification of oocytes.

Although data are very limited, the birth weights of children conceived through oocyte cryopreservation were within the normal range.

On the whole, very limited data have been reported on pregnancy outcomes after oocyte cryopreservation, therefore further studies are necessary to evaluate the

Table 10.1. Data from oocyte cryopreservation births "series reports"

Parameter	Cryopreservation method		
	Slow freezing	Vitrification	Both
Number of embryo transfers	1974	834	19
Number of oocytes thawed/warmed	11890	5435	271
Number of oocytes that survived	8056	4392	244
% of oocyte survival	68 (range: 22–90)	81 (range: 69–99)	90
% of 2-pronucleate fertilization	73 (range: 50–86)	79 (range: 59–93)	81
Number of live-born babies	282	285	12
Baby gender (gender information available for 168 slow freezing, 189 vitrification, and 12 for both methods)	99 female, 69 male	86 female, 103 male	8 female, 4 male
Birth defects	1 ventricular septal defect, 1 choanal atresia, 1 Rubinstein–Taybi syndrome	2 ventricular septal defects, 1 biliary atresia, 1 clubfoot, 1 skin hemangioma	None

n = 35 reports: 23 slow freezing, 9 vitrification, 3 both cryopreservation methods. (Noyes et al., 2009 [31].)

Table 10.2. Birth anomalies in cases of natural conception versus oocyte cryopreservation, listed from the most common to the most rare

Birth anomaly	Approximate incidence in natural conception births	Incidence in total of 936 oocyte cryopreservation births (n)
All	One in 33	12 (one in 78)
Skin hemangioma	One in 50–225	1
Cardiac defects	One in 125	3
Neural tube defects	One in 385	0
Cleft lip and palate	One in 710	1
Clubfoot	One in 735	3
Arnold–Chiari syndrome	One in 1200	1
Choanal atresia	One in 7000	1
Biliary atresia	One in 10 000–15 000	1
Rubinstein–Taybi syndrome	One in 100 000–125 000	1

(Noyes et al., 2009 [31].)

Table 10.3. Obstetric and perinatal outcomes and incidence of congenital malformations in children conceived after oocyte vitrification

Characteristics	All pregnancies (n = 165)	Singleton pregnancies (n = 137)	Multiple gestation pregnancies (n = 28)
Mean gestational age (weeks + days)	37 + 1	37 + 3	35 + 5
Number of deliveries at 34–37 weeks (%)	46 (30)	30 (22)	16 (57)
Number of deliveries at <34 weeks	10 (6)	6 (4)	4 (14)
	All newborns (n = 200)	**Singleton newborns (n = 141)**	**Multiple gestation newborns (n = 59)**
Birth weight (mean +/–SEM) (g)	2784+/–37	2920+/–37	2231+/–55
Number of LBW (%)	68 (34)	24 (17)	44 (74)
Number of VLBW (%)	4 (2)	1 (0.7)	3 (5)
Median Apgar score at 1 min	8	9	8
Median Apgar score at 5 min	10	10	10
Incidence of congenital anomalies			
Biliary atresia	1	0	1
Clubfoot	1	1	0

Table 10.3. (cont.)

Characteristics	All pregnancies (n = 165)	Singleton pregnancies (n = 137)	Multiple gestation pregnancies (n = 28)
Skin hemangioma	1	1	0
Ventricular septal defect	2	0	2
Total (%)	5 (2.5%)	2 (1.4%)	3 (5.1%)

SEM, standard error of mean; LBW, low birth weight (1500–2500 g); VLBW, very low birth weight (<1500 g). (Chian et al., 2008 [32].)

characteristics of pregnancies and the long-term follow-up of the children. It is a particularly urgent need because of the experimental connotation of this technique. In order to follow up the outcomes and evaluate the efficacy and safety of oocyte cryopreservation techniques, a registry was recently adopted in the U.S. as a national five-year prospective, multicenter, observational study (HOPE: "The Human Oocyte Preservatione Experience") [34].

Embryo cryopreservation

Cryopreservation of human embryos is now an established procedure that has been practiced for more than 25 years. Since the early 1970s, Wilmut and Whittingham [35,36] independently developed methods for cryopreservation of mouse embryos using dimethyl sulfoxide (DMSO) as the cryoprotectant. Currently most used solutions include freezing DMSO, ethylene glycol, 1,2-propanediol, and glycerol; these solutions are frequently added to glucose or sucrose. Since the 1980s, the freezing of human embryos has been introduced as a routine procedure in ART, and in 1980 Trounson and Mohr [37] reported the first pregnancy achieved by thawing and transfer of an embryo of eight cells, which had been stored for four months in liquid nitrogen. The first pregnancy was obtained by thawing of blastocysts, and was presented by Cohen et al. [38]. Rall and Fahy, in the same year, introduced a new technique for freezing mouse embryos called vitrification [39].

Freezing of embryos may help in avoiding multiple pregnancy, increasing cumulative pregnancy rate, and preventing ovarian hyperstimulation syndrome. Cryopreservation of embryos seems to be advantageous from the economical point of view because a cycle of cryopreserved embryo transfer costs about one fifth that of a conventional cycle of in vitro fertilization [40].

Embryos can be cryopreserved by using a slow-freezing protocol or vitrification. The slow-freezing method provides a slow decrease in temperature (0.1–0.3 C° /min) after exposure of embryos to low concentrations of cryoprotectants. The most used is the cryoprotectant propanediol, which shows higher permeability and is less toxic than DMSO. In the standard protocol, 1,2-propanediol is used in combination with serum and sucrose.

Vitrification is a process of freezing that prevents intracellular ice formation through the use of high concentrations of cryoprotectants and extremely high cooling rates (15 000–30 000°C/min). Vitrification is, however, still an experimental technique that could be burdened by a potential toxicity of cryoprotectants used in high doses. The use of new devices, which further increase the cooling rate, seems to correlate with good clinical results [40]. The increase in cooling rate can be achieved through a reduction in the volume of vitrification solution, which also has the advantage of reducing the risk of formation of ice crystals. The most recently introduced method of vitrification, which uses minimum volumes of vitrification solution is the Cryotop, which achieves good results with a survival rate of 90%–100% [41].

As regards the clinical efficiency of cryopreservation of embryos, in 2005 in Europe a total of 72 347 cycles of thawing and 70 150 frozen embryo transfer cycles were performed, which led to 13 719 pregnancies [42]. The overall rate of pregnancy for thawing and transfer was 19% and 19.6%, respectively. The percentage of deliveries for thawing varies greatly among countries: Italy, 7.9%; Spain, 7.2%; U.K., 15.9%; and Sweden, 15.4%.

U.S. data published by the CDC for 2006 [43] appear significantly better than those in Europe. In particular, in the U.S., where 121 000 transfer cycles of patients' own frozen embryos were made, the percentage of live births per transfer was 28.9%. The same parameter evaluated in transfer cycles of fresh embryo is 35.4%. The transfer cycles of frozen embryos derived from donor oocytes were a total of 14 000, with a percentage of live births per transfer of 32.1%, compared to 53.7% with the transfer of fresh embryos.

Vitrification seems to be associated with a significantly higher survival rate after thawing compared to slow freezing, as reported in a recent meta-analysis (OR 15.57, 95% CI: 3.68–65.82) [44].

The stage of embryonic development at the moment of cryopreservation has an undoubted impact on its clinical efficiency. Cryopreservation of pronuclear stage embryos (zygotes) has an advantage; in this stage there is not the meiotic spindle and nuclear material, which is poorly organized, and it is protected by the pronuclear membrane. Some features of zygotes, such as the position of the two pronuclei, which should preferably be at the center of the oocyte, the number and distribution of nucleoli, and the characteristics of the cytoplasm, can guide the selection of embryos for cryopreservation. The survival rate for the zygotes is around 70% (56%–93%) and the pregnancy rate per transfer is 17%–31%.

The evaluation of the embryos at early stages of division is simpler than that of the zygote, and is based primarily on the degree of fragmentation and distribution of the fragments. An embryo of good quality is made up of four cells on day 2 and six to eight cells on day 3. Fragmentation should be less than 15% and should not be present in multinuclear blastomeres. The survival rate of embryos in this stage after thawing is about 70% (11%–93%) and the pregnancy rate per transfer does not exceed 20%. The potential for implantation of frozen embryos in an early stage of division is closely related to the survival rate of blastomeres.

The data in the literature appear to be controversial; however, the freezing of embryos at a multicellular stage allows a more accurate selection if compared to the freezing of the zygote. The best results are obtained with the freezing of eight-cell embryos. Intracytoplasmic spermatozoon injection seems to have a negative impact on the freezing of embryos in the early stages, probably due to damage to the zona pellucida. However, in both stages of development, it seems to be advisable to thaw the embryos a few hours before the transfer in order to observe the dynamic parameters of the embryo after thawing and make an additional selection. Reports in the literature of the overall percentage of live births after freezing of zygotes and embryos at the early stage vary from 3.1% to 3.8% to 7% in different series for zygotes and 3.4% to 6% in the early stages of division.

Cryopreservation of the blastocyst has several advantages, therefore it is currently practiced in many centers. The extended duration of in vitro culture allows a better selection of embryos; the blastocyst is also easier to freeze because of the higher ratio of nucleus/cytoplasm. The higher number of cells allows for survival of the embryo in the event of partial cell damage. Glycerol is one of the most suitable cryoprotectants for freezing of the blastocyst.

The freezing of the blastocyst is associated with embryo implantation rates to approximately two times greater than that observed for embryos at an early stage and with 11.3% of live births (39 children out of 278 embryos transferred). The success rates of freezing of blastocysts vary considerably in different series, however, especially in relation to the use of different methods of embryo culture [45].

Although embryos can, theoretically, be cryopreserved for an indefinite time, there are still doubts about what is the maximum period of freezing without compromising success rates. In the literature, there are examples of births after cryopreservation of embryos for several years. Quintans et al. published a report of the birth of a healthy baby after transfer of four embryos that were cryopreserved for 8.9 years to the uterus of a recipient patient aged 43 years [46]. Similarly, Lopez and colleagues report the birth of a healthy baby after transfer to the uterus of three embryos that had been cryopreserved for 13 years [47].

The impact of the duration of freezing on embryo survival and the percentage of implantation and pregnancy rates were recently estimated from 11 768 frozen embryos through a retrospective study [48]. The study includes patients with donors and recipients who undergo at least one embryo thaw cycle between 1986 and 2007. The duration of freezing (ranging from 30 to 5665 days) was not found to be correlated significantly with the survival rate of embryos, both for the frozen embryos at the zygote stage and for those cryopreserved at the multicellular stage. The rate of clinical pregnancy, abortion, and planting, "as the percentage of live births were not, likewise, related to the duration of freezing" (Tables 10.4 and 10.5) [48].

Frydman et al. [49] published the first descriptive study on obstetric and perinatal results of 50 pregnancies after embryo cryopreservation. This study was performed over a two-year period. One pregnancy was terminated at 22 weeks' gestation for a severe fetal malformation, one delivery was premature, and a high incidence of breech presentation (12%) in singleton pregnancies occurred.

Table 10.4. Characteristics for in vitro fertilization patients in cycles of embryo cryopreservation

Variable	All cycles	ZG*-only stage	CLE**-only stage
Freeze cycles			
N	1553	968	435
Patient's age (years)	34.0 ± 4.0	34.1 ± 3.8	34.0 ± 4.5
Embryos frozen	6.2 ± 4.5	6.0 ± 5.0	5.9 ± 3.1
Thaw cycles			
N	1927	1236	537
Patient's age (years)	34.8 ± 4.1	34.8 ± 3.9	34.7 ± 4.4
Storage time (days)	420.2 ± 497.9	419.4 ± 496.2	400.5 ± 495.0
Viable embryos	2.97 ± 1.6	2.9 ± 1.6	3.1 ± 1.5
Survival proportion	0.71 ± 0.29	0.71 ± 0.29	0.73 ± 0.28
Transfer cycles			
N	1709	1090	474
Embryos transferred	2.92 ± 1.1	2.9 ± 1.2	2.9 ± 1.0
Live birth rate (%)	16.9	16.9	15.4
Clinical pregnancy rate (%)	21.8	22.6	18.9
Other clinical outcomes			
Miscarriage rate (%)	23.9 (n = 373)	25.5 (n = 247)	22.2 (n = 90)
Implantation rate (%)	10.2 (n = 5217)	10.1 (n = 3305)	10.0 (n = 1459)

* ZG, zygote;** CLE, cleavage stage embryos. (Riggs et al., 2008 [48].)

Table 10.5. Live birth rates in ZG*-only and CLE**-only groups, stratified by length of storage time of cryopreserved embryos, in in vitro fertilization cycles and oocyte donation cycles

	IVF			Oocyte donation		
Length of storage time (days)	CLE** only	ZG* only	P	CLE** only	ZG*only	P
30–100	14.2 (21/148)	18.8 (57/304)	0.229	22.8 (13/57)	10.8 (6/57)	0.079
101–365	16.3 (29/178)	13.9 (60/432)	0.445	26.8 (26/97)	21.6 (11/51)	0.485
366–730	16.4 (9/55)	15.9 (24/151)	0.935	24.3 (9/37)	25.0 (5/20)	0.955
731–1095	15.3 (9/59)	18.8 (22/117)	0.560.	31.6 (6/19)	25.0 (2/8)	0.732
> 1095	24.4 (21/86)	24.4 (21/86)	0.245	16.7 (4/24)	11.8 (2/17)	0.662

* ZG, zygote;** CLE, cleavage stage embryos. (Riggs et al., 2008 [48].)

A retrospective study [50] considered 232 babies conceived from cryopreserved embryos between 1985 and 1991 and an equivalent number of babies born after standard IVF programs used as controls. In the two groups, mean gestational age, birth weight, and perinatal mortality rates were similar, and major malformations were found to be even lower in the cryopreserved group than in the control group. It is possible that a "filtering" effect occurred by not counting "chemical" pregnancies and early spontaneous abortions as a sign of congenital abnormality.

An observational study was performed by Heijnsbroek et al. [51] on 30 pregnancies, following transfer of frozen-thawed embryos. All babies presented an over-average birth weight (45% of singletons weighing more than the 75th percentile); no major congenital anomalies except for two minor malformations (clubfeet and an undescended testicle), a low prematurity rate (4%), and a high-breech presentation rate (14%) were found in singleton pregnancies as well.

Sutcliffe et al. [52] compared a group of 91 children (68 singletons, 20 twins, and 3 triplets) conceived after cryopreservation with a control group of 83 normally conceived children between 1989 and 1994. In the study group, a higher incidence of perinatal problems was noted, such as longer periods spent in special care baby units and the presence of three children with major congenital abnormalities. However, the frequency of minor and major congenital anomalies was similar between the two groups (31.9% versus 21.7% and 3.3% versus 2.4%, respectively), and the relative risk in the cryopreserved embryo group compared with the control group was 1.7 for minor congenital anomalies and 1.4 for major congenital anomalies. The minor congenital malformations included nevi and hemangiomas in both groups; the major congenital anomalies were Down's syndrome, Beckwith–Wiedemann syndrome, and hypophosphatemic rickets in the cryopreserved embryos, and hydronephrosis and gastroschisis in the controls (Table 10.6).

Table 10.6. Outcomes of infants born after embryo cryopreservation and infants naturally conceived

	Cryopreserved embryo			Controls
	Singleton (n = 68)	**Multiple birth (n = 23)**	**Total (n = 91)**	**(n = 83)**
Mean (SD) birth weight (g)	328.6 (672.8)+++	2649.7 (649.2)	3122.6 (721.4) ***	3538.4 (553.4)
Mean (SD) gestational age (weeks)	38.59 (2.36)++	37.09 (1.62)	38.38 (2.33)***	39.67 (1.96)
Mode of delivery				
Vaginal	34	10	4	72
Cesarean section	34	13	47***	11
SCBU admissions	11	2	13	5
• Hyaline membrane disease	1	0	1	0
• Transient tachypnea	2	1	3	2
• Hypothermia (temperature < 36°C)	4	0	4	0
• Failure to feed	1	1	2	1
• Vomiting	1	0	1	0
• Small for gestational age	2	0	2	2
Boys/girls	39/29	11/12	50/41	40/43
Social class (%)				
0 (unemployed)			1 (1.1)	2 (2.4)
1			21 (23.1)	29 (34.9)
2			31 (34.1)	34 (41.0)
3			28 (30.8)	16 (19.3)
4			10 (11.0)	2 (2.4)

Levels of significance: total (cryopreserved embryo) vs. controls:
***, $P < 0.001$; singleton (cryopreserved embryo) vs. multiple births (cryopreserved embryo):
+++, $P < 0.001$ and
++, $P < 0.01$; SCBU, special care baby unit. (Sutcliffe et al., 1995 [52].)

Table 10.7. Perinatal outcomes of 82 children aged one- to nine years old conceived from cryopreserved embryos

Pregnancies	Singleton (75)	Twin (7)	Total (82)
Premature deliveries			
<37 wa	14.7 (11)	85.7 (6)	20.7 (17)
36 wa	8.0 (6)	28.6 (2)	9.8 (8)
<31 wa	1.3 (1)	0 (0)	1.2 (1)
Children (n)	75	14	89
SFGA (<10th percentile)	8.0 (6)	28.6 (4)	11.2 (10)
Weight			
<2500 g	9.3 (7)	64.3 (9)	18.0 (16)
<1500 g	2.7 (2)	0 (0)	1.1 (1)
Perinatal mortality	1.3 (1)	0 (0)	1.1 (1)

Wa, weeks of amenorrhoea; SFGA, small for gestational age. (Olivennes et al., 1996) [53].)

The same results were confirmed by a study of 89 children born after transfer of cryopreserved-thawed embryos without controls [53]. This study showed a high incidence of multiple births and premature births (14.7% for singleton pregnancies and 85.7% for twin pregnancies), whereas the malformation rate (1.1% with only one child with a short ureter) was comparable to that observed in the general population, even considering the two therapeutic abortions that occurred for Down's syndrome and polymalformation (3.4%) (Table 10.7).

Wennerholm et al. [54] evaluated the obstetric and neonatal outcomes in 270 children (163 singleton pregnancies, 98 bigeminy, 9 triplets) born from pregnancies obtained after cryopreservation of embryos, compared with two control groups made up of those born following the application of fresh techniques and spontaneous pregnancies. The main variables examined, such as the duration of gestation, birth weight, and the incidence of malformations and perinatal mortality, were comparable in the three study groups. In particular, the incidence of major malformations in the study group was 2.7%, which is comparable to that of the general Swedish population (Tables 10.8 and 10.9).

Kallen et al. [55] published results concerning a series of 1055 children born from frozen embryos in 890 deliveries. The data obtained largely confirm what has already been observed in previous studies; no significant differences in the risk of preterm delivery, low birth weight, and infant mortality were observed among the different techniques of IVF. The risk of preterm delivery, low birth weight, and low Apgar score shown, however, tends to be lower among children born after embryo freezing. The incidence of multiple pregnancy is less frequent in cycles of embryo cryopreservation, both in association with the use of standard IVF (18.1%) and in combination with ICSI (21.8%), compared with fresh IVF cycles (24.4 %) (Table 10.10) [55].

The finding of differences in birth weight among newborns from different IVF techniques has led Shih and coworkers to deepen the study of factors associated with low birth weight as a result of IVF techniques [56]. The mean birth weight was significantly lower in the case of fresh techniques (IVF, ICSI, GIFT) if compared to embryo freezing. In addition, the rate of preterm birth and low birth weight were lower in the thawing cycles. Several explanations have been suggested to justify these figures: the freezing may allow better selection of embryos and exclusively promote the survival of the most suitable embryos; moreover, the cryoprotectants, according to some authors, could have a protective effect with respect to imprinting defects. Although several hypotheses seem plausible, it can be stated that the low birth weight of the singletons born by ART is not attributable to individual laboratory procedures involved in IVF and ICSI, but rather to ovarian stimulation or, more likely, to anesthesia or oocyte pick-up, which occur only in fresh cycles [56].

Table 10.8. Weight at birth in the three groups (cryopreserved embryos, standard in vitro fertilization, spontaneous)

	Cryopreserved		Standard IVF		Spontaneous	
	n	%	n	%	n	%
Singleton	(n = 160)		(n = 160)		(n = 160)	
>2500 g	152	95.0	148	92.5	154	96.3
1000–2499 g	7	4.4	12	7.5	6	3.7
<1000 g	1	0.6	0	0	0	0
SGA<=22%	7	4.4	9	5.6	6	3.7
Mean birth weight +/– SD	3476+/–616		3407+/–637		3459+/–523	
Twin:	(n = 98)		(n = 98)		(n = 98)	
>2500 g	58	59.2	56	57.1	67	68.4
1000–2499 g	40	40.8	38	38.8	28	28.6
<1000 g	0	0	4	4.1	3	3.1
SGA<=22%	21	21.4	20	20.4	21	21.4
Mean birth weight +/– SD	2574+/–560		2441+/–666a		2673+/–647b	

IVF, in vitro fertilization; SGA, small for gestational age (<=2SD) according to the Swedish reference values for birth weight (Marsal et al, 1996); a versus b: P = 0.014, unpaired t-test. (Wennerholm et al., 1997 [54].)

Table 10.9. Children in the three groups (cryopreserved embryos, standard in vitro fertilization, spontaneous) with major malformations

	Cryopreserved (n = 258) N = 7 (2.7 %)	Standard IVF (n = 258) N = 8 (3.1%)	Spontaneous (n = 258) N = 8 (3.1%)
Major malformations	Trisomy 13	Trisomy 21	Achondroplasia
	Trisomy 21	Translocation	VSD
	Trisomy 21	A	VSD, ASD
	VSD	VSD	ASD
	ASD	VSD	ASD
	Cleft palate	ASD	Aplasia of one
	Hypospadia	ASD	ear
	Limb	Hypospadia	Onfalocele
	malformation	Onfalocele	

IVF, in vitro fertilization; VSD, ventricular septal defect; ASD, atrial septal defect; A, unbalanced translocation. (Wennerholm et al., 1997 [54].)

Table 10.10. Preterm birth (<37 wk), low birth weight (<2500 g), and Apgar score (<7 at 5 min) among singletons in fresh in vitro fertilization cycles, frozen embryo in vitro fertilization cycles, fresh intracytoplasmic spermatozoon injection cycles, frozen embryo intracytoplasmic spermatozoon injection cycles

IVF method	Preterm birth		Low birth weight		Low Apgar score	
	OR	95% CI	OR	95% CI	OR	95% CI
Standard fresh IVF	1.00	Reference	1.0	Reference	1.0	Reference
Standard frozen IVF	0.69	0.50–0.95	0.49	0.02–0.75	1.05	0.73–1.50
Fresh ICSI	0.96	0.80–1.15	0.98	0.79–1.19	1.05	0.73–1.50
Frozen ICSI	0.97	0.55–1.38	0.99	0.59–1.66	0.98	0.42–2.31

IVF, in vitro fertilization; ICSI, intracytoplasmic spermatozoon injection.
Note: odds ratios with 95% CIs are adjusted for year of birth, maternal age, parity, smoking, and years of involuntary childlessness. (With permission from Kallen et al., 2005 [55].)

A recent Belgian prospective cohort study found similar results in terms of outcomes among babies born after embryo freezing and those born after the application of fresh techniques. In particular, individuals born from cryopreservation showed a trend toward a higher mean birth weight, while the rates of low birth weight and multiple pregnancies were comparable in the two groups. No statistically significant differences were found between the incidence of new chromosomal abnormalities in the study group (3.2%) and control group (1.7%). The major malformations were significantly higher in children born after cryopreservation of embryos (6.4%) than those born from fresh techniques (3.4%). A further comparison was made within the group of offspring of cryopreservation, between the outcomes in children born from embryos fertilized through IVF or through ICSI. The results in the two groups were comparable, except that the rate of major malformations appeared higher in the group of children born from cryopreserved embryos after ICSI (Tables 10.11 and 10.12) [57].

A systematic review of all studies performed on neonatal outcomes and characteristics of children born after embryo, blastocyst, and oocyte freezing from 1984 to 2008 was recently published by Wennerholm et al. [33]. The 21 studies related to the freezing of embryos at an early stage showed, overall, obstetric outcomes assessed in terms of mean birth weight and incidence of preterm delivery that were better, or at least comparable, in children born after freezing than in children born from IVF fresh cycles.

The rate of preterm birth for singleton pregnancies ranged from 9.2% to 12% in the cycles of embryo cryopreservation and from 7.4% to 14% in fresh pregnancies, while the rate of low birth weight was from 6.2% to 10.5% among children born after cryopreservation and 7.2% to 13.6% among those born after fresh cycles. The perinatal mortality was reported in only two studies and was similar among children born after embryo freezing and after fresh cycles. The incidence of congenital malformations varied from 0.7% to 8.6% in the cycles of embryo cryopreservation, and from 0.7% to 8.7% in the fresh cycles. The physical and mental development in the first two years of life and the incidence of chronic cancer showed no significant differences between the progeny born after cryopreservation and spontaneous pregnancies. Overall, the data regarding children born from frozen embryos by slow freezing appear reassuring; however, further and more extensive follow-up studies are necessary [33].

Pinborg et al. [58] recently published data on the singletons born from embryo cryopreservation in Denmark in the period between 1995 and 2006, as taken from national registers. The study group consisted of 957 children born in singleton pregnancies achieved with cryopreservation of embryos, and the two control groups were formed by all children born from IVF or ICSI in the same period and a random sample of births in singleton spontaneous pregnancies, respectively. The mean birth weight was higher for infants born after cryopreservation (3578 g, SD 625) than those born by fresh techniques (average weight: 3373 g, SD 648) and those born by natural conception (average weight: 3537 g, SD 572). In the study group a lower incidence of low birth weight (<2500 g) and

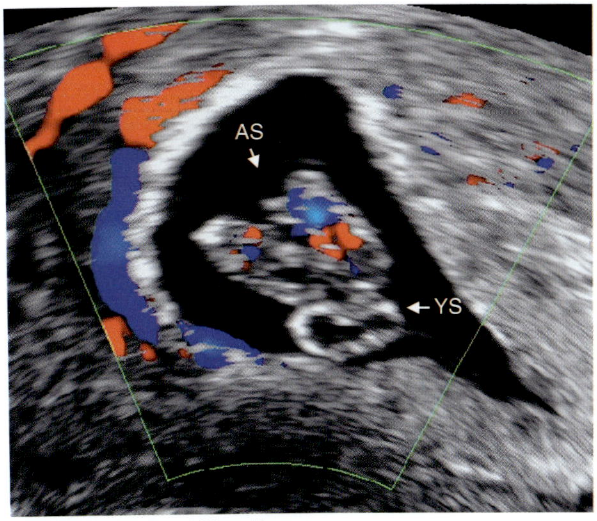

AS, amniotic sac; YS, yolk sac.

Figure 3.4. Ultrasound findings of a monochorionic and monoamniotic pregnancy: one gestational sac, one amniotic sac, one yolk sac, and two embryos.

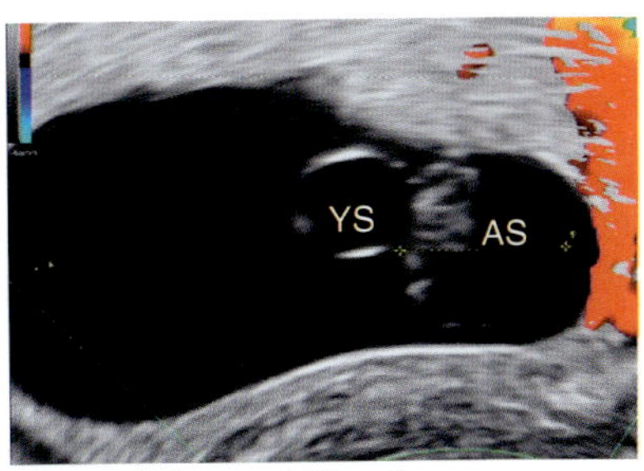

AS, amniotic sac; YS, yolk sac.

Figure 3.5. Ultrasound features associated with a higher likelihood of miscarriage: yolk sac and amniotic sac without a viable embryo.

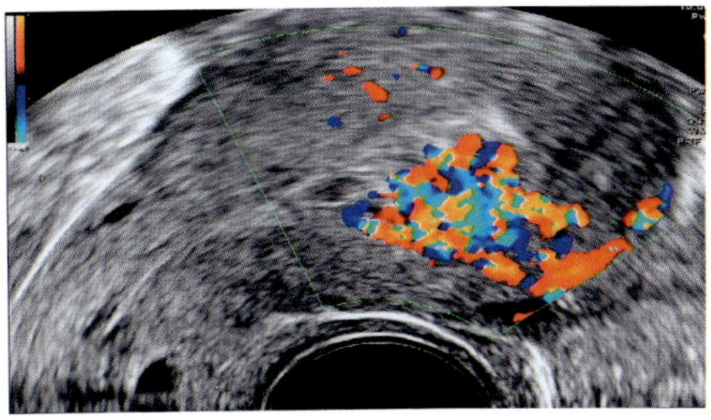

Figure 3.7. Ultrasound appearance of retained products of conception: high vascularity on Doppler examination.

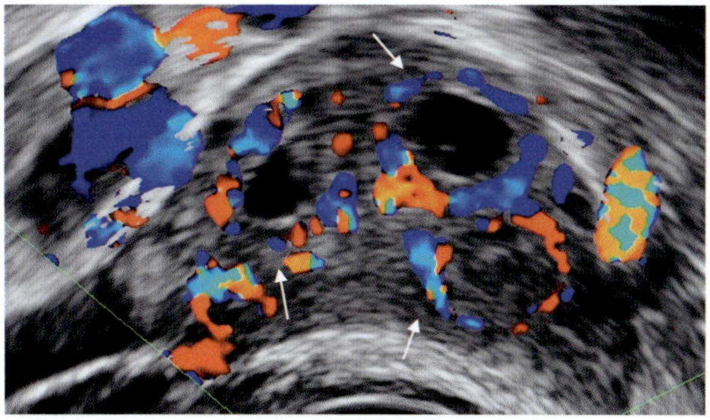

Figure 3.11. Doppler assessment demonstrates multiple "rings of fire" (arrows) surrounding four corpus lutea in an ovary.

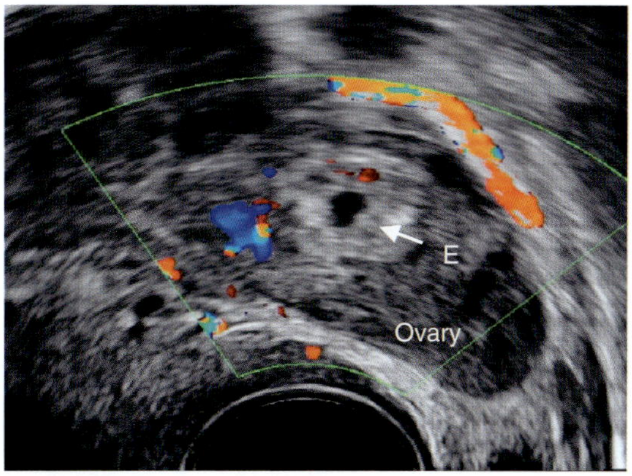

Figure 3.12. Ultrasound features of non-tubal ectopic pregnancy: ovarian ectopic.

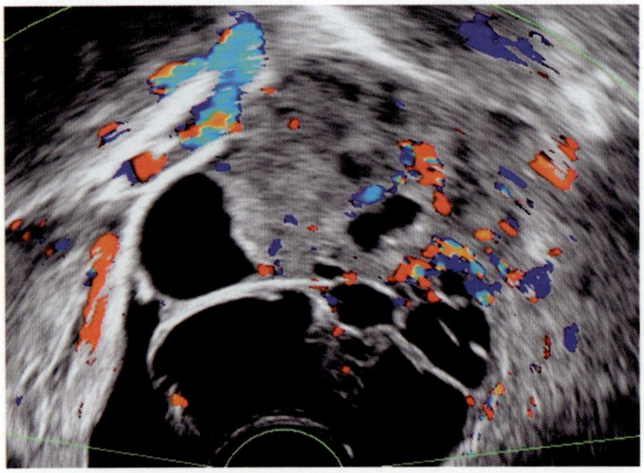

Figure 3.18. Ultrasound appearance of a malignant ovarian tumor.

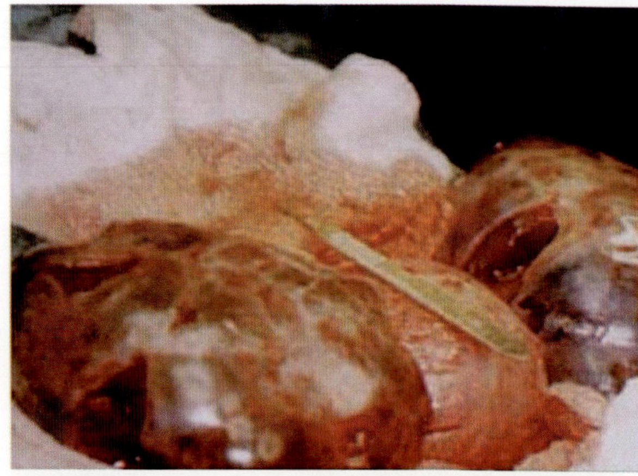

Figure 4.1. Hyperstimulated ovaries. (Reproduced with permission from Serour G. (In: Gerris J, Delvigne A, Olivennes F, eds. *Ovarian Hyperstimulation Syndrome*. London, UK: Informa Press, 2006.)

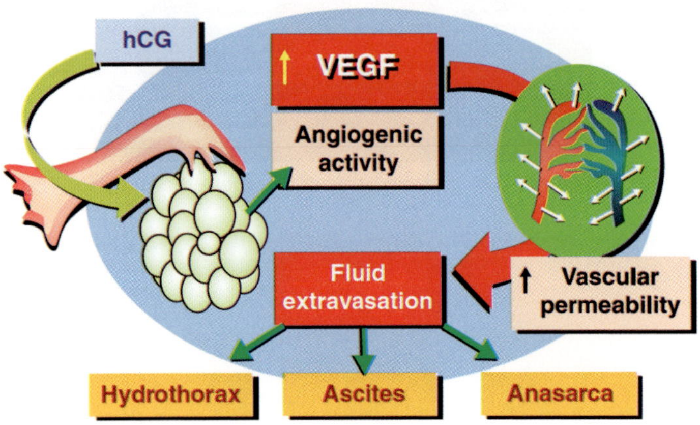

Figure 4.7. Diagrammatic representation of increased vascular permeability and ascites formation in ovarian hyperstimulation syndrome. (Reproduced with permission from Rizk B, ed. *Ultrasonography in Reproductive Medicine and Infertility*. Cambridge, UK: Cambridge University Press, 2010; 306.)

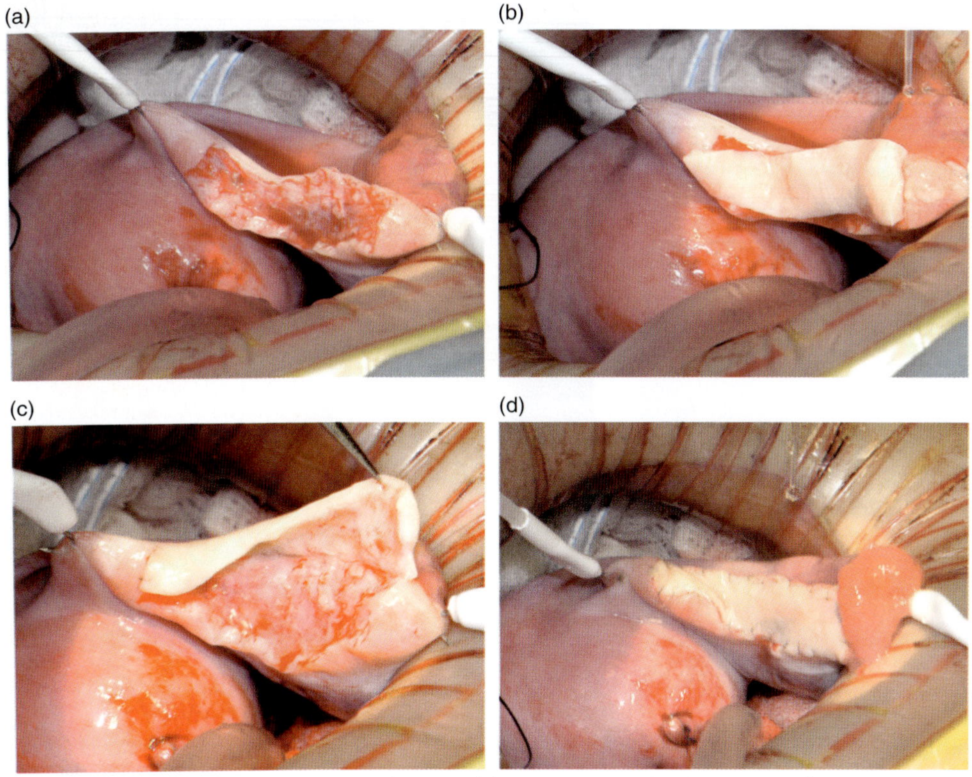

Figure 12.1. (a): the depleted "menopausal" cortex of the recipient ovary has been removed, exposing the medulla; (b): the slice of donor ovarian tissue is placed on top of the recipient medulla; (c): the donor cortical slice is being sutured microsurgically to the medulla of the recipient with 9–0 nylon interrupted sutures after good hemostasis is secured; (d): the completed ovarian tissue transplant.

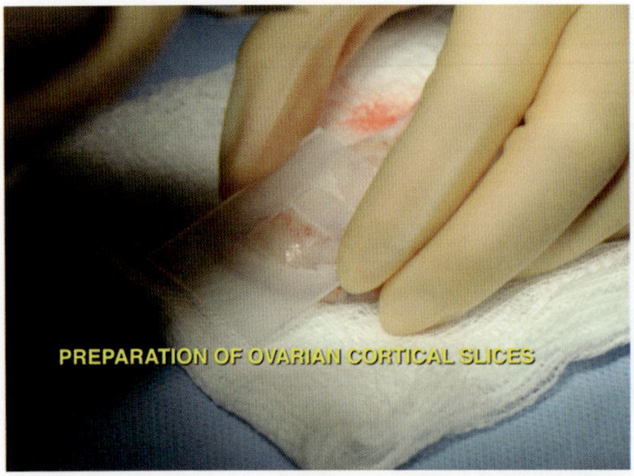

Figure 12.2. "Cryotissue" device (Kitazato, Japan), used to prepare ultrathin slices of cortex for vitrification.

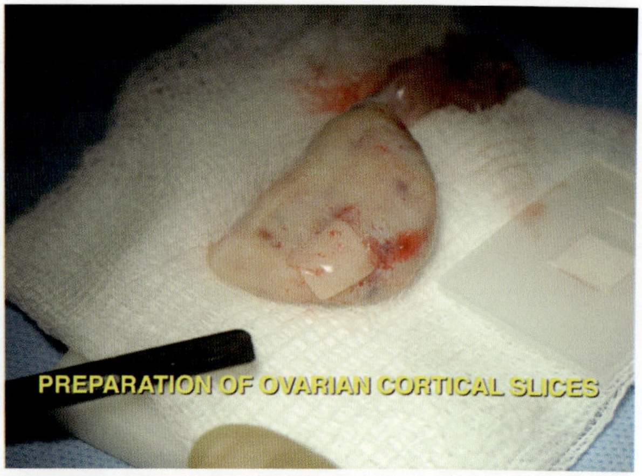

Figure 12.3. Thin slice of ovarian cortex prepared for cryopreservation.

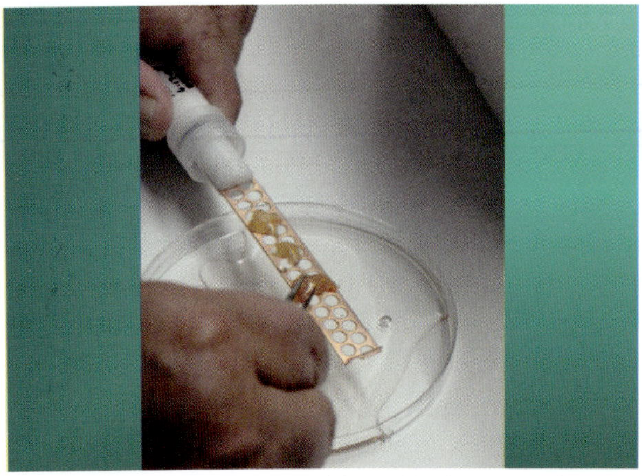

Figure 12.4. Thin ovarian cortical slices placed onto a perforated copper grid.

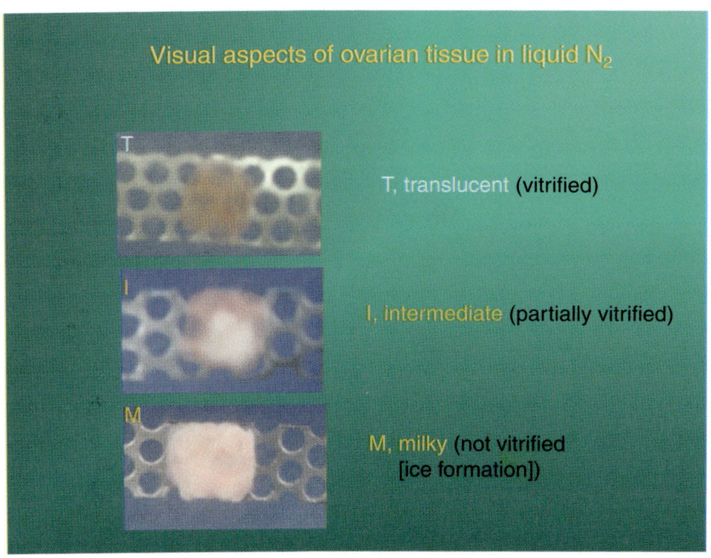

Figure 12.5. The tissue at the top had 40% cryoprotectant and was safely vitrified. The tissue at the bottom had 30% cryoprotectant and was destroyed by freezing. The tissue in the middle was vitrified in 35% cryoprotectant.

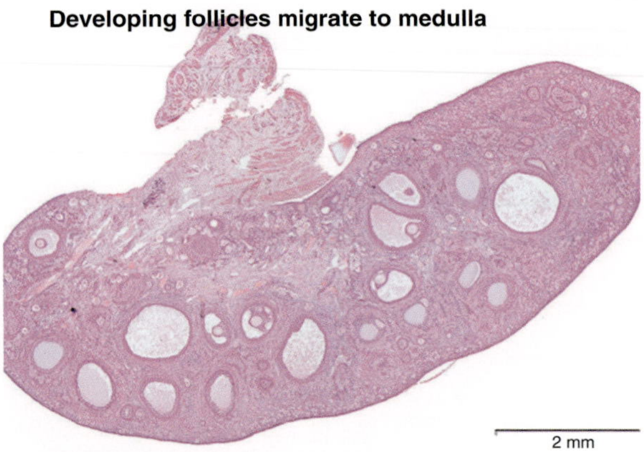

Figure 12.6. All of the resting primordial follicles are located in the fibrous outer cortex. In order to develop over four months into primary and secondary, and finally mature follicles, they must migrate into the softer medulla.

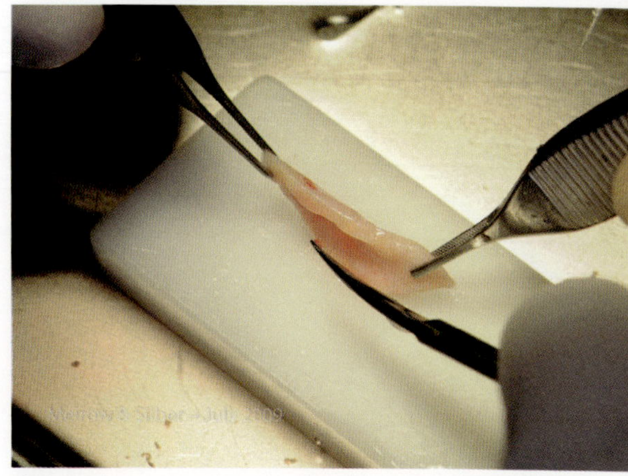

Figure 12.7. 1 mm thin slice of ovarian cortex ready for transplantation.

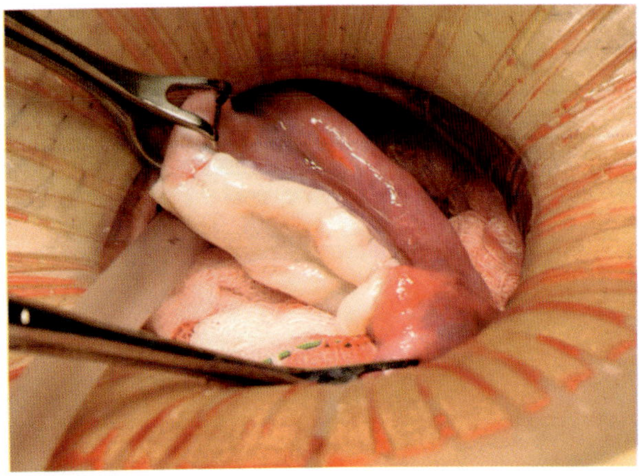

Figure 12.8. Completed first fresh ovarian tissue transplant.

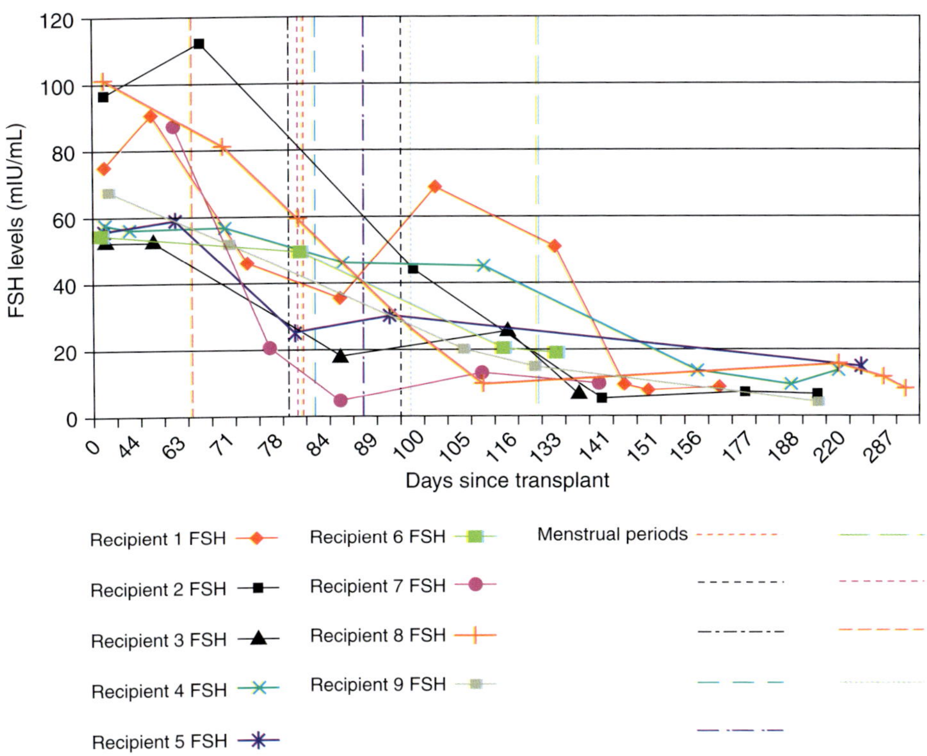

Figure 12.9. Graph showing the return of menstrual cycling and decline of follicle stimulating hormone (FSH) levels in the first nine cases of fresh ovarian transplantation.

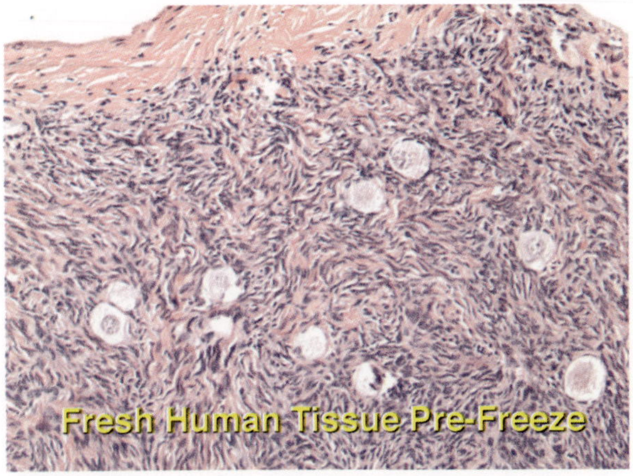

Figure 12.10. This figure and Figure 12.11 show no difference between fresh ovarian tissue and frozen (vitrification) ovarian tissue.

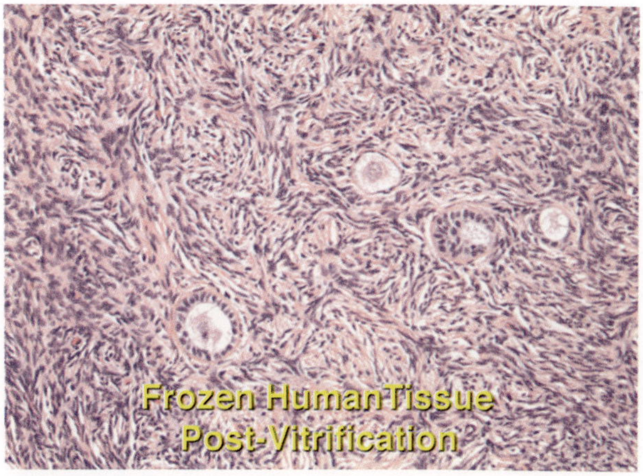

Figure 12.11. This figure and Figure 12.10 show no difference between fresh ovarian tissue and frozen ovarian tissue using vitrification.

Table 10.11. Chromosome abnormalities pre- and postnatally in frozen embryo intracytoplasmic spermatozoon injection cycles versus frozen embryo in vitro fertilization cycles and fresh intracytoplasmic spermatozoon injection cycles

	ICSI			IVF	
	Cryo ICSI N (%)	Fresh ICSI N (%)	OR (95% CI) cryo ICSI versus fresh ICSI	Cryo IVF N (%)	OR (95% CI) cryo ICSI versus cryo IVF
Prenatal	N = 200	N = 1586		N = 72	
De novo	7 (3.5)	25 (1.5)	2.27 (0.97–5.31)	1(1.4)	2.51 (0.30–20.71)
Gender-related		10			
Klinefelter	3				
Autosomal numerical		8			
Trisomy 18					
Trisomy 21	3				
Autosomal structural	1	7			
Inherited	1 (0.5)	22 (1.4)			0.35 (0.02–5.62)
Prenatal total	8 (4)	47 (2.9)			1.42 (0.29–6.84)
Postnatal	N = 81	N = 338			
De novo	2	7			
Gender-related		2			
Autosomal numerical		3			
Trisomy 21	1				
Autosomal structural	1	2			
Inherited	1	6			
Postnatal total	3 (3.7)	13 (3.8)			3.60 (0.18–71.21)
Overall (prenatal and postnatal anomalies in tested group)	N = 281	N = 1924			
De novo	9 (3.2)	32(1.7)			3.68 (0.46–29.33)
Total	11 (3.9)	60(3.1)			2.24 (0.49–10.28)

ICSI, intracytoplasmic spermatozoon injection; IVF, in vitro fertilization; cryo, cryopreserved. (Belva et al., 2008 [57].)

preterm delivery (between 34 and 37 weeks) than those born to other techniques of IVF were also detected. Comparable data were obtained between children born to cryopreservation and children born from natural conception. However, the perinatal mortality was double in the study group (1.6%) than that of those born naturally (0.8%); an increase in the rate of severe prematurity (<34 weeks) and admission to neonatal intensive care unit were also detected. There were no statistically significant differences among the three study groups in relation to congenital malformations, neurological sequelae, cancer, and diseases related to imprinting (Table 10.13) [58].

Taken together, information derived from the various studies are in part reassuring but partly points toward further investigations to ascertain whether freezing in itself may be a potential hazard to children's health.

Table 10.12. Birth characteristics of children born after transfer of cryopreserved and fresh embryos

	ICSI					IVF				
	Cryo ICSI		Fresh ICSI		P	Cryo IVF		Fresh IVF		P
	N	Mean (SD)	N	Mean (SD)		N	Mean (SD)	N	Mean (SD)	
Mean birth weight										
Total group	539	3067.9 (666.6)	2799	2806.7 (719.1)	<0.001	384	3023.8 (689.1)	2920	2765.3 (725.0)	<0.001
Singletons	381	3301.2 (571.9)	1476	3224.3 (581.9)	0.059	281	3269.7 (535.2)	1523	3176.4 (582.6)	0.046
Twins	155	2505.3 (533.2)	1211	2394.5 (522.0)	0.013	98	2365.6 (623.7)	1251	47.7 (3.7)	0.776

ICSI, intracytoplasmic spermatozoon injection; IVF, in vitro fertilization; cryo, cryopreserved. (With permission from Belva et al., 2008 [57].)

Table 10.13. Odds ratios (95% CI) for different outcomes in the different groups (frozen embryo intracytoplasmic spermatozoon injection cycles, frozen embryo in vitro fertilization cycles, fresh in vitro fertilization cycles, fresh intracytoplasmic spermatozoon injection cycles, spontaneous pregnancies)

Outcome measure*	Cryo vs. fresh	Cryo vs. non-ART	IVF cryo vs. fresh	ICSI cryo vs. fresh	Fresh ICSI vs. IVF
LBW	0.63 (0.45–0.87)	1.03 (0.88–1.28)	0.67 (0.47–0.98)	0.47 (0.22–1.01)	0.87 (0.73–1.03)
VLBW	0.66 (0.33–1.29)	1.119 (0.79–1.80)	0.67 (0.31–1.44)	0.36 (0.05–2.64)	0.71 (0.49–1.02)
PTB	0.70 (0.53–0.92)	1.12 (0.96–1.32)	0.68 (0.49–0.95)	0.66 (0.36–1.19)	0.75 (0.49–1.02)
VPTB	0.81 (0.52–1.27)	1.35 (1.02–1.65)	0.72 (0.42–1.25)	0.89 (0.36–2.23)	0.70 (0.54–0.92)
NICU	0.89 (0.72–1.09)	1.30 (1.02–1.65)	0.91 (0.71–1.16)	0.83 (0.54–1.27)	0.91 (0.80–1.03)
Malformations, all	0.92 (0.71–1.19)	0.83 (0.73–1.31)	0.89 (0.65–1.22)	0.91 (0.54–1.51)	1.0 (0.86–1.18)
Stillbirth + perinatal mortality	0.83 (0.36–1.90)	1.69 (0.73–1.31)	0.75 (0.27–2.08)	0.96 (0.58–1.56)	0.86 (0.52–1.40)

* multiple logistic regression analyses were performed with adjustment for maternal age and parity, and childhood year of birth and gender; cryo, cryopreserved; IVF, in vitro fertilization; ICSI, intracytoplasmic spermatozoon injection; ART, assisted reproductive technology; LBW, low birth weight (< 2500 g); VLBW, very low birth weight (<1500 g); PTB, preterm birth (<37 wk); VTPB, very preterm birth (<34 wk); NICU, neonatal intensive care units. (Pinborg et al., 2010 [58].)

Conclusion

Cryopreservation of oocytes and embryos has reached greater importance in recent years, due to the increasing request for fertility preservation in patients at risk of premature ovarian failure and with the wish to postpone pregnancy. A growing proportion of the children born after ART are born after cryopreservation cycles (25% worldwide in 2004) [59].

The most important concerns of all ART are the safety of the patients and the birth of healthy babies, which particularly must be evaluated in cryopreservation cycles where the effect of freezing and thawing represent a potential source of additional damage. Slow-freezing embryo cryopreservation has been performed for 25 years and can be considered a well-founded technique; data concerning pregnancy and postnatal outcomes after embryo cryopreservation are numerous and appear reassuring. In some reports outcomes obtained in embryo cryopreservation cycles seem to be even better in terms of birth weights and preterm births if compared with fresh IVF/ICSI cycles. These surprising results cannot be explained easily, but there has been an argument for an adverse effect of therapy for ovarian stimulation in fresh cycle IVF and a better quality of embryos surviving freezing and thawing.

Oocyte cryopreservation is still considered an experimental technique, although the pregnancy rates achieved with the technique are comparable with those registered after embryo cryopreservation, and the number of centers offering oocyte freezing is rapidly expanding. In the current situation of conservative attitudes toward oocyte cryopreservation, the evaluation of the outcomes of children born after oocyte cryopreservation is of crucial importance in order to include oocyte cryopreservation in the well-established ARTs, particularly for women diagnosed with malignancy and requiring cytotoxic therapy.

Data reported are encouraging because they refer to a large series and do not show an increase in congenital malformation in children born after oocyte cryopreservation if compared with naturally conceived infants. The creation of a registry of oocyte cryopreservation could be an efficient method to assure the safest development of the technology.

References

1. Chen C. Pregnancy after human oocyte cryopreservation. *Lancet* 1986; **1**: 884–886.
2. Porcu E, Fabbri R, Seracchioli R, et al. Birth of a healthy female after intracytoplasmic sperm injection of cryopreserved human oocytes. *Fertil Steril* 1997; **68**: 724–726.
3. Allan J. Re: case report: Pregnancy from intracytoplasmic injection of a frozen-thawed oocyte. *Aust N Z J Obstet Gynaecol* 2004; **44**: 588.
4. Antinori S, Dani G, Selman HA, et al. Pregnancies after sperm injection into cryopreserved human oocytes. *Hum Reprod* 1998; **13**: 157–158.
5. Borini A, Bonu MA, Coticchio, et al. Pregnancies and births after oocyte cryopreservation. *Fertil Steril* 2004; **82**: 601–605.
6. Borini A, Lagalla C, Bonu MA, et al. Cumulative pregnancy rates resulting from the use of fresh and frozen oocytes: 7 years' experience. *Reprod Biomed Online* 2006; **12**: 481–486.
7. Chen SU, Lien YR, Tsai YY, et al. Successful pregnancy occurred from slowly freezing human oocytes using the regime of 1.5 mol/l 1,2-propanediol with 0.3 mol/l sucrose. *Hum Reprod* 2002; **17**: 1412–1413.
8. Huttelova R, Becvarova V, Brachtlova T. More successful oocyte freezing. *J Assist Reprod Genet* 2003; **20**: 293.
9. Miller KA, Elkind-Hirsch K, Levy B, et al. Pregnancy after cryopreservation of donor oocytes and preimplantation genetic diagnosis of embryos in a patient with ovarian failure. *Fertil Steril* 2004; **82**: 211–214.
10. Notrica J, Kanzepolsky L, Divita A, Neuspiller F, Polak de Fried E. A healthy female born after ICSI of a cryopreserved oocyte and cryopreserved spermatozoa banked prior to radiotherapy in a patient with a seminoma: a case report. *Fertil Steril* 2003; **80**: S149.
11. Porcu E, Fabbri R, Petracchi S, Ciotti PM, Flamingni C. Ongoing pregnancy after intracytoplasmic injection of testicular spermatozoa into cryopreserved human oocytes. *Am J Obstet Gynecol* 1999; **180**: 1044–1045.
12. Porcu E, Fabbri R, Damiano G, et al. Clinical experience and application of oocyte cryopreservation. *Mol Cell Endocrinol* 2000; **169**: 33–37.
13. Porcu E, Fabbri R, Ciotti P, et al. Four healthy children from frozen human oocytes and frozen human sperms. *Fertil Steril* 2001; **76**: S76.
14. Porcu E, Fabbri R, Ciotti P, et al. Oocytes or embryo storage. *Fertil Steril* 2002; **78**: S15.
15. Tucker M, Wright G, Morton P, et al. Preliminary experience with human oocyte cryopreservation using 1,2- propanediol and sucrose. *Hum Reprod* 1996; **11**: 1513–1515.
16. Tucker MJ, Wright G, Morton PC, Massey JB. Birth after cryopreservation of immature oocytes with subsequent in vitro maturation. *Fertil Steril* 1998; **70**: 578–579.
17. Bianchi V, Coticchio G, Distratis V, et al. Differential sucrose concentration during dehydration (0.2 mol/l) and rehydration (0.3 mol/l) increases the implantation rate of frozen human oocytes. *Reprod Biomed Online* 2007; **14**: 64–71.
18. Fabbri R, Porcu E, Marsella T, et al. Human oocyte cryopreservation: new perspectives regarding oocyte survival. *Hum Reprod* 2001; **16**: 411–416.
19. Kuwayama M, Vajta G, Kato O, Leibo SP. Highly efficient vitrification method for cryopreservation of human oocytes. *Reprod Biomed Online* 2005; **11**: 300–308.
20. Lucena E, Bernal DP, Lucena C, et al. Successful ongoing pregnancies after vitrification of oocytes. *Fertil Steril* 2006; **85**: 108–111.

21. Selman H, Angelini A, Barnocchi N, et al. Ongoing pregnancies after vitrification of human oocytes using a combined solution of ethylene glycol and dimethyl sulfoxide. *Fertil Steril* 2006; **86**: 997–1000.

22. Ciotti PM, Porcu E, Notarangelo L et al., Meiotic spindle recovery is faster in vitrification of human oocyte compared to slow freezing. *Fertil Steril* 2009; **91**: 2399–2407.

23. Huang JY, Chen HY, Park JY, Tan SL, Chian RC. Comparison of spindle and chromosome configuration in in vitro- and in vivo-matured mouse oocytes after vitrification. *Fertil Steril* 2008; **90**: 1424–1432.

24. Borini A, Levi Setti PE, Anserini P, et al. Multicenter observational study on slow-cooling oocyte cryopreservation: clinical outcome. *Fertil Steril* 2010; **94**: 1662–1668.

25. Practice Committee of The American Society of Reproductive Medicine 2006; Practice Committee of the Society for Assisted Reproductive Technology. Ovarian tissue and oocyte cryopreservation. *Fertil Steril* 2006; **86**: S142–S147.

26. Bonduelle M, Wennerholm UB, Loft A, et al. A multi-centre cohort study of the physical health of 5-year-old children conceived after intracytoplasmic sperm injection, in vitro fertilization and natural conception. *Hum Reprod* 2005; **20**: 413–419.

27. McDonald SD, Han Z, Mulla S, et al. Preterm birth and low birth weight among in vitro fertilization singletons: a systematic review and meta-analyses. *Eur J Obstet Gynecol Reprod Biol* 2009; **146**: 138–148.

28. Porcu E, Fabbri R, Seracchioli R, et al. Obstetric, perinatal outcome and follow up of children conceived from cryopreserved oocytes. *Fertil Steril* 2000; **74**: S48.

29. Porcu E. Cryopreservation of oocytes: indications, risks and outcomes. *Hum Reprod* 2005; **20**: S50.

30. Borini A, Cattoli M, Mazzone S, et al. Survey of 105 babies born after slow cooling oocyte cryopreservation. *Fertil Steril* 2007; **88**: S13.

31. Noyes N, Porcu E, Borini A. Over 900 oocyte cryopreservation babies born with no apparent increase in congenital anomalies. *Reprod Biomed Online* 2009; **18**: 769–776.

32. Chian RC, Huang JY, Tan SL, et al. Obstetric and perinatal outcome in 200 infants conceived from vitrified oocytes. *Reprod Biomed Online* 2008; **16**: 608–610.

33. Wennerholm UB, Söderström-Anttila V, Bergh C, et al. Children born after cryopreservation of embryos or oocytes: a systematic review of outcome data. *Hum Reprod* 2009; **24**: 2158–2172.

34. Ezcurra D, Rangnow J, Craig M, Schertz J. The Human Oocyte Preservation Experience (HOPE): a phase IV, prospective, multicenter, observational oocyte cryopreservation registry. *Reprod Biol Endocrinol* 2009; **7**: 53.

35. Wilmut I. The effect of cooling rate, warming rate, cryoprotective agent and stage of development on survival of mouse embryos during freezing and thawing. *Life Sci II* 1972; **11**: 1071–1079.

36. Wilmut I. The low temperature preservation of mammalian embryos. *J Reprod Fertil* 1972; **31**: 513–514.

37. Trounson A, Mohr L. Human pregnancy following cryopreservation, thawing and transfer of an eight-cell embryo. *Nature* 1983; **305**: 707–709.

38. Cohen J, Simons RF, Edwards RG, Fehilly CB, Fishel SB. Pregnancies following the frozen storage of expanding human blastocysts. *J In Vitro Fert Embryo Transf* 1985; **2**: 59–64.

39. Rall WF, Fahy GM. Ice-free cryopreservation of mouse embryos at −196 degrees C by vitrification. *Nature* 1985; **313**: 573–575.

40. Michelmann HW, Nayudu P. Cryopreservation of human embryos. *Cell Tissue Bank* 2006; **7**: 135–141.

41. Kuwayama M. Highly efficient vitrification for cryopreservation of human oocytes and embryos: the Cryotop method. *Theriogenology* 2007; **67**: 73–80.

42. ESHRE. The European IVF monitoring programme (EIM), for the European Society of Human Reproduction and Embryology (ESHRE). Assisted reproductive technology in Europe,2004. Results generated from European Registers by ESHRE. *Hum Reprod* 2009; **24**: 1267–1287.

43. U.S. Department of Health and Human Services Centers for Disease Control and Prevention. Assisted Reproductive Technology Success Rates – National Summary and Fertility Clinic Reports, 2006.

44. Loutradi KE, Kolibianakis EM, Venetis CA, et al. Cryopreservation of human embryos by vitrification or slow freezing: a systematic review and meta-analysis. *Fertil Steril* 2008; **90**: 186–193.

45. Menezo Y. Cryopreservation of IVF embryos: which stage? *Eur J Obstet Gynecol Reprod Biol* 2004; **113**: S28–S32.

46. Quintans CJ, Donaldson MJ, Bertolino MV, Godoy H, Pasqualini RS. Birth of a healthy baby after transfer of embryos that were cryopreserved for 8.9 years. *Fertil Steril* 2002; **77**: 1074–1076.

47. Lopez Teijon M, Serra O, Olivares R, et al. Delivery of a healthy baby following the transfer of embryos cryopreserved for 13 years. *Reprod Biomed Online* 2006; **13**: 821–822.

48. Riggs R, Mayer J, Dowling-Lacey D, et al. Does storage time influence postthaw survival and pregnancy outcome? An analysis of 11,768 cryopreserved human embryos. *Fertil Steril* 2010; **93**: 109–115.
49. Frydman R, Forman RG, Belaisch-Allart J, et al. An obstetric analysis of fifty consecutive pregnancies after transfer of cryopreserved human embryos. *Am J Obstet Gynecol* 1989; **160**: 209–213.
50. Wada I, Macnamee MC, Wick K, Bradfield JM, Brinsden PR. Birth characteristics and perinatal outcome of babies conceived from cryopreserved embryos. *Hum Reprod* 1994; **9**: 543–546.
51. Heijnsbroek I, Helmerhorst FM, van den Bergh-Helder AF, et al. Follow-up of 30 pregnancies after embryo cryopreservation. *Eur J Obstet Gynecol Reprod Biol* 1995; **59**: 201–204.
52. Sutcliffe AG, D'Souza SW, Cadman J, et al. Outcome in children from cryopreserved embryos. *Arch Dis Child* 1995; **72**: 290–293.
53. Olivennes F, Schneider Z, Remy V, et al. Perinatal outcome and follow-up of 82 children aged 1–9 years old conceived from cryopreserved embryos. *Hum Reprod* 1996; **11**: 1565–1568.
54. Wennerholm UB, Hamberger L, Nilsson L, et al. Obstetric and perinatal outcome of children conceived from cryopreserved embryos. *Hum Reprod* 1997; **12**: 1819–1825.
55. Kallen B, Finnstrom O, Nygren KG, Olausson PO. In vitro fertilization (IVF) in Sweden: risk for congenital malformations after different IVF methods. *Birth Defects Res* 2005; **73**: 162–169.
56. Shih W, Rushford DD, Bourne H, et al. Factors affecting low birthweight after assisted reproduction technology: difference between transfer of fresh and cryopreserved embryos suggests an adverse effect of oocyte collection. *Hum Reprod* 2008; **23**: 1644–1653.
57. Belva F, Henriet S, Van den Abbeel E, et al. Neonatal outcome of 937 children born after transfer of cryopreserved embryos obtained by ICSI and IVF and comparison with outcome data of fresh ICSI and IVF cycles. *Hum Reprod* 2008; **23**: 2227–2238.
58. Pinborg A, Loft A, Aaris Henningsen AK, Rasmussen S, Andersen AN. Infant outcome of 957 singletons born after frozen embryo replacement: the Danish National Cohort Study 1995–2006. *Fertil Steril* 2010; **94**: 1320–1327;.
59. ICMART (International Committee Monitoring ART). Presentation of preliminary data for 2004. 24th Annual Meeting of ESHRE. Barcelona, Spain, 2008.

Chapter 11

Pregnancy after fertility preservation

Ephia Yasmin and Melanie C. Davies

Introduction

Fertility preservation is primarily considered for men and women in the reproductive age group, but also for children and adolescents where the condition and/or treatment are/is likely to render them infertile. The need for fertility preservation is increasing because of more cancer survivors and improved prognosis of treatment of cancers. Fertility preservation for social reasons is also on the rise with women considering fertility preserving options as an insurance policy against delayed child-bearing.

There are an estimated 12.7 million cancer cases around the world every year. Cancer in the female population ranges from 182/100 000 to 325/100 000 [1]. Worldwide, 10.9 % of cancers in women are breast cancers and 10% are cervical cancers [1]. The lifetime risk for breast cancer is 1 in 10 for women in developed countries, although 80% occur in women over 50 years of age [2]. The incidence of cervical cancer is highest for women in the reproductive age group (25–40 years). Cancer of the endometrium is on the rise but usually present in the postmenopausal age group. Hodgkin's lymphoma is one of the most common cancers in children and adolescents. The prognosis for Hodgkin's lymphoma is increasing with 78% of patients surviving 10 years or more [1] Leukemias account for a third of all cancers diagnosed in children. More than 80% of children with leukemia survive for at least five years after diagnosis [1]. In men, the incidence of testicular cancer appears to be rising.

Fertility is an extremely emotive issue with significant implications for quality of life with men and women who survive cancer. Adolescents and individuals in the reproductive age group need counseling and information about the options available to preserve their fertility, the success rates with different fertility preserving techniques, the outcome of pregnancy following cancer, and risks to offspring [3].

Effects of cancer treatment on fertility

The risk of infertility is generally related to the tissues or organs involved in the cancer and the specific treatment used. Surgery and radiotherapy (RT) have local effects. Chemotherapy affects fertility depending on the type, dose, and combination of cytotoxic therapy. In addition, age at treatment, gender, and likely genetic factors also influence the risk of infertility. Tables 11.1 and 11.2 list the gonadotoxic chemotherapeutic agents and doses of RT, respectively.

Chemotherapy

Chemotherapy causes depletion of the ovarian pool of follicles [4]. The severity of damage depends on the dose, age of the patient, and type of cytotoxic agent used. Increasing age makes women more vulnerable to loss of ovarian function compared with younger patients. Most chemotherapeutic drugs affect mainly the dividing cells such as granulosa and theca cells. The most cytotoxic agents are alkylating agents such as cyclophosphamide, which can destroy primordial follicles [5]. Although most chemotherapy agents target dividing cells, cyclophosphamide is not cell cycle specific and can therefore damage the resting primordial follicles, which compromises ovarian reserve [5]. Resulting amenorrhea may be temporary or permanent. It has been suggested that destruction of maturing follicles causes temporary amenorrhea while destruction of primordial follicles causes permanent amenorrhea [6]. Depending on the nature of chemotherapy and age at chemotherapy, menstrual function and fertility may return variably after the cessation of

Pregnancy After Assisted Reproductive Technology, ed. Eric R. M. Jauniaux and Botros R. M. B. Rizk. Published by Cambridge University Press.

Table 11.1. Gonadotoxicity of different chemotherapeutic agents

Low risk	Intermediate risk	High risk
Methotrexate	Cisplatin	Alkylating agents
5-Fluorouracil	Adriamycin	Cyclophosphamide
Actinomycin D		Busulfan
Bleomycin		Melphalan
Vincristine		Nitrogen mustard
6-Mercaptopurine		

Table 11.2. Gonadotoxicity of radiotherapy

Study	Number of pregnancies	Site of irradiation	Adverse outcome	Risk of adverse outcome
Green et al., 2003 [21] Childhood cancer survival study	4029 pregnancies, 1970–1986	Cranial irradiation	Miscarriage	RR 1.4, 95% CI: 1.02–1.94, P = 0.04
		Craniospinal irradiation	Miscarriage	RR 3.63, 95% CI: 1.70–7.78, p < 001
		Pelvic irradiation	Miscarriage	RR 1.84, 95% CI: 1.07–3.18, P = 0.03
Signorello et al., 2006 [20] Childhood cancer survival study	2201 pregnancies, 1968–2002	Pelvic irradiation	Preterm delivery	OR 3.5, 95% CI: 1.5–8.0, P = 0.003
			Low birth weight	OR 6.8, 95% CI: 2.1–22.2, P = 0.001
Green et al., 2002 [18] National Wilm's tumor study group	427 pregnancies, 1969–1999	Flank irradiation	Preterm delivery	P = 0.03
			Low birth weight	P = 0.02
			Fetal malposition	P = 0.007
Chiarelli et al., 2000 [19] Ontario Cancer Registry	594 pregnancies, 1964–1988	Abdomino-pelvic irradiation	Low birth weight	OR 3.64, 95% CI 1.33–9.96
			Preterm delivery	OR 3.29, 95% CI: 0.97–11.1

therapy in the case of temporary damage to the ovarian follicles [7].

The testis is very sensitive to the detrimental effects of chemotherapy at any age. The germinal epithelium is more sensitive than the Leydig cells, and therefore oligospermia and azoospermia occur even if testosterone production continues.

Radiotherapy

Improvement in technology has permitted customization of radiation doses to conform to the tumor and spare normal tissues. The dose tolerance of the ovary is dependent on several factors including the volume irradiated, the total radiation dose, the fractionation schedule, and the patient's age at the time of treatment [8]. The ovarian follicles are remarkably vulnerable to DNA damage from ionizing radiation, resulting in a significant reduction in the ovarian follicle pool. The follicles are at risk of undergoing induced apoptosis under the effect of RT. The ovaries of women in their later reproductive life seem to be more vulnerable as they have a smaller pool than the prepubertal ovaries [9]. It has been estimated that a total radiation exposure of 20 Gy fractionated over six weeks in younger women and children produces sterility with 95% confidence [10]. In males, radiation doses of 0.1 to 1.2 Gy can impair spermatogenesis and doses of >4 Gy can cause permanent azoospermia [11].

Craniospinal irradiation has been found to cause gonadal toxicity, because the ovaries lie close to the midline at the caudal limit of the radiation field [12]. Doses to the ovaries exceeding 24 Gy invariably produce permanent ovarian ablation [13]. Using the best available model for follicle decline, Wallace et al. reported their calculation of the radiosensitivity of the human oocyte in terms of LD50 [9]. Radiation is more toxic when given in a single dose compared with fractionated doses [14]. Two studies indicated that the breakpoint for radiation-induced ovarian failure is approximately 300 cGy to the ovaries. Only 11%–13% of patients experienced ovarian failure with doses below 300 cGy versus 60%–63% above that threshold value [15]. It is estimated that less than 2 Gy is enough to destroy 50% of the oocyte population (LDL50 2 Gy) [9].

Conversely, chemotherapy does not appear to have any direct deleterious effects on the uterus and uterine receptivity [16]; pelvic irradiation may cause reduced uterine volume, impaired uterine distensibility due to myometrial fibrosis, uterine vasculature damage, and endometrial injury [17]. Pelvic irradiation may increase the risk for pregnancy-related complications, including spontaneous miscarriages, preterm labor and delivery, low birth weight (LBW), and placental abnormalities such as placenta accreta [18–20].

In males, testicular cancer and chemotherapy and RT can cause sterilization as can hemoglobinopathies requiring bone marrow transplantation and autoimmune disorders such as rheumatoid arthritis. Most patients will develop azoospermia two to three months after starting chemotherapy [21,22]. Azoospermia may be encountered especially in patients with testicular cancer. Azoospermia rates of 18% have been observed in men sent for cryopreservation prior to cancer treatment [23].

Strategies for preservation of fertility

Different methods have evolved over recent decades in an attempt to preserve fertility. A brief description is presented in this chapter. The methods used are pharmacological, cryopreservation of spermatozoa, oocytes, and embryos, and preservation of ovarian tissue.

Gonadal suppression with gonadotrophin releasing hormone agonists

Suppression of ovarian function through manipulation of the hypothalamic–pituitary–gonadal axis concurrent with systemic therapy has been postulated for preservation of ovarian function [24]. The background to this strategy is the observation that the prepubertal ovary seems to be less susceptible to the damaging side effects of chemotherapy. Destruction of follicles by chemotherapeutic agents causes a rise in follicle-stimulating hormone (FSH), which in turn stimulates more follicles to enter the maturation pathway, rendering them more susceptible to the toxic effects of chemotherapy. The use of a concurrent gonadotrophin releasing hormone (GnRH) agonist helps to prevent follicles from entering into the recruitment and maturation pathway and therefore may offer protection [24]. Animal studies have shown that GnRH agonists could protect the ovary against cyclophosphamide-induced damage. Blumenfeld et al. reported several studies on the potential protective actions of GnRH-agonists against the deleterious effects of chemotherapeutic agents [25]. All the reports demonstrated a diminished incidence of ovarian failure in patients who received a GnRH-agonist before starting chemotherapy. The protective effect of GnRH-agonists have been questioned by other authors, who have pointed out that primordial follicles are independent of gonadotrophins and the reason the prepubertal ovary is more resistant to the depletion of oocytes is because of their higher number of follicles [26].

The incidence of ovarian failure or resumption of ovulation demonstrated a statistically significant difference in favor of the GnRH-agonist co-treatment [27]. The same group observed only three spontaneous pregnancies from their cohort. The occurrence of spontaneous pregnancy, however, showed no statistically significant difference between GnRH-agonist co-treatment and the control groups [28]. At the time of writing, there were two randomized controlled trials examining fertility preservation with concurrent GnRH-agonist treatment in breast cancer (the OPTION trial in the U.K. and the Southwestern oncology group trial); results are awaited.

Cryopreservation of embryos

Controlled ovarian stimulation, oocyte retrieval and in vitro fertilization (IVF), and cryopreservation of embryos represent an established method of fertility preservation with the highest success rate and with long-term data [29]. Cryopreservation of the human embryo has been achieved successfully at the zygote (day 1), cleavage (day 2/3), and blastocyst (day 5) stages; however, each stage presents specific advantages and disadvantages. During the past decades, two major methods have been applied: slow freezing (equilibrium procedure) and vitrification (nonequilibrium procedure).

The overwhelming majority of published data prove that the latest vitrification methods induce less cellular trauma and are a more effective cryopreservation technique for human embryos than any other versions of slow freezing [30]. Cytotoxic therapy may need to be delayed in order to complete a stimulation cycle. The human embryo is found to be resistant to damage from cryopreservation. The post-thaw survival rate of embryos ranges between 35% and 90%, and if multiple embryos are available for cryopreservation, cumulative pregnancy rates can be more than 60% [31]. Delivery rates per embryo transfer utilizing cryopreserved embryos are reported by the Society for Assisted Reproductive Technology to be in the range of 36.5% [32]. There are no published data showing successful pregnancy rates after IVF carried out as an emergency procedure in patients with cancer. There are concerns over safety of this method, particularly in women with breast cancer. The appropriateness of ovarian stimulation with resultant supraphysiological levels of estrogen in women with hormonally responsive ER/PR positive tumors has been called into question [31].

Protocols have been developed to induce follicle development while minimizing estrogen production. One is the addition of tamoxifen, which results in increased gonadotrophin secretion while reducing the exposure of the tumor to estrogen [33]. The other is the addition of the aromatase inhibitor letrozole, which results in a lower peak level of estradiol without affecting the success rates [34]. The embryo cryopreservation option is not suitable for prepubertal or adolescent girls, and women without a partner.

Cryopreservation of oocytes

Human oocyte cryopreservation began in the 1980s with sporadic reports of successful pregnancies [35]. Before 2004, only 100 births were reported from frozen oocytes [36]. Variations to cryopreservation methods such as changes in sucrose [37,38] and sodium [39] concentrations in slow-freezing media, and most significantly, the first report of successful oocyte vitrification [40] have improved the outcome in fertilization and pregnancy rates. Vitrification is known to establish a glass-like solid state during the cooling process. The high concentration of cryoprotectants and an extremely rapid rate of cooling are responsible for the formation of the solid state, and also prevent formation of intracellular ice crystals. Hence, in theory, vitrification should minimize cryoinjuries, and therefore has great promise for oocyte and embryo cryopreservation [41]. A birth rate of 5%–6% per thawed oocyte after vitrification has been reported [42].

Oocyte survival was significantly higher following vitrification–warming (81%) compared with freezing–thawing (67%) [43]. Fertilization was more successful in oocytes vitrified-warmed compared with frozen-thawed. Fertilized oocytes from vitrification–warming had significantly better cleavage rates (84%) compared with freezing–thawing (71%) and resulted in embryos with significantly better morphology. Although similar numbers of embryos were transferred, embryos resulting from vitrified oocytes had significantly enhanced clinical pregnancy rates (38%) compared with embryos resulting from frozen oocytes (13%). Miscarriage and/or spontaneous abortion rates were similar [44].

Results of recent studies suggest that vitrification–warming is currently the most efficient means of oocyte cryopreservation in relation to subsequent success in establishing pregnancy [45,46]. Cobo et al. performed a study of oocyte donors in which oocytes from a given donor were either inseminated fresh, or were frozen by vitrification for a minimum of one hour and then thawed, inseminated, and cultured along with the fresh oocytes from that same donor cycle. They found no differences in fertilization or cleavage rates, or in the assigned embryo quality scores of the fresh and vitrified oocyte groups. In 23 cycles, embryos from frozen-thawed oocytes were transferred, resulting in a 65.2% pregnancy, 40.8% implantation, and a 47.8% ongoing pregnancy rate, similar to what was obtained with fresh oocytes [47].

Over the past decade, more than 500 live births have been reported [48–50]. The majority of these have been in the past three years, renewing interest in the technology. Prior reported pregnancy rates after ovum freezing range from 8% to 33% [43,49]. A meta-analysis in 2006 reported an overall 21.6% live birth rate per embryo transfer over an 11-year period [48].

Cryopreservation of ovarian tissue

Unlike a suspended single cell, tissue cryopreservation presents serious physical constraints related to heat and mass transfer and the potential formation of ice crystals, which is responsible for the freeze-thaw injury. Consequently, better survival is expected from primordial follicles because of their smaller size and lack of follicular fluid. Baird and associates pioneered the sheep ovarian transplantation model [51]. Using cryopreserved-thawed ovarian cortical strips, they showed follicular survival and endocrine function, as well as restoration of fertility after transplantation of frozen-thawed ovarian cortical strips. Subsequent work has developed human ovarian tissue regrafting and achieved restoration of endocrine and ovulatory function, albeit of relatively short duration [52]. The advantages of ovarian tissue storage are that it can be performed quickly by laparoscopic surgery at any stage of the menstrual cycle, and is applicable to children and adolescents as well as the reproductive age-group. However, further surgery is required for re-implantation and success rates are not yet established. The potential risk of re-grafting tissue in women with hormone-sensitive cancers or with hematological malignancies (as tissue could harbor leukemic cells [53]) has led to research on the extraction of primordial follicles and their maturation in vitro. However, this is far from being achieved with human oocytes.

Oktay and coworkers developed three different surgical techniques of ovarian cortical strip transplantation: orthotopic transplant into the pelvis or heterotopically into the arm or abdominal wall [54]. The orthotopic transplant was in a patient with benign disease who required oophorectomy and subsequently underwent transplant of the strips into the pelvis. Ovarian function ceased within the first nine months. In two cases of heterotopic transplant to the arm (brachioradialis muscle) with fresh ovarian cortical strips, ovarian function ceased after three years. Giacalone et al. first reported a case of ovulation induction and oocyte retrieval performed on a transposed ovary [55]. Dolmans et al. studied nine women in whom 21 oocyte retrieval attempts were made [56]. At least one oocyte was collected in 15 cases, giving an empty follicle rate per retrieval of 29% (6/21). Sixteen oocytes were recovered, of which six were abnormal or immature (38%) and 10 (62%) were in metaphase II (MII). Three MII oocytes failed to fertilize, two showed abnormal fertilization, and five normal MII oocytes successfully fertilized with subsequent normal embryo development (Grade 2), yielding an embryo transfer rate of 24% per retrieval. However, no pregnancy occurred. Several case reports have revealed live births following ovarian tissue cryopreservation and transplantation (Table 11.3). Worldwide, 15 have been born as a result of transplanting frozen-thawed ovarian tissue [57,58].

Ovarian transposition and oophoropexy

For some patients subjected to gonadotoxic RT, ovarian function could be maintained by transposing the ovaries out of the field of irradiation. The radiation dose to the ovary after transposition is reduced to approximately 5%–10% of that of *in situ* ovaries in abdominal radiation [59]. Ovarian transposition involves the division of the utero-ovarian ligaments and tubes and the ovaries moved to the paracolic gutters so that they would lie 3 cm above the upper border of the field. Bidziński et al. confirmed that ovarian function was preserved if they were transposed at least 3 cm from the upper border of the field [60].

Oophoropexy involves fixing the ovary to the round ligaments or uterosacral ligaments to move the ovaries away from the field of maximum irradiation. Oophoropexy may protect against radiation-induced ovarian failure in girls receiving spinal radiation. A high risk of ovarian dysfunction was seen in patients who did not undergo oophoropexy compared with patients who did, where a lower rate of ovarian dysfunction was observed [61]. In a study of oophoropexy in 11 adolescents prior to pelvic irradiation for Hodgkin's lymphoma, 14 pregnancies were recorded among these 11 women, with 12 live births (one twin birth) and three miscarriages [62].

Cryopreservation of spermatozoa

Spermatozoon cryopreservation is an established and successful technique for fertility preservation in the adult male. Spermatozoon preservation has been available since the late 1970s [63]. Cryopreservation of spermatozoa is quick with easy access to centers

Table 11.3. Live births after fertility preservation techniques

Method	Evidence	Live births
Embryo cryopreservation	Wennerholm et al., 2009 [67]	>350,000**
Oocyte cryopreservation	Trokoudes et al., 2011 [68]	>500
	Grynberg et al., 2011 [69]	
Ovarian tissue cryopreservation and re-grafting	Donnez et al., 2011 [70]	15 reported
	Meirow et al., 2005 [71]	
	Demeestere et al., 2007 [72]	
	Anderson et al., 2008 [73]	
	Silber et al., 2008 [74]	
	Sánchez-Serrano et al., 2010 [75]	
	Roux et al., 2010 [76]	
Ovarian transposition and oophoropexy	Bisharah and Tulandi, 2003 [77]	Not quantified
	Kuohung et al., 2008 [61]	
	Terenziani et al., 2009 [62]	
Ovarian suppression with GnRH	Badaiwy et al., 2009 [28]	Not quantified
	Guiseppe et al., 2007 [78]	
	Nitzschke et al., 2010 [79]	

GnRH, gonadotrophin releasing hormone;
**, $P = 0.01$

of cryopreservation with no delay in starting chemotherapy or RT. Spermatozoon banking in adolescents and children poses few difficulties. The ability to bank spermatozoa successfully in 16- to 17-year-olds has been found to be 86% [64], and with sensitive handling and counseling, can be offered to adolescents as young as 14 years of age. Methods of procuring semen for spermatozoon cryopreservation are masturbation for those sufficiently mature, penile vibratory stimulation or rectal electrostimulation under general anesthesia. If spermatogenesis is established, testicular or epididymal spermatozoon aspiration can be performed. With IVF and intracytoplasmic spermatozoon injection (ICSI), success rates are good even with relatively poor-quality spermatozoa [65]. A report from the Netherlands found that relatively few men return to use samples; 7.5% requested use and 5% requested disposal [66]. The clinical pregnancy rates using cryopreserved spermatozoa were 30.1% for IVF, 25% for ICSI, and 14.3 % for intrauterine insemination (IUI). Altogether, 54% of users achieved a successful pregnancy [66].

Spontaneous pregnancy in cancer survivors

It has to be borne in mind that many cancer survivors retain their fertility with resulting spontaneous pregnancies. Nearly 50% of young women have intermittent ovarian follicle function and 16% of these cases may exhibit sporadic ovulatory cycles after the diagnosis of premature ovarian failure (POF) [80]. A postal survey of 2083 childhood cancer survivors of reproductive age, performed by Hawkins and Smith (1989), reported that 22% of those exposed to abdominal irradiation and 41% of those unexposed were found to have live births [81]. In the Danish population study by Winther and colleagues conducted between 1977 and 2003, 1479 pregnancies with 1497 fetuses were reported among 1688 cancer survivors, with an average of 0.9 pregnancies per woman [82]. The average number of pregnancies per women who were ever pregnant was found to be 2.3 for survivors. Of 1915 female cancer survivors, 4029 pregnancies were reported with 63% live births in the U.S. and Canada Childhood Cancer Survivor Study [83]. In a study by Salooja and co workers, out of 19 412 allogenic and 17 950 autologous transplant patients, 232 (0.6%) were found to have conceived, which was lower than the national average of 1.7/1000 [84]. Similarly in the British Childhood Cancer Survivor Study survey, which was completed by 10 483 survivors, 7300 pregnancies were reported. The study noted that the number of live births observed from all female survivors was two thirds of that expected (O/E: 0.64; 95% CI: 0.62–0.66) and lowest among survivors treated with brain (O/E: 0.52; 95% CI: 0.48–0.56) and abdominal RT [85].

Pregnancy outcome in cancer survivors

Miscarriage, preterm labor, and low birth weight

Pregnancy outcomes that are most often evaluated are rates of miscarriage, LBW, preterm delivery, and stillbirth. Virtually all series reported to date are retrospective and therefore subject to recall bias. Under-reporting is particularly an issue with early miscarriage.

The postal survey by Hawkins and Smith has revealed that females having undergone direct abdominal irradiation (exposed), particularly for Wilms' tumor, have an increased risk of several adverse pregnancy outcomes as compared with female survivors of the same types of tumor who had not undergone direct abdominal irradiation (unexposed) [81]. Among female survivors, 22% of those exposed and 41% of those unexposed have children. The percentages of first pregnancies reported as ending in miscarriage were 9/40 or 22% (exposed mothers) and 11/174 or 6% (unexposed mothers). The mean birth weight of first singleton children born to exposed mothers was over 300 g less than the corresponding value for unexposed mothers. We conclude that radiation is probably involved in the mechanism producing these effects. The findings have implications for counseling survivors, monitoring their pregnancies, and treating future patients.

An increased incidence of miscarriage, LBW babies, and neonatal deaths has been described for women with Wilms tumor who had received at least 20 Gy abdominal radiation [83]. Hodgkin's disease survivors who had received both radiation and chemotherapy (but not either alone) also appear to be at increased risk of miscarriage. Swerdlow et al. confirmed that there was no excess of stillbirths, LWB, congenital malformations, abnormal karyotypes, or cancer in the offspring of women treated for Hodgkin's disease [86]. However, Fenig et al. [87] cited an increase in LWB and miscarriage, especially if conception occurred less than a year after radiation exposure. A delay in pregnancy of one to two years is advisable after RT.

The Childhood Cancer Survivor Study (CCSS) compared pregnancy outcome (i.e., live birth, miscarriage, birth weight) in female five-year survivors, who were younger than 21 years old at diagnosis, with outcomes in their sibling controls [88]. Over 1900 females reported 4029 pregnancies (63% live births, 1% stillbirths, 15% miscarriages, 17% abortions, and 3% unknown or in gestation). There were no significant differences in pregnancy outcome between patients who had received chemotherapy and controls. However, women who had undergone pelvic irradiation were significantly more likely to have infants weighing less than 2500 g at birth. Study limitations included survey design with possible recall bias. The CCSS study also noted that the risk of stillbirth and neonatal death in the offspring of men who were fertile after gonadal irradiation was low. Green et al. reported that malposition of the fetus and early or threatened labor were more frequent among female Wilms' tumor survivors who received abdominal irradiation than among those who did not, with the frequency rising with increasing abdominal radiation dose. In addition, the frequency of both LBW (<2500 g) and early gestational age (<36 weeks) rose with increasing abdominal radiation dose. No effect of abdominal irradiation on pregnancy outcome was observed in the partners of irradiated male Wilms tumor survivors or in their offspring [89].

The mechanism responsible for LWB in these studies is unclear. The research of Critchley et al. suggested that damage to both the uterine vasculature and myometrium contributed to restricted fetal growth and early birth. They demonstrated that uterine length was significantly less in 10 women with ovarian failure who had been treated with whole abdomen irradiation. Endometrial thickness, based on weekly ultrasound examinations, did not increase in response to hormone replacement therapy in three women. No blood flow was detectable with Doppler ultrasound through either uterine artery of five women and through only one uterine artery in three additional women [90].

In the study of bone marrow transplant survivors by Salooja and coworkers the Cesarean section rate was 42%, the preterm delivery rate was 20%, and the LBW rates were 23% in survivors compared with 16%, 6%, and 6% in the female population, respectively [84].

Congenital and chromosomal abnormalities

The risk of congenital malformations, genetic disorders, and cancer appears to be low, with the exception of the cancer risk in offspring born to survivors with germline cancer-predisposing mutations. Based on several thousand survivor offspring, there is no overall increased risk of either congenital malformations or childhood cancer. Further studies will define the outcome of offspring of cancer survivors treated in the modern era [91]. No significant increases in genetic or congenital defects were seen in an international survey of 25 000 survivors (3.7% and 4% in survivors and sibling controls) [92]. Similar statistics are reported by other large studies of offspring of cancer survivors [92]. However, a trend toward increased congenital malformations has been found in survivors of Wilms' tumor [89].

Risk of cardiotoxicity

Irradiation of a substantial volume of the heart to a sufficiently high dose can damage virtually any component of the heart, including the pericardium, myocardium, heart valves, coronary arteries, capillaries, and conducting system. Among the serious complications that have been reported are arrhythmias, myocardial necrosis causing a dilated cardiomyopathy, vasospasm or vasoocclusion resulting in angina or myocardial infarction, and pericarditis. Pericarditis is the typical acute manifestation of radiation injury, while chronic pericardial disease, coronary artery disease, cardiomyopathy, valvular disease, and conduction abnormalities can manifest years or decades after the original treatment and cause significant morbidity or mortality [93,94].

Cancer patients receiving chemotherapy have an increased risk of developing cardiovascular complications, and the risk is even greater if there is a known history of heart disease. A wide range of chemotherapy agents have been associated with cardiotoxicity, of which the anthracyclines and related compounds (doxorubicin, daunorubicin, idarubicin, epirubicin, and the anthraquinone, mitoxantrone) are some of the most frequently implicated agents [95].

The data on the late cardiovascular toxicity of RT come primarily from survivors of breast cancer and Hodgkin's lymphoma, diseases in which RT is a frequent component of the initial management and in which survival is often prolonged. Similar effects may be present in other cancer survivors who receive thoracic RT, although data are more limited. An awareness of the potential cardiotoxicity of RT led to the application of improved RT techniques that minimize irradiation to the heart. Contemporary techniques that minimize irradiation to the heart appear to have substantially decreased the incidence of delayed complications, although whether there still is some residual risk remains uncertain.

Prenatal advice to cancer survivors

The optimal timing of a subsequent pregnancy after cancer is unclear and depends on the patient's prognosis, age, and personal situation. The usual advice is to delay pregnancy for at least three years after chemotherapy. In addition, prognosis must be taken into account; in cancers where early relapse is a risk, allow sufficient time for follow-up (typically 1–2 years). Meirow and Schiff postulated that patients who recover from ovarian failure after high-dose chemotherapy or RT treatments should not delay child-bearing for too many years [96]. These patients should try to conceive after a disease-free interval of a few years, but not less than six to twelve months after the treatment, owing to the possible toxic effects of the therapy on growing oocytes. A delay of two to three years after cancer treatment is conventionally recommended, so that the period associated with the greatest risk of recurrence has passed before a pregnancy [97]. In patients with hormone-positive breast cancers, tamoxifen and GnRH analogues do not cause permanent amenorrhea, but this treatment can last up to five years, during which time a pregnancy is contraindicated [97].

Patients at risk of cardiotoxicity should have prenatal advice and echocardiography for their cardiac function, and those at risk of nephrotoxicity should have renal function testing prior to pregnancy.

Pregnancy after breast cancer

Pregnancy after breast cancer does not seem to increase the risk of recurrence or to adversely affect maternal outcome [98]. Moreover, no increased risk for congenital malformations in children conceived after completion of chemotherapy has been found [99]. However, breast cancer survivors who become pregnant may be a self-selected group and may not be representative of the larger population of women, as those having a high risk of tumor recurrence may have chosen not to get pregnant. Timing a pregnancy after a diagnosis of breast cancer is also a complex issue, but in general, patients are advised to delay pregnancy attempts for at least two years after the diagnosis, mainly because the risk of recurrence is greatest during this period [98]. For patients prescribed tamoxifen, pregnancy is usually considered safe after completion of the five-year treatment period. Tamoxifen has a similar structure to diethylstilbestrol, and pregnancy while on tamoxifen treatment is discouraged because of the potential teratogenic effects of this drug during pregnancy [100].

Although a pregnancy is considered safe for most breast cancer survivors, gestational surrogacy may be suitable for breast cancer survivors with a high risk for recurrence or who have to be on lifelong therapy with tamoxifen or aromatase inhibitors [101]. In women with *BRCA1* or *BRCA2* gene mutations, the risk of pregnancy is less well established. A gestational carrier may be indicated in patients who have undergone salpingo-oophorectomy with the aim of reducing endogenous estrogen production and therefore the risk of cancer recurrence [102].

Pregnancy after cervical cancer

For cervical cancer cases with a low risk of relapse who wish to maintain their fertility, radical trachelectomy is an alternative to radical hysterectomy. Over 900 cases of radical trachelectomy have been reported [103]. Most have been carried out vaginally (radical vaginal trachelectomy and laparoscopic pelvic node dissection). A smaller number have been performed abdominally. There have been over 300 pregnancies reported with 196 live births. There has been a significant prematurity rate with 10% of births occurring prior to 32 weeks of gestation. In this series, there were 31 recurrences (4%) and 16 deaths (2%). Most women are advised to wait six to twelve months after conization or trachelectomy before attempting to become pregnant [104]. Even if a woman waits to attempt pregnancy, there is a risk of pregnancy complications and/or infertility after cervical cancer treatment. There is an increased risk of difficulty in becoming pregnant if the cervix or lower uterus becomes scarred or narrowed as a result of the conization or radical trachelectomy. This can be overcome with an infertility treatment, such as IUI. Women who have had cervical conization or radical trachelectomy may be at an increased risk of cervical insufficiency. A review of 212 patients followed up after radical trachelectomy showed 60 pregnancies in 50 women of which 8.3% had a first-trimester miscarriage, 5.0% delivered prematurely before the 28th week of gestation, 25% delivered between 28 and 36 weeks, and 45% reached full term [105].

Conclusion

There has been a tremendous improvement in cancer survival rates, particularly in childhood and adolescence, as well as in the reproductive age group. Therefore, the demand for fertility preservation is increasing. Fertility preservation is also on the rise for social reasons in women wishing to retain fertility for delayed child-bearing. It is important to provide accurate and up-to-date information on the techniques available and also on the prognosis of the different options. Different strategies will be appropriate for different situations. For example, ovarian tissue cryopreservation and transplantation may be the only option in children while oocyte cryopreservation is available to single women. Women planning a pregnancy after cancer must be advised of the appropriate waiting times, and informed of the implications of their illness and treatment for spontaneous and assisted pregnancies. Specific prenatal counseling and advice need to be available and the pregnancy monitored for increased risk of LBW and preterm labor.

References

1. Ferlay J, Shin H-R, Bray F, et al. Estimates of worldwide burden of cancer in 2008: GLOBOCAN 2008. *Int J Cancer* 2010; **127**: 2893–2917.

2. Sasieni PD, Shelton J, Ormiston-Smith N, Thomson CS, Silcocks PB. What is the lifetime risk of developing cancer?: the effect of adjusting for multiple primaries. *Br J Cancer* 2011; **105**: 460–465.

3. Huyghe E, Matsuda T, Thonneau P. Increasing incidence of testicular cancer worldwide: a review. *J Urol* 2003; **170**: 5–11.

4. Schilsky RL, Lewis BJ, Sherins RJ, Young RC. Gonadal dysfunction in patients receiving chemotherapy for cancer. *Ann Intern Med* 1980; **93**: 109–114.

5. Nicosia SV, Matus-Ridley M, Meadows AT. Gonadal effects of cancer therapy in girls. *Cancer* 1985; **55**: 2364–2372.

6. Falcone T, Attaran M, Bedaiwy MA, Goldberg JM. Ovarian function preservation in the cancer patient. *Fertil Steril* 2004; **81**: 243–257.

7. Minisini AM, Menis J, Valent F, et al. Determinants of recovery from amenorrhea in premenopausal breast cancer patients receiving adjuvant chemotherapy in the taxane era. *Anticancer Drugs* 2009; **20**: 503–507.

8. Wallace WH, Anderson RA, Irvine DS. Fertility preservation for young patients with cancer: who is at risk and what can be offered? *Lancet Oncol* 2005; **6**: 209–218.

9. Wallace WH, Thomson AB, Saran F, Kelsey TW. Predicting age of ovarian failure after radiation to a field that includes the ovaries. *Int J Radiat Oncol Biol Phys* 2005; **62**: 738–744.

10. Lushbaugh CC, Casarett GW. The effects of gonadal irradiation in clinical radiation therapy: a review. *Cancer* 1976; **37**: 1111–1120.

11. Wallace WH. Oncofertility and preservation of reproductive capacity in children and young adults. *Cancer* 2011; **117**: 2301–2310.

12. Chow EJ, Friedman DL, Yasui Y, et al. Timing of menarche among survivors of childhood acute lymphoblastic leukemia: a report from the Childhood Cancer Survivor Study. *Pediatr Blood Cancer* 2008; **50**: 854–858.

13. Grigsby PW, Russell A, Bruner D, et al. Late injury of cancer therapy on the female reproductive tract. *Int J Radiat Oncol Biol Phys* 1995; **31**: 1281–1299.

14. Meirow D, Nugent D. The effects of radiotherapy and chemotherapy on female reproduction. *Hum Reprod Update* 2001; **7**: 535–543.

15. Husseinzadeh N, Nahhas WA, Velkley DE, Whitney CW, Mortel R. The preservation of ovarian function in young women undergoing pelvic radiation therapy. *Gynecol Oncol* 1984; **18**: 373–379.

16. Critchley HOD, Wallace WHB, Mamtora H, et al. Abdominal irradiation in childhood; the potential for pregnancy. *Br J Obstet Gynaecol* 1992; **99**: 392–394.

17. Larsen EC, Schmiegelow K, Rechnitzer C, et al. Radiotherapy at a young age reduces uterine volume of childhood cancer survivors. *Acta Obstet Gynecol Scand* 2004; **83**: 96–102.

18. Green DM, Peabody EM, Nan B, et al. Pregnancy outcome after treatment for Wilms tumor: a report from the National Wilm's Tumor Study Group. *J Clin Oncol* 2002; **20**: 2506–2513.

19. Chiarelli AM, Marrett LD, Darlington GA. Pregnancy outcomes in females after treatment for childhood cancer. *Epidemiology* 2000; **11**: 161–166.

20. Signorello LB, Cohen SS, Bosetti C, et al. Female survivors of childhood cancer: preterm birth and low birth weight among their children. *J Natl Cancer Inst* 2006; **98**: 1453–1461.

21. Green DM, Whitton JA, Stovall M, et al. Pregnancy outcome of partners of male survivors of childhood cancer: a report from the Childhood Cancer Survivor Study. *J Clin Oncol* 2003; **21**: 716–721.

22. Schrader M, Müller M, Straub B, Miller K. The impact of chemotherapy on male fertility: a survey of the biologic basis and clinical aspects. *Reprod Toxicol* 2001; **15**: 611–617.

23. Lass A, Akagbosu F, Abusheikha N, et al. A programme of semen cryopreservation for patients with malignant disease in a tertiary infertility centre: lessons from 8 years' experience. *Hum Reprod* 1998; **13**: 3256–3261.

24. Meistrich ML, Shetty G. Hormonal suppression for fertility preservation in males and females. *Reproduction* 2008; **136**: 691–701.

25. Blumenfeld Z. How to preserve fertility in young women exposed to chemotherapy? The role of GnRH agonist cotreatment in addition to cryopreservation of embrya, oocytes, or ovaries. *Oncologist* 2007; **12**: 1044–1054.

26. Gerber B, Dieterich M, Müller H, Reimer T. Controversies in preservation of ovary function and fertility in patients with breast cancer. *Breast Cancer Res Treat* 2008; **108**: 1–7.

27. Recchia F, Saggio G, Amiconi G, et al. Gonadotropin-releasing hormone analogues added to adjuvant chemotherapy protect ovarian function and improve clinical outcomes in young women with early breast carcinoma. *Cancer* 2006; **106**: 514–523.

28. Badaiwy A, Elnashar A, El-Ashry M, Shahat M. Gonadotropin-releasing hormone agonists for prevention of chemotherapy-induced ovarian damage: prospective randomized study. *Fertil Steril* 2009; **91**: 694–697.

29. Andersen AN, Erb K. Register data on assisted reproductive technology (ART) in Europe including a detailed description of ART in Denmark. *Int J Androl* 2006; **29**: 12–16.

30. Capalbo A, Rienzi L, Buccheri M, et al. The worldwide frozen embryo reservoir: methodologies to achieve optimal results. Efficiency of oocyte cryopreservation: a meta-analysis. *Ann N Y Acad Sci* 2011; **1221**: 32–39.

31. Son WY, Yoon SH, Yoon HJ, Lee SM, Lim JH. Pregnancy outcome following transfer of human blastocysts vitrified on electron microscopy grids after induced collapse of the blastocoele. *Hum Reprod* 2003; **18**: 137–139.

32. American Society of Reproductive Medicine, Annual meeting, 2008.

33. Oktay K, Buyuk E, Davis O, et al. Fertility preservation in breast cancer patients: IVF and embryo cryopreservation after ovarian stimulation with tamoxifen. *Hum Reprod* 2003; **18**: 90–95.

34. Oktay K, Hourvitz A, Sahin G, et al. Letrozole reduces estrogen and gonadotropin exposure in women with breast cancer undergoing ovarian stimulation before chemotherapy. *J Clin Endocrinol Metab* 2006; **91**: 3885–3890.

35. Chen C. Pregnancies after human oocyte cryopreservation. *Ann N Y Acad Sci* 1988; **541**: 541–549.

36. Stachecki JJ, Cohen J. An overview of oocyte cryopreservation. *Reprod Biomed Online* 2004; **9**: 152–163.

37. Bianchi V, Cottichio G, Distratis V, et al. Differential sucrose concentration during dehydration (0.2 Mol/L) and rehydration (0.3 Mol/L) increases the implantation rate of frozen human oocytes. *Reprod Biomed Online* 2007; **14**: 64–71.

38. De Santis L, Cino I, Rabelloti E, et al. Oocyte cryopreservation: clinical outcome of slow-cooling protocols differing in sucrose concentration. *Reprod Biomed Online* 2007; **14**: 57–63.

39. Quintans CJ, Donaldson MJ, Bertolino M, Pasqualini R. Birth of two babies using oocytes that were cryopreserved in a choline based freezing medium. *Hum Reprod* 2002; **17**: 3149–3152.

40. Kuleshova LL, Lopata A. Vitrification can be more favorable than slow cooling. *Fertil Steril* 2002; **78**: 449–454.

41. Yoon TK, Chung HM, Lim JM, et al. Pregnancy and delivery of healthy infants developed from vitrified oocytes in a stimulated in vitro fertilization-embryo transfer program. *Fertil Steril* 2000; **734**: 180–181.

42. Porcu E, Bazzocchi A, Notarangelo L, et al. Human oocyte cryopreservation in infertility and oncology. *Curr Opin Endocrinol Diabetes Obes* 2008; **15**: 529–535.

43. Borini A, Bonu MA, Coticchio G, et al. Pregnancies and births after oocyte cryopreservation. *Fertil Steril* 2004; **82**: 601–605.

44. Smith GD, Serafini PC, Fioravanti J, et al. Prospective randomized comparison of human oocyte cryopreservation with slow-rate freezing or vitrification. *Fertil Steril* 2010; **94**: 2088–2095.

45. Grifo JA, Noyes N. Delivery rate using cryopreserved oocytes is comparable to conventional in vitro fertilization using fresh oocytes: potential fertility preservation for female cancer patients. *Fertil Steril* 2010; **93**: 391–396.

46. Cobo A, Domingo J, Pe´ rez S, et al. Vitrification: an effective new approach to oocyte banking and preserving fertility in cancer patients. *Clin Transl Oncol* 2008; **10**: 268–273.

47. Cobo A, Meseguer M, Remohí J, Pellicer A. Use of cryo-banked oocytes in an ovum donation programme: a prospective, randomized, controlled, clinical trial. *Hum Reprod* 2010; **25**: 2239–2246.

48. Oktay K, Cil A, Bang H. Efficacy of oocyte cryopreservation: a meta-analysis. *Fertil Steril* 2006; **86**: 70–80.

49. Yoon TK, Lee DR, Cha SK, et al. Survival rate of human oocytes and pregnancy outcome after vitrification using slush nitrogen in assisted reproductive technologies. *Fertil Steril* 2007; **88**: 952–956.

50. Chian RC, Huang JY, Gilbert L, et al. Obstetric outcomes following vitrification of in vitro and in vivo matured oocytes. *Fertil Steril* 2009; **91**: 2391–2398.

51. Baird DT, Webb R, Campbell BK, Harkness LM, Gosden RG. Long-term ovarian function in sheep after ovariectomy and transplantation of autografts stored at −196°C. *Endocrinology* 1999; **140**: 462–471.

52. Radford J. Restoration of fertility after treatment for cancer. *Horm Res* 2003; **59**: 21–23.

53. Kim SS, Radford J, Harris M, et al. Ovarian tissue harvested from lymphoma patients to preserve fertility may be safe for autotransplantation. *Hum Reprod* 2001; **16**: 2056–2060.

54. Oktay K, Tilly J. Livebirth after cryopreserved ovarian tissue autotransplantation. *Lancet* 2004; **364**: 2091–2092.

55. Giacalone PL, Laffargue F, Bénos P, Dechaud H, Hédon B. Successful in vitro fertilization-surrogate pregnancy in a patient with ovarian transposition who had undergone chemotherapy and pelvic irradiation. *Fertil Steril* 2001; **76**: 388–389.

56. Dolmans MM, Donnez J, Camboni A, et al. IVF outcome in patients with orthotopically transplanted ovarian tissue. *Hum Reprod* 2009; **24**: 2778–2787.

57. Ernst E, Bergholdt S, Jørgensen JS, Andersen CY. The first woman to give birth to two children following transplantation of frozen/thawed ovarian tissue. *Hum Reprod* 2010; **25**: 1280–1281.

58. Schmidt KT, Rosendahl M, Ernst E, et al. Autotransplantation of cryopreserved ovarian tissue in 12 women with chemotherapy-induced premature

ovarian failure: the Danish experience. *Fertil Steril* 2011; **95**: 695–701.

59. Howell SJ, Shalet SM. Fertility preservation and management of gonadal failure associated with lymphoma therapy. *Curr Oncol Rep* 2002; **4**: 443–452.
60. Bidziński M, Lemieszczuk B, Zieliński J. Evaluation of the hormonal function and features of the ultrasound picture of transposed ovary in cervical cancer patients after surgery and pelvic irradiation. *Eur J Gynaecol Oncol* 1993; **14**: 77–80.
61. Kuohung W, Ram K, Cheng DM, et al. Laparoscopic oophoropexy prior to radiation for pediatric brain tumor and subsequent ovarian function. *Hum Reprod* 2008; **23**: 117–121.
62. Terenziani M, Piva L, Meazza C, et al. Oophoropexy: a relevant role in preservation of ovarian function after pelvic irradiation. *Fertil Steril* 2009; **91**: 935.e15–e16.
63. Ragni G, Somigliana E, Restelli L, et al. Sperm banking and rate of assisted reproduction treatment: insights from a 15-year cryopreservation program for male cancer patients. *Cancer* 2003; **97**: 1624–1629.
64. Bahadur G, Spoudeas H, Davies MC, Ralph D. Factors affecting sperm banking for adolescent cancer patients. *Arch Dis Child* 2006; **91**: 715–716.
65. Neal MS, Nagel K, Duckworth J, et al. Effectiveness of sperm banking in adolescents and young adults with cancer: a regional experience. *Cancer* 2007; **110**: 1125–1129.
66. van Casteren NJ, van Santbrink EJ, van Inzen W, Romijn JC, Dohle GR. Use rate and assisted reproduction technologies outcome of cryopreserved semen from 629 cancer patients. *Fertil Steril* 2008; **90**: 2245–2250.
67. Wennerholm U-B, Soderstrom-Anttila V, Bergh C, et al. Children born after cryopreservation of embryos or oocytes: a systematic review of outcome data. *Hum Reprod* 2009; **24**: 2158–2172.
68. Trokoudes KM, Pavlides C, Zhang X. Comparison outcome of fresh and vitrified donor oocytes in an egg-sharing donation program. *Fertil Steril* 2011; **95**: 1996–2000.
69. Grynberg M, Hesters L, Bénard J, et al. In vitro maturation of oocytes: an option for fertility preservation in women. *J Gynecol Obstet Biol Reprod (Paris)* 2011; **40**: 103–108.
70. Donnez J, Squifflet J, Pirard C, et al. Live birth after allografting of ovarian cortex between genetically non-identical sisters. *Hum Reprod* 2011; **26**: 1384–1388.
71. Meirow D, Levron J, Eldar-Geva T, et al. Pregnancy after transplantation of cryopreserved ovarian tissue in a patient with ovarian failure after chemotherapy. *N Engl J Med* 2005; **353**: 318–321.
72. Demeestere I, Simon P, Emiliani S, Delbaere A, Englert Y. Fertility preservation: successful transplantation of cryopreserved ovarian tissue in a young patient previously treated for Hodgkin's disease. *Oncologist* 2007; **12**: 1437–1442.
73. Anderson RA, Wallace WH, Baird DT. Ovarian cryopreservation for fertility preservation: indications and outcomes. *Reproduction* 2008; **136**: 681–689.
74. Silber SJ, Grudzinskas G, Gosden RG. Successful pregnancy after microsurgical transplantation of an intact ovary. *N Engl J Med* 2008; **359**: 2617–2618.
75. Sánchez-Serrano M, Crespo J, Mirabet V, et al. Twins born after transplantation of ovarian cortical tissue and oocyte vitrification. *Fertil Steril* 2010; **93**: 268.e11–e13.
76. Roux C, Amiot C, Agnani G, et al. Live birth after ovarian tissue autograft in a patient with sickle cell disease treated by allogeneic bone marrow transplantation. *Fertil Steril* 2010; **93**: 2413.e15–e19.
77. Bisharah M, Tulandi T. Laparoscopic preservation of ovarian function: an underused procedure. *Am J Obstet Gynecol* 2003; **188**: 367–370.
78. Giuseppe L, Attilio G, Edoardo DN, et al. Ovarian function after cancer treatment in young women affected by Hodgkin disease (HD). *Hematology* 2007; **12**: 141–147.
79. Nitzschke M, Raddatz J, Bohlmann MK, et al. GnRH analogs do not protect ovaries from chemotherapy-induced ultrastructural injury in Hodgkin's lymphoma patients. *Gynecol Obstet* 2010; **282**: 83–88.
80. van Kasteren YM, Schoemaker J. Premature ovarian failure: a systematic review on therapeutic interventions to restore ovarian function and achieve pregnancy. *Hum Reprod Update* 1999; **5**: 483–492.
81. Hawkins MM, Smith RA. Pregnancy outcomes in childhood cancer survivors: probable effects of abdominal irradiation. *Int J Cancer* 1989; **43**: 399–402.
82. Winther JF, Boice JD Jr, Frederiksen K, et al. Radiotherapy for childhood cancer and risk for congenital malformations in offspring: a population-based cohort study. *Clin Genet* 2009; **75**: 50–56.
83. Green DM, Whitton JA, Stovall M, et al. Pregnancy outcome of female survivors of childhood cancer: a report from the Childhood Cancer Survivor Study. *Am J Obstet Gynecol* 2002; **187**: 1070–1080.
84. Salooja N, Szydlo RM, Socie G, et al. Pregnancy outcomes after peripheral blood or bone marrow transplantation: a retrospective survey. *Lancet* 2001; **358**: 271–276.
85. Reulen RC, Zeegers MP, Wallace WH, et al. Pregnancy outcomes among adult survivors of childhood cancer in the British Childhood Cancer Survivor Study.

Cancer Epidemiol Biomarkers Prev 2009; **18**: 2239–2247.

86. Swerdlow AJ, Jacobs PA, Marks A, et al. Fertility, reproductive outcomes, and health of offspring, of patients treated for Hodgkin's disease: an investigation including chromosome examinations. *Br J Cancer* 1996; **74**: 291–296.
87. Fenig E, Mishaeli M, Kalish Y, Lishner M. Pregnancy and radiation. *Cancer Treat Rev* 2001; **27**: 1–7.
88. Signorello LB, Mulvihill JJ, Green DM, et al. Stillbirth and neonatal death in relation to radiation exposure before conception: a retrospective cohort study. *Lancet* 2010; **376**: 624–630.
89. Green DM, Lange JM, Peabody EM, et al. Pregnancy outcome after treatment for Wilms tumor: a report from the national Wilms tumor long-term follow-up study. *J Clin Oncol* 2010; **28**: 2824–2830.
90. Critchley HO, Wallace WH, Shalet SM, et al. Abdominal irradiation in childhood; the potential for pregnancy. *Br J Obstet Gynaecol* 1992; **99**: 392–394.
91. Blatt J. Pregnancy outcome in long-term survivors of childhood cancer. *Med Pediatr Oncol* 1999; **33**: 29–33.
92. Boice JD Jr, Tawn EJ, Winther JF, et al. Genetic effects of radiotherapy for childhood cancer. *Health Phys* 2003; **85**: 65–80.
93. Floyd JD, Nguyen DT, Lobins RL, et al. Cardiotoxicity of cancer therapy. *J Clin Oncol* 2005; **23**: 7685–7696.
94. Chen MH, Colan SD, Diller L. Cardiovascular disease: cause of morbidity and mortality in adult survivors of childhood cancers. *Circ Res* 2011; **108**: 619–628.
95. Dempsey KS. Chemotherapy-induced cardiotoxicity in women. *Heart Fail Clin* 2011; **7**: 427–435.
96. Meirow D, Schiff E. Appraisal of chemotherapy effects on reproductive outcome according to animal studies and clinical data. *J Natl Cancer Inst Monogr* 2005; **34**: 21–25.
97. Du X, Freeman JL, Goodwin JS. Information on radiation treatment in patients with breast cancer: the advantages of the linked medicare and SEER data. Surveillance, Epidemiology and End Results. *J Clin Epidemiol* 1999; **52**: 463–470.
98. Valachis A, Tsali L, Pesce LL, et al. Safety of pregnancy after primary breast carcinoma in young women: a meta-analysis to overcome bias of healthy mother effect studies. *Obstet Gynecol Surv* 2010; **65**: 786–793.
99. Langagergaard V. Birth outcome in women with breast cancer, cutaneous malignant melanoma, or Hodgkin's disease: a review. *Clin Epidemiol* 2010; **3**: 7–19.
100. Phillips DH. Understanding the genotoxicity of tamoxifen? *Carcinogenesis* 2001; **22**: 839–849.
101. Hulvat MC, Jeruss JS. Maintaining fertility in young women with breast cancer. *Curr Treat Options Oncol* 2009; **10**: 308–317.
102. Krychman ML, King T. Pregnancy after breast cancer: a case study resolving the reproductive challenge with a gestational surrogate. *Breast J* 2006; **12**: 363–365.
103. Milliken DA, Shepherd JH. Fertility preserving surgery for carcinoma of the cervix. *Curr Opin Oncol* 2008; **20**: 575–580.
104. Fagotti A, Gagliardi ML, Moruzzi C, et al. Excisional cone as fertility-sparing treatment in early-stage cervical cancer. *Fertil Steril* 2011; **95**: 1109–1112.
105. Speiser D, Mangler M, Köhler C, et al. Fertility outcome after radical vaginal trachelectomy: a prospective study of 212 patients. *Int J Gynecol Cancer* 2011; **21**: 1635–1639.

Chapter 12

Pregnancy after ovarian transplantation

Sherman J. Silber

Introduction

A successful series of human ovarian tissue transplantations between monozygotic (MZ) twin sisters discordant for premature ovarian failure (POF) was first reported in 2005 [1–4]. Menstrual cycles resumed after four months, and spontaneous pregnancy usually occurred, leading to the birth of healthy babies. Altogether there have been eight healthy babies born as a result of fresh human ovary transplantation (out of nine transplants), all demonstrating ovulatory cycles with normalized serum follicle-stimulating hormone (FSH) levels [2,3]. Spare ovarian cortical tissue from the donor ovary was cryopreserved for future grafting as a backup in case the first transplant became depleted of follicles and ceased to function. In one case, a different technique (direct microvascular anastomosis of ovarian artery and vein rather than the simpler cortical grafting technique) was used, with microvascular transplantation of a whole ovary, and this also led to a prompt return of normal cycles, pregnancy by natural conception, and the delivery of a healthy child [4]. To date, nine healthy babies have resulted from fresh ovary transplantation, none of whom required immunosuppression.

Despite this apparent success, there has been concern whether ovarian tissue grafts, either fresh or cryopreserved, have only transient function, and whether frozen-thawed grafts would fare worse than fresh ovary grafts [5–7]. There have been only a few successful cases reported of thawed autotransplanted ovarian tissue in former cancer patients [8–13] and no large series, while information about graft longevity is sparse and successes were only sporadic case reports. Our present report represents a long-term follow-up of the duration of function of fresh and frozen human ovarian grafts in a large series so as to estimate the degree of follicle loss from ischemia and from cryopreservation.

One solution to ischemic oocyte loss, microsurgical transplantation of an intact whole ovary, is technically much more difficult and risky than cortical grafting [4,14–16]. It would be preferable and simpler if a cortical grafting technique and freezing could minimize oocyte loss.

A long-term follow-up of our series of MZ twins offered an unusual opportunity to study the duration of function of fresh ovarian cortical grafts to evaluate oocyte loss from the transplant itself without the confusion created by cryopreservation, and to try to improve results with cryopreservation by vitrification [17]. We now have evidence of long-term ovarian function in the current twin series, suggesting that a substantial reserve of follicles survives in fresh cortical grafts despite being subjected to lengthy ischemia compared with vascular transplantation. We have also found that slow freezing causes significant loss of oocyte viability compared with the vitrification technique, which results in virtually no loss. This has resulted in two additional healthy babies born from frozen-thawed ovarian cortical grafts, a total of 11 babies from just one center.

Patient population and surgery for fresh transplants

Nine pairs of female MZ twins, in which one sister had either idiopathic [8] or iatrogenic [1] POF and the other had normal reproductive function, underwent fresh ovarian transplantation. Each donor had a unilateral oophorectomy by laparoscopy or minilaparotomy under general anesthesia. The ovary was transferred immediately to a Petri dish with Leibovitz L-15 medium cooled over a dish of saline ice slush. The following surgical principles were strictly adhered to: (i) the cortex was trimmed down to a bare 0.75–1.0 mm thickness to promote rapid revascularization; (ii) perfect hemostasis

Pregnancy After Assisted Reproductive Technology, ed. Eric R. M. Jauniaux and Botros R. M. B. Rizk. Published by Cambridge University Press.

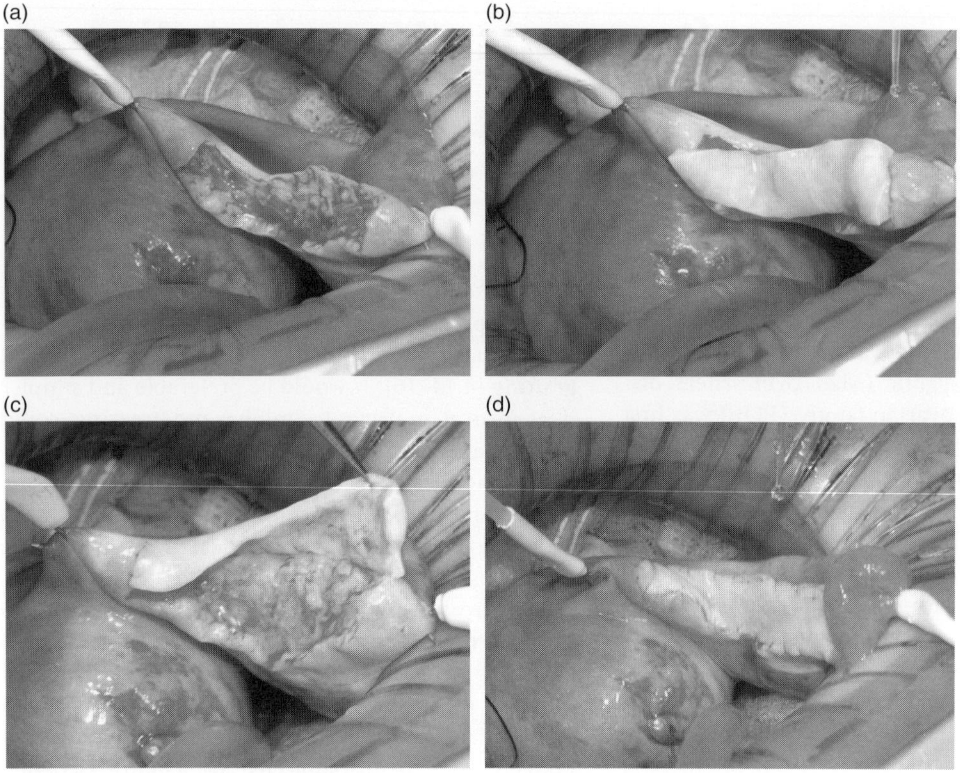

Figure 12.1. (a):the depleted "menopausal" cortex of the recipient ovary has been removed, exposing the medulla; (b): the slice of donor ovarian tissue is placed on top of the recipient medulla; (c): the donor cortical slice is being sutured microsurgically to the medulla of the recipient with 9–0 nylon interrupted sutures after good hemostasis is secured; (d): the completed ovarian tissue transplant. (See color plate section for colored image.)

of the graft bed was assured using microbipolar forceps; (iii) 9–0 nylon interrupted sutures were used to prevent microhematoma formation under the graft; (iv) the grafts were applied to the highly vascular ovarian medulla; and (v) continual pulsatile irrigation with heparinized saline was applied to the graft surface to prevent adhesion formation (Figure 12.1).

A quarter to a third of the donor ovary was transplanted as a cortical slice, the remaining tissue being cryopreserved as a backup for replacing the primary graft if necessary. Because the ovaries and tubal ampullae were congenitally absent in case #3, donor tissue was grafted onto the peritoneum of the denuded Fallopian tube isthmus, without any expectation of natural fertility, and as expected, this patient underwent in vitro fertilization (IVF) to become pregnant. In one of these nine cases a fresh intact microvascular whole ovary was transplanted, but the subject of this chapter is ovarian cortical transplants, and there was no difference between the results of this patient and those of the ovarian cortical grafts.

Frozen ovarian transplants

In addition to these nine fresh transplants described, two patients underwent a transplantation of frozen cortical tissue. In both cases, the tissue had been cryopreserved by the slow-freezing protocol. One of these frozen tissue transplants was for a 31-year-old woman who, 11 years earlier, had her tissue frozen because of Hodgkin's lymphoma, and she subsequently underwent several cycles of chemotherapy and radiation before having a bone marrow transplant. After more than eight years she was considered to be cancer free, although menopausal, had married, and had gained approval from her oncologist for her frozen ovarian tissue to be transplanted back.

The other frozen tissue recipient was from the identical twin series, one of whom (case #1) had undergone a successful fresh ovary transplant in 2004 leading to two spontaneous pregnancies and the delivery of a healthy child. After more than three years, she became menopausal again and had a second transplant of spare donor sibling tissue that had been cryopreserved at the time of the original fresh transplant. She became pregnant and delivered her second baby from this frozen transplant, became menopausal again one and a half years later, and then underwent a second frozen tissue transplant.

Cryopreservation: slow freezing versus vitrification

For slow freezing, after enucleating medullary tissue with sharp scalpel dissection, the cortex was pared down manually to an ultrathin translucent shell with a thickness of ≤1 mm. Tissue for cryopreservation was divided into multiple strips and transferred to 1.5 mL cryovials after equilibration in 1.5 mol/L 1,2-propanediol and 0.1 mol/L sucrose at 37°C for 30 min, followed by 1.5 mol/L 1,2-propanediol and 0.2 mol/L sucrose for 5 min, and then cooled at a controlled rate 0.3°C/min, as described previously [18–20]. Thawing was achieved rapidly by agitating the vials in a warmed water bath. If tissue had thickened by contraction after thawing, it was pared down again to<1 mm under an operating microscope with microsurgical scissors before transplantation.

Vitrification procedure: the cryotissue method

Cortex slices from the ovary were cut into pieces 1 × 10 ×10 mm. The precise 1 mm tissue thickness was guaranteed with a tissue slicer designed explicitly for this purpose (Figures 12.2 and 12.3). The tissue slicer plate has a 1 × 10 × 10 mm cubic space. The tissue slicer was put on the surface of the ovary. Then another plate was placed over the tissue slicer, and the ovary was cut between the slicer and the surface of the ovary using a sharp edge. The cortical ovarian tissue was thus cut into 1 × 10 × 10 mm pieces. The ultra-thinness of the tissue was thought to be crucial, not just for the cryopreservation, but also for the rapidity of revascularization after grafting.

Ovarian tissues were initially equilibrated in 7.5% ethylene glycol (EG) and 7.5% dimethyl sulfoxide (DMSO) in handling medium [HM; HEPES-buffered TCM-199 solution supplemented with 20% (v/v) synthetic serum substitute (SSS; Irvine Scientific, Santa Ana, CA, U.S.)] for 25 min, followed by a second equilibration in 20% EG and 20% DMSO with 0.5 mol/L sucrose for 15 min. Ovarian tissues were then

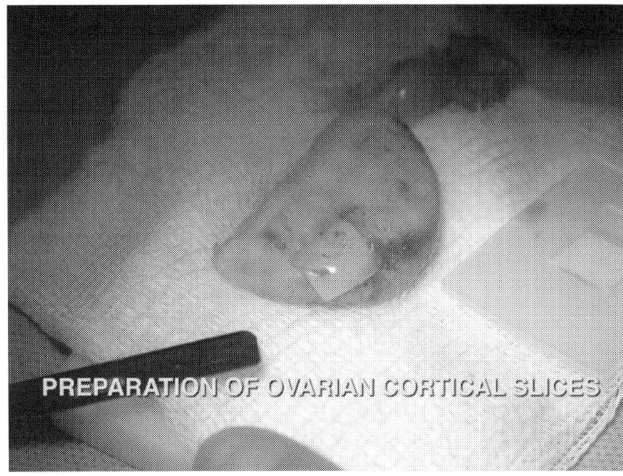

Figure 12.3. Thin slice of ovarian cortex prepared for cryopreservation. (See color plate section for colored image.)

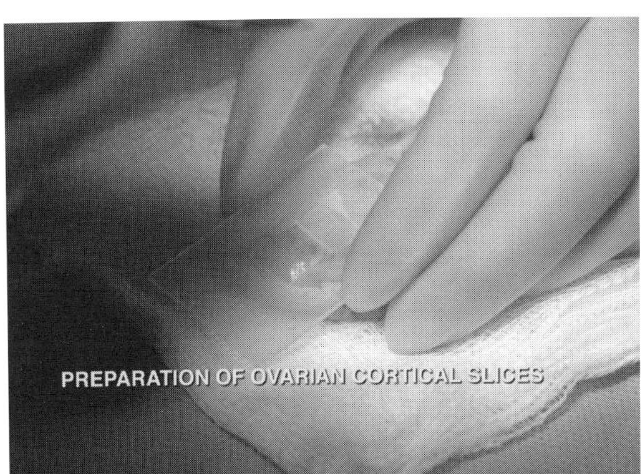

Figure 12.2. "Cryotissue" device (Kitazato, Japan), used to prepare ultrathin slices of cortex for vitrification. (See color plate section for colored image.)

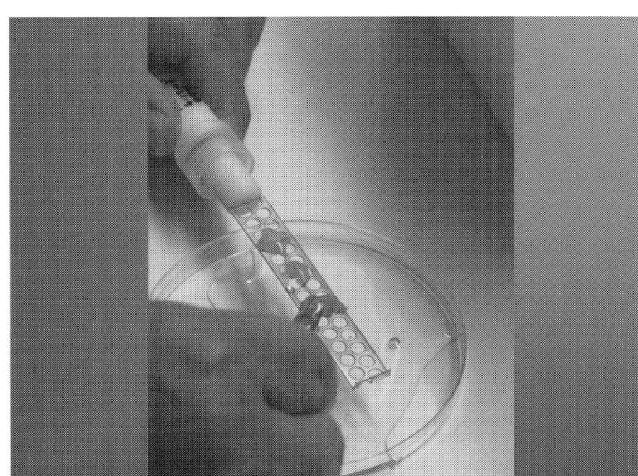

Figure 12.4. Thin ovarian cortical slices placed onto a perforated copper grid. (See color plate section for colored image.)

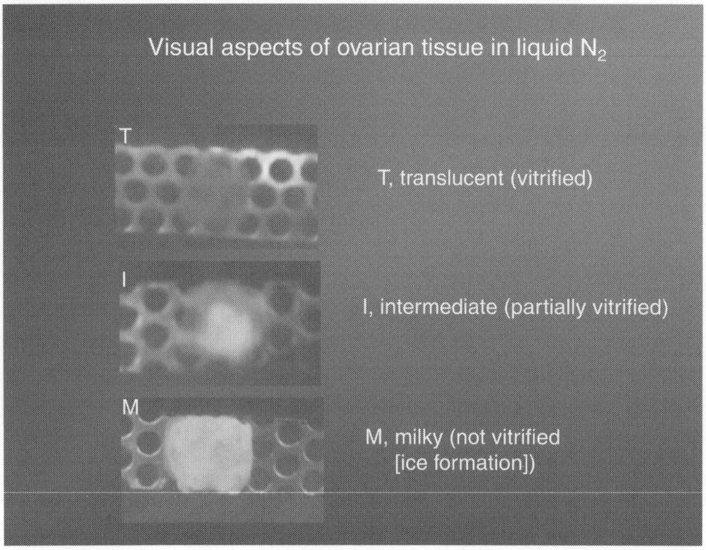

Figure 12.5. The tissue at the top had 40% cryoprotectant and was safely vitrified. The tissue at the bottom had 30% cryoprotectant and was destroyed by freezing. The tissue in the middle was vitrified in 35% cryoprotectant. (See color plate section for colored image.)

placed in a minimum volume of solution onto a thin metal strip (Figure 12.4), and submerged directly into sterile liquid nitrogen, following which the strip was inserted into a protective container and placed into a liquid nitrogen storage tank. For warming, the protective cover was removed and the Cryotissue metal strip was immersed directly into 40 mL of 37°C HM solution supplemented with 1.0 mol/L sucrose for 1 min. Then, ovarian tissues were transferred into 15 mL of 0.5 mol/L sucrose HM solution for 5 min at room temperature, and washed twice in HM solution for 10 min before viability analysis or transplantation. No ice crystal formation was observed during any of the procedures. Prior experiments have shown that lesser concentrations of cryoprotectant than 40% will not be adequate for tissue vitrification (Figure 12.5). For viability testing, tissues were incubated and pipetted in type I collagenase (1 mg/mL) for 10 min to isolate the small follicles and visualize their oocytes. The cells were briefly incubated in Hoechst 33342 and propidium iodide, then washed before viewing by fluorescence microscopy, for a total of 2301 oocytes from 16 patients. Transmission electron microscopy was also used to analyze ovarian tissue that had been either cryopreserved by slow freezing or vitrified by ultrarapid freezing [21].

Cancer patients tissue study

A total of 16 cancer patients requesting fertility preservation by ovarian banking consented to an oocyte viability test and histological review of a small (10%) of their fresh or preserved tissue. In eight cases, the tissue had been preserved by vitrification, six by a slow-freezing protocol, and in two only fresh tissue was analyzed. The total of this section was to determine which method produced a higher cell survival rate.

Transplant results

The principle behind ovarian cortical transplantation is that all primordial resting follicles are located in the outer one millimeter of the otherwise fibrous ovarian cortex (Figure 12.6). As the follicles go through their three to four month development from a resting follicle to a mature Graafian follicle, they migrate inward

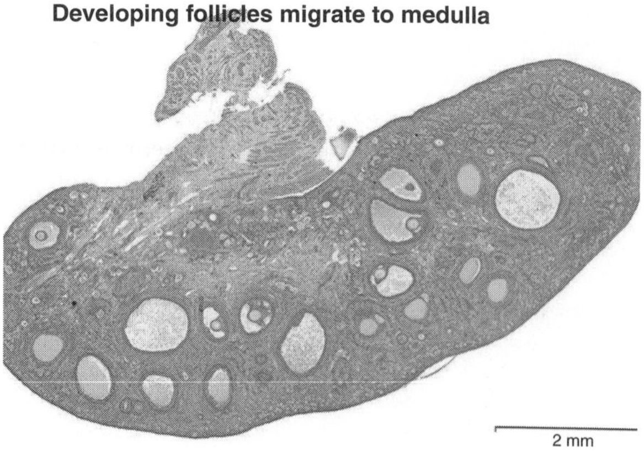

Figure 12.6. All of the resting primordial follicles are located in the fibrous outer cortex. In order to develop over four months into primary and secondary, and finally mature follicles, they must migrate into the softer medulla. (See color plate section for colored image.)

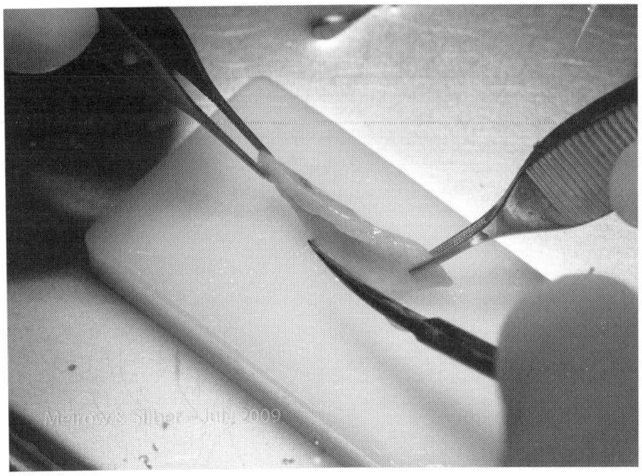

Figure 12.7. 1 mm thin slice of ovarian cortex ready for transplantation. (See color plate section for colored image.)

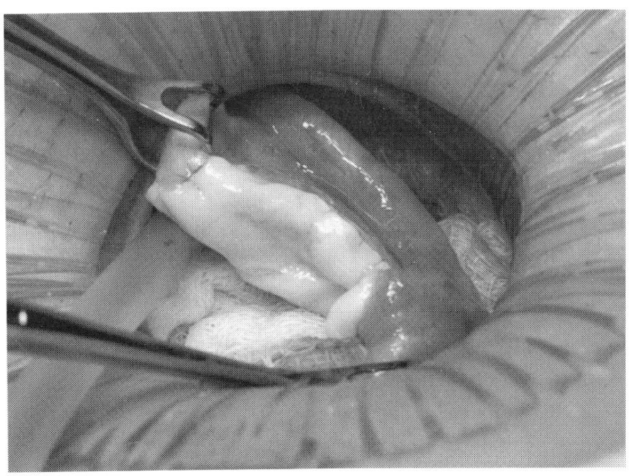

Figure 12.8. Completed first fresh ovarian tissue transplant. (See color plate section for colored image.)

toward the softer tissue of the ovarian medulla (Figure 12.6). At any given time, it is the primordial follicles that represent 99% of the ovary's ovum supply. Therefore, a simple cortical grafting procedure, akin to a full thickness skin graft, should be able to completely transfer its whole ovarian reserve to a recipient medulla (Figures 12.7 and 12.8). However, for this "skin grafting" type of technique to work properly, full attention must be paid to standard plastic surgery principles for skin grafting [1–4]. These principles have not always been followed in previous publications [5].

The grafted tissue must be very thin to allow rapid revascularization to avoid ischemic injury. Furthermore, there must be no microhematoma formation between the graft and the graft bed, for the same reason. Thus, a bloodless operation is required, and tiny 9–0 nylon sutures must firmly anchor the graft to avoid any tiny accumulations of blood under the graft. Finally, there must be continuous pulsatile irrigation with heparinized saline by the assistant to avoid adhesion formation around the graft.

The pregnancy and endocrine data of all nine cases of ovarian transplantation in the identical twin series are summarized in Table 12.1 and Figure 12.9. All nine returned to regular menses and ovulatory cycles by 60–130 days after surgery. Six of the eight who had normal Fallopian tubes delivered eight healthy babies after natural conception, and cases #1, #4, #7, and #9 had one early miscarriage each. Case #5 had not become pregnant but continued to cycle for more than four years. Serum FSH levels on day 3 of the cycles had begun to decline by three months after surgery in all cases and reached normal baseline levels in every recipient by five months (Figure 12.9). There was no difference in the rate of decline of FSH between fresh and frozen grafts.

Case #1 became menopausal again at a little over three years after surgery. A retransplantation of frozen-thawed donor tissue then led to a prompt decline in FSH levels again, and she became pregnant and delivered another healthy child. She then became menopausal once more one and a half years later, had a second frozen graft, and then once more conceived and was carrying her third child at the time of the study. The other case involving a frozen transplant (who had undergone unilateral oophorectomy and ovarian cortex freezing for Hodgkin's lymphoma many years earlier) followed a similar course after transplantation, with serum FSH falling to normal levels by four months and becoming pregnant without the need for further medical assistance. She had a healthy ongoing pregnancy (20 weeks) and delivered a healthy baby boy at 38 weeks.

In the identical twin series, Case #2, who had a transplant at the age of 38 years, became pregnant after five months and delivered a healthy girl the following year. She then became pregnant again four years later from the same fresh graft and delivered a healthy boy at the age of 42 years. Case #7, from the identical twin series, miscarried the first pregnancy after transplantation, but three years later became pregnant again from the same graft and delivered a healthy baby. Thus, two of the healthy babies from spontaneous pregnancies were born to women who had undergone prior pelvic irradiation.

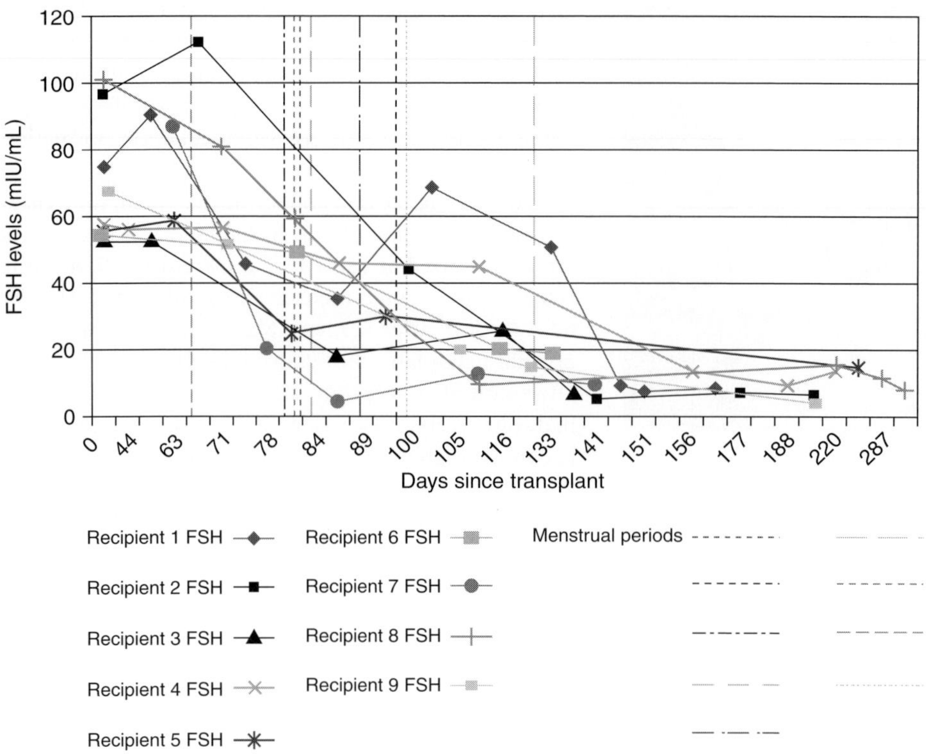

Figure 12.9. Graph showing the return of menstrual cycling and decline of follicle-stimulating hormone (FSH) levels in the first nine cases of fresh ovarian transplantation. (See color plate section for colored image.)

In summary, among 10 women with complete ovarian failure, there were 12 transplants. Nine were fresh ovarian transplants from one identical twin to another. Three were auto-transplants of ovarian tissue that had been frozen prior to ovarian failure. Eight cases were for idiopathic premature ovarian failure, and two were for ovarian failure in cancer patients resulting from chemotherapy, radiation, and bone marrow transplant.

Fresh and frozen transplants in these 10 patients resulted in 14 pregnancies and 11 healthy babies with three miscarriages. Nine babies resulted from fresh transplants and two babies were from two different frozen transplants. It is important to know that two of the patients had pelvic radiation and bone marrow transplants, and each of them had a spontaneous pregnancy and a normal live birth.

On average, it required four and a half months for the return of menstruation and normal ovarian function with a normal day 3 FSH level (Figure 12.9). There was usually more than five years of continuous ovarian function from ovarian grafts, which represented about one third of one ovary or one sixth of ovarian reserve, and which would indicate minimal oocyte loss from ischemia. Furthermore, viability of oocytes and follicles from fresh control ovarian tissue compared to vitrified ovarian tissue showed no loss of oocyte viability, whereas ovarian tissue that had undergone slow freezing exhibited a 60% loss of viability.

A longer duration of transplant function was associated with a larger ovarian reserve expressed either by the antral follicle count (AFC) or the relative density of primordial follicles. Six of the eight fresh cortical grafts functioned for five years or more, one lasted for only two years and another transplant was still functioning at the time of writing, less than three years after surgery. The six with five or more years of ovarian function had an AFC per ovary of nine follicles or greater, and histological examination revealed abundant primordial follicles (+++). The two with less than three years of cycling had an AFC of less than five and few small follicles (+ or ++).

Table 12.1. Summary table of the ovarian transplant results with the first nine fresh and three frozen ovary transplants

Patient	Age	Preop FSH	Postop FSH	Initial Postop Menses intervals	Pregnancy	Babies Delivered	Years of Graft Function
1	24	75	7.1	2nd baby: FROZEN	3	2	4
2	38	96	5.2	93, 42, 24, 27, 25 . . .	3	3	>7
3	25	112	6.8	76, 23, 30, 26, 25, 26, 21, 24, 27, 34, 25, 27, 51, 30, 27, 26, 28, 19 . . .	1	2	>6
4	34	58	9.4	81, 22, 47, 26, 21, 20, 27, 26 . . .	2	1	4
5	40	60	6.8	86, 29, 38, 34, 28, 28, 31, 35, 24, 28, 33, 35, 30 . . .	0	0	4
6	26	101	7.5	64, 20, 39, 40, 32, 26, 29, 26, 26, 41 . . .	1	1	2
7	34	86	4.4	83, 22, 29, 29 . . .	3	2	>6
8	37	86	7.4	100, 17, 39, 29, 27, 22, 23, 20, 34, 25, 26, 29 . . .	1	1	>4
9	35	54	4.2	128, 42, 18, 25 . . .	1	0	2
10	31	78	3.4	FROZEN	1	1	2
11	33	85	8.6	FROZEN	1	1	>1

* *Note: each graft represents only 1/3 of one ovary or 1/6 of entire ovarian reserve.* FSH, follicle-stimulating hormone.

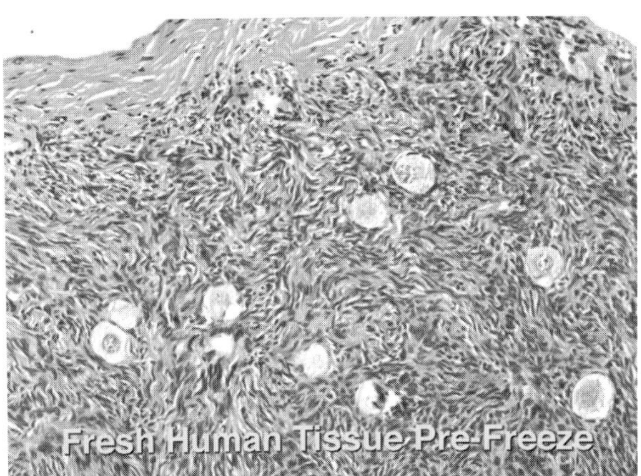

Figure 12.10. This figure and Figure 12.11 show no difference between fresh ovarian tissue and frozen (vitrification) ovarian tissue. (See color plate section for colored image.)

Cryoinjury

Most of the stroma cells in the slow freeze-cryopreserved specimen were lysed and their nuclei compressed between dense bundles of extracellular fibers. The same cells were generally intact after vitrification. Small follicles were found in each specimen, all of which were intact within their basement membranes. The high viability (92%) of oocytes in control (fresh) specimens indicated that disaggregation per se had only caused minimal damage to this cell type. Overall, 2301 oocytes were examined from 16 specimens. Results within each of the three groups were consistent and revealed no significant difference overall between fresh and vitrified tissue, although the viability of slow freeze-cryopreserved tissue was less than a half (42%) and highly significant (Figures 12.10 and 12.11).

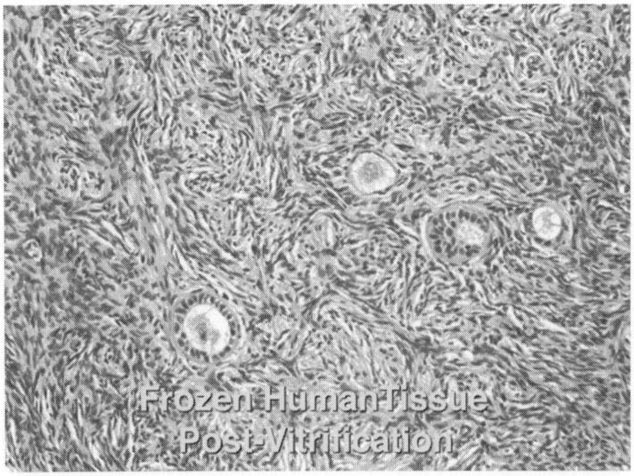

Figure 12.11. This figure and Figure 12.10 show no difference between fresh ovarian tissue and frozen ovarian tissue using vitrification. (See color plate section for colored image.)

Discussion of success with ovarian transplantation

The chief significance of this long-term study of ovarian tissue transplantation is not so much for MZ twins who are discordant for POF, which will always be rare, but for young cancer patients needing fertility preservation. Ovarian tissue banking for a future transplantation provides another fertility option for these patients, and sometimes the only one available.

At least 1/250 women of reproductive age is a cancer survivor, and nowadays 90% of them become long-term survivors depending on the type of disease [22–24]. However, their treatment is likely to reduce their fertility or render them completely sterile [25–28]. Most such women with cancer are anxious to preserve their potential for having children genetically related to them rather than resorting to ova from an unrelated donor or to adoption, which are not always available or desirable options [29,30]. Another indication for fertility preservation is aging, particularly for women with a family history of POF, but also for those with normal ovaries who are increasingly postponing child-bearing [31–37]. The uterus does not seem to play a significant role in this age-related decline, as evidenced by the high pregnancy rates in women of advanced reproductive age who use oocytes donated by younger women [38]. Whereas the MZ twin series involved histo-compatible donor tissue instead of an autograft, and healthy individuals rather than cancer patients, this is the largest series of ovarian transplants to date with the largest number of pregnancies and live births. It provides rare information for guiding fertility preservation practices and counseling patients about the likelihood of success.

It is difficult to draw inferences about the impact of ischemia except from a series of fresh human ovarian transplantation such as this. Ischemia time is reduced from an estimated two to four days with cortical tissue slices to only one to two hours for restoring perfusion after microvascular surgery, which provides the most physiological approach [39]. Yet data from this MZ twin series provide striking proof of the effectiveness and safety of fresh cortical transplants. Eight healthy babies were born to six women from fresh cortical grafts, and all frozen cortical grafts also resulted in healthy pregnancies. Assisted reproductive technology was not required, natural conception occurring often within the first year after surgery and in one instance after the first ovulation. Early conception is not a rule, however; one woman conceived after three years and another had her second child more than four years after her transplant. It is not surprising that at 40 years old, the oldest recipient (case #5) had not become pregnant by the time of writing. Nevertheless, her primordial follicle density and AFC were both relatively high, which probably accounted for the transplant maintaining normal menstrual cycles for more than four years.

Menstrual cycles were reinitiated within two to four months in all cases and continued from one to over four years, with seven of eight women still cycling regularly from their fresh cortical transplant, and without any negative impact reported by the ovary donors. Maximizing the number of ovulatory cycles is obviously desirable for the opportunity that many ovulations provide for conception. The number of cycles to viable conception was one, two, five, seven, eight, eleven, sixteen, and thirty. Nevertheless, if the quality of oocytes is high and coitus is carefully synchronized at midcycle, even short-lived transplants can be effective, as with case #6, who conceived in the first year, gave birth to a child, and then once again became menopausal. Pregnancy results after frozen transplantation were as robust as after fresh, but duration of function after slow freezing, as would be expected, was shorter. Ovarian transplantations involve a single operation with a relatively low surgical burden and low cost, with the advantages of no further medicalization of reproduction and, thus far, only singleton pregnancies. There have been few miscarriages, no birth defects, or obstetric complications associated with transplantation, to date.

We surmise that careful preparation of the donor tissue as a very thin wafer, avoiding microhematoma formation beneath the highly vascular graft bed, and closely apposing the graft all contributed to the success of the present series by promoting rapid revascularization. The orthotopic location may also be important, not only for natural conception but possibly for avoiding pressure from neighboring tissues, which in some heterotopic sites might conceivably distort growing follicles and affect their physiology. Future technical advances may further improve clinical outcomes through significantly reducing ischemia time and accelerating angiogenesis [40,41].

However, the long-term function of these fresh ovarian cortical grafts indicates that follicle reserve was well preserved. If a sterile recipient was given a whole ovary transplant from a 40-year-old donor, and no follicles were lost in the process, a simple model of follicle dynamics predicts that function will last for approximately eight years [42]. It was impressive, therefore, to find that both case #2 and case #5, who were 38 and 40 years old, respectively, at the time of their transplantation, were still cycling after four years, which is halfway to their theoretical limit. Furthermore, if one expects 20 years of remaining ovarian function in the average 30-year-old woman with two ovaries, then one third of one ovary might be anticipated to function perhaps not so much longer than what we have observed in our younger patients whose donor had good ovarian reserve.

Viability markers indicated that less than 50% of human oocytes survived the slow-freezing protocol, which has been the standard method for ovarian tissue since the pioneering studies in sheep [18,19,43–50]. Our studies have revealed that vitrification may produce results superior to standard cryopreservation [17]. Because most centers, including our own, have used mainly the slow-freezing cryopreservation protocol, it is reassuring that three viable pregnancies were obtained in the present study as well as five others for cancer patients in other centers [8,10–13]. The percentage of viable oocytes in vitrified tissue was remarkably similar to that of fresh tissue controls, suggesting that vitrification might provide even better results after transplantation than slow-freeze cryopreservation, although this cannot be stated definitively without long-term studies.

Conclusion

What is the future for women whose ovaries were frozen before undergoing treatment for leukemia or breast cancers that might have already metastasized to the ovary [51–60]? Hodgkin's disease is the safest cancer for transplanting ovarian tissue back to the patient. But what can be done with frozen ovarian tissue of the leukemia survivor if there happens to have been leukemic cells in that tissue? Culturing that tissue to obtain mature follicles for IVF in these patients is currently the subject of intense research efforts [61–63]. Culturing of primordial follicles may still be a distant goal [64–68], but progress is now being made with three-dimensional culturing of secondary follicles, because one mechanism controlling follicle maturation in the ovarian cortex may be physical pressure and tissue rigidity [69–72]. Using this concept, remarkable progress has been made in

Table 12.2. Summary table of worldwide frozen ovarian cortex tissue transplant pregnancies

Case	Diagnosis	Babies	Where
1	Hodgkins	1	Donnez
2	Neuro Tumor	1	Donnez
3	Non-Hodgkins	1	Meirow
4	Hodgkins	1	Demeestere
5	Ewings	3	Andersen
6	Hodgkins	1	Andersen
7	POF	1	Silber
8	Hodgkins	2	Silber
9	Polyangiitis	1	Piver
10	Breast Cancer	2	Pellicer
11	Sickle Cell	1	Piver
12	Hodgkins	2	Revel
Totals: 12 patients		**17 Babies**	**8 Centers**
Fresh + **Frozen**		**28 Babies**	Silber – **14 Babies**

POF, premature ovarian failure.

culturing ovarian tissue and maturing secondary follicles in vitro. But for patients in whom there is no significant risk of ovarian metastasis, ovarian tissue transplantation may now be ready for clinical use. In fact, at the time of writing, 22 babies had already been born from ovarian transplantation worldwide, and 13 of those from frozen ovarian tissue (Table 12.2) [73,74].

References

1. Silber SJ, Lenahan KM, Levine DJ, et al. Ovarian transplantation between monozygotic twins discordant for premature ovarian failure. *N Engl J Med* 2005; **353**: 58–63.
2. Silber SJ, Gosden RG. Ovarian transplantation in a series of monozygotic twins discordant for ovarian failure. *N Engl J Med* 2007; **356**: 1382–1384.
3. Silber SJ, DeRosa M, Pineda J, et al. A series of monozygotic twins discordant for ovarian failure: ovary transplantation (cortical versus microvascular) and cryopreservation. *Hum Reprod* 2008; **23**: 1531–1537.
4. Silber SJ, Grudzinskas G, Gosden RG. Successful pregnancy after microsurgical transplantation of an intact ovary. *N Eng J Med* 2008; **359**: 2617–2618.
5. Oktay K, Karikaya G. Ovarian function after transplantation of frozen, banked autologous ovarian tissue. *N Eng J Med* 2000; **342**: 1919.
6. Radford JA, Lieberman BA, Brison DR, et al. Orthotopic reimplantation of cryopreserved ovarian cortical strips after high-dose chemotherapy for Hodgkin's lymphoma. *Lancet* 2001; **357**: 1172–1175.
7. Sanchez M, Alama P, Gadea B, et al. Fresh human orthotopic ovarian cortex transplantation; long-term results. *Hum Reprod* 2007; **22**: 786–791.
8. Donnez J, Dolmans MM, Demylle D, et al. Livebirth after orthotopic transplantation of cryopreserved ovarian tissue. *Lancet* 2004; **364**: 1405–1410.
9. Donnez J, Dolmans MM, Demylle D, et al. Restoration of ovarian function after orthotopic (intraovarian and periovarian) transplantation of cryopreserved ovarian tissue in a woman treated by bone marrow transplantation for sickle cell anaemia: case report. *Hum Reprod* 2006; **21**: 183–188.
10. Meirow D, Levron J, Eldar-Geva T, et al. Pregnancy after transplantation of cryopreserved ovarian tissue in a patient with ovarian failure after chemotherapy. *N Engl J Med* 2005; **353**: 318–321.
11. Demeestere I, Simon P, Buxant F, et al. Ovarian function and spontaneous pregnancy after combined heterotopic and orthotopic cryopreserved ovarian tissue transplantation in a patient previously treated with bone marrow transplantation: case report. *Hum Reprod* 2006; **21**: 2010–2014.
12. Demeestere I, Simon P, Emiliani S, Delbaere A, Englert Y. Fertility preservation: successful transplantation of cryopreserved ovarian tissue in a young patient previously treated for Hodgkin's disease. *Oncologist* 2007; **12**: 1437–1442.
13. Andersen CY, Rosendahl M, Byskov AG, et al. Two successful pregnancies following autotransplantation of frozen/thawed ovarian tissue. *Hum Reprod* 2008; **23**: 2266–2272.
14. Baird DT, Webb R, Campbell BK, Harkness LM, Gosden RG. Long-term ovarian function in sheep after ovariectomy and transplantation of autografts stored at −196°C. *Endocrinology* 1999; **140**: 462–471.
15. Bedaiwy MA, Falcone T. Harvesting and autotransplantation of vascularized ovarian grafts: approaches and techniques. *Reprod Biomed Online* 2007; **14**: 360–371.
16. Arav A, Revel A, Nathan Y, et al. Oocyte recovery, embryo development and ovarian function after cryopreservation and transplantation of whole sheep ovary. *Hum Reprod* 2005; **20**: 3554–3559.
17. Kagawa N, Silber S, Kuwayama M. Successful vitrification of bovine and human ovarian tissue. *Reprod Biomed Online* 2009; **18**: 568–577.
18. Gosden RG, Baird DT, Wade JC, Webb R. Restoration of fertility to oophorectomized sheep by ovarian autografts stored at −196 degrees C. *Hum Reprod* 1994; **9**: 597–603.
19. Newton H, Aubard Y, Rutherford A, Sharma V, Gosden R. Low temperature storage and grafting of human ovarian tissue. *Hum Reprod* 1996; **11**: 1487–1491.
20. Gook DA, Edgar DH, Stern C. Effect of cooling rate and dehydration regimen on the histological appearance of human ovarian cortex following cryopreservation in 1,2-propanediol. *Hum Reprod* 1999; **14**: 2061–2068.
21. Keros V, Xella S, Hultenby K, et al. Vitrification versus controlled-rate freezing in cryopreservation of human ovarian tissue. *Hum Reprod* 2009; **24**: 1670–1683.
22. Bleyer WA. The impact of childhood cancer on the United States and the world. *CA Cancer J Clin* 1990; **40**: 355–367.
23. Ries LAG, Smith MA, Gurney JG, et al. eds. *Cancer Incidence and Survival among Children and Adolescents: United States SEER Program 1975–1995*. Bethesda, MD: National Cancer Institute, SEER Program, 1999.
24. Jeruss JS, Woodruff TK. Preservation of fertility in patients with cancer. *N Engl J Med* 2009; **360**: 902–911.

25. Anderson RA, Themmen AP, Al-Qahtani A, Groome NP, Cameron DA. The effects of chemotherapy and long-term gonadotrophin suppression on the ovarian reserve in premenopausal women with breast cancer. *Hum Reprod* 2006; **21**: 253–259.

26. Anderson RA, Cameron DA. Assessment of the effect of chemotherapy on ovarian function in women with breast cancer. *J Clin Oncol* 2007; **25**: 1630–1632.

27. Larsen EC, Muller J, Schmiegelow K, Rechnitzer C, Andersen AN. Reduced ovarian function in long-term survivors of radiation and chemotherapy-treated childhood cancer. *J Clin Endocrinol Metab* 2003; **88**: 5307–5314.

28. Lee SJ, Schover LR, Partridge AH, et al. American Society of Clinical Oncology recommendations on fertility preservation in cancer patients. *J Clin Oncol* 2006; **24**: 2917–2931.

29. Schover LR, Rybicki LA, Martin BA, Bringelsen KA. Having children after cancer. A pilot survey of survivors' attitudes and experiences. *Cancer* 1999; **86**: 697–709.

30. Schover LR, Brey K, Lichtin A, Lipshultz LI, Jeha S. Knowledge and experience regarding cancer, infertility, and sperm banking in younger male survivors. *J Clin Oncol* 2002; **20**: 1880–1889.

31. Leridon H. Can assisted reproduction technology compensate for the natural decline in fertility with age? A model assessment. *Hum Reprod* 2004; **19**: 1548–1553.

32. Lampic C, Svanberg AS, Karlstrom P, Tyden T. Fertility awareness, intentions concerning childbearing, and attitudes toward parenthood among female and male academics. *Hum Reprod* 2006; **21**: 558–564.

33. Maheshwari A, Porter M, Shetty A, Bhattacharya S. Women's awareness and perceptions of delay in childbearing. *Fertil Steril* 2008; **90**: 1036–1042.

34. Te Velde ER, Pearson PL. The variability of female reproductive ageing. *Hum Reprod Update* 2002; **8**: 141–154.

35. Devroey P. Female age predicts embryonic implantation after ICSI: a case-controlled study. *Hum Reprod* 1996; **11**: 1324–1327.

36. Silber SJ, Nagy Z, Devroey P, Camus M, Van Steirteghem AC. The effect of female age and ovarian reserve on pregnancy rate in male infertility: treatment of azoospermia with sperm retrieval and intracytoplasmic sperm injection. *Hum Reprod* 1997; **12**: 2693–2700.

37. Fretts RC. Effect of advanced age on fertility and pregnancy in women. *Up To Date Online* 2007. (Available at: http://www.uptodate.com)

38. SART. Assisted reproductive technology success rates. *National Summary and Fertility Clinic Reports.* Atlanta, GA: Centers for Disease Control and Prevention, 2005.

39. Yin H, Wang X, Kim SS, et al. Transplantation of intact rat gonads using vascular anastomosis: effects of cryopreservation, ischaemia and genotype. *Hum Reprod* 2003; **18**: 1165–1172.

40. Candy CJ, Wood MJ, Whittingham DG. Restoration of a normal reproductive lifespan after grafting of cryopreserved mouse ovaries. *Hum Reprod* 2006; **15**: 1300–1304.

41. Israely T, Dafni H, Granot D, et al. Vascular remodeling and angiogenesis in ectopic ovarian transplants: a crucial role of pericytes and vascular smooth muscle cells in maintenance of ovarian grafts. *Biol Reprod* 2003; **68**: 2055–2064.

42. Faddy MJ, Gosden RG, Gougeon A, Richardson SJ, Nelson JF. Accelerated disappearance of ovarian follicles in mid-life: implications for forecasting menopause. *Hum Reprod* 1992; **7**: 1342–1346.

43. Aubard Y, Piver P, Cogni Y, et al. Orthotopic and heterotopic autografts of frozen-thawed ovarian cortex in sheep. *Hum Reprod* 1999; **14**: 2149–2154.

44. Salle B, Lornage J, Demirci B, et al. Restoration of ovarian steroid secretion and histologic assessment after freezing, thawing, and autograft of a hemi-ovary in sheep. *Fertil Steril* 1999; **72**: 366–370.

45. Lee DM, Yeoman RR, Battaglia DE, et al. Live birth after ovarian tissue transplant. *Nature* 2004; **428**: 137–138.

46. Kim S, Battaglia DE, Soules MR. The future of human ovarian cryopreservation and transplantation: fertility and beyond. *Fertil Steril* 2001; **75**: 137–138.

47. Kim SS, Yang HW, Kang HG, et al. Quantitative assessment of ischemic tissue damage in ovarian cortical tissue with or without antioxidant (ascorbic acid) treatment. *Fertil Steril* 2004; **82**: 679–685.

48. Kim SS, Radford J, Harris M, et al. Ovarian tissue harvested from lymphoma patients to preserve fertility may be safe for autotransplantation. *Hum Reprod* 2001; **16**: 2056–2060.

49. Kim SS. DEBATE: Ovarian tissue banking for cancer patients – To do or not to do? *Hum Reprod* 2003; **18**: 1759–1761.

50. Kim SS, Kang HG, Kim NH, Lee HC, Lee HH. Assessment of the integrity of human oocytes retrieved from cryopreserved ovarian tissue after xenotransplantation. *Hum Reprod* 2005; **20**: 2502–2508.

51. Falcone T, Attaran M, Bedaiwy MA, Goldberg JM. Ovarian function preservation in the cancer patient. *Fertil Steril* 2004; **81**: 243–257.

52. Gadducci A, Cosio S, Genazzani AR. Ovarian function and childbearing issues in breast cancer survivors. *Gynecol Endocrinol* 2007; **23**: 625–631.

53. Jemal A, Siegel R, Ward E, et al. Cancer statistics. *CA Cancer J Clin* 2008; **58**: 71–96.

54. Lobo RA. Potential options for preservation of fertility in women. *N Engl J Med* 2005; **353**: 64–73.

55. Colgan TJ, Murphy J, Cole DE, Narod S, Rosen B. Occult carcinoma in prophylactic oophorectomy specimens: prevalence and association with BRCA germline mutation status. *Am J Surg Pathol* 2001; **25**: 1283–1289.

56. Elizur SE. Detection of microscopic metastasis of solid tumors and hematological malignancies in cryopreserved ovaries. *Fertil Steril* 2004; **82**: S116.

57. Meirow D, Hardan I, Dor J, et al. Searching for evidence of disease and malignant cell contamination in ovarian tissue stored from hematologic cancer patients. *Hum Reprod* 2008; **23**: 1007–1013.

58. Nakayama K. Gonadal failure after treatment of hematologic malignancies: from recognition to management for health-care providers. *Natl Clin Pract Oncol* 2008; **5**: 78–89.

59. Schroder CP, Timmer-Bosscha H, Wijchman JG, et al. An in vitro model for purging of tumour cells from ovarian tissue. *Hum Reprod* 2004; **19**: 1069–1975.

60. Sklar CA, Mertens AC, Mitby P, et al. Premature menopause in survivors of childhood cancer; a report from the childhood cancer survivor study. *J Natl Cancer Inst* 2006; **98**: 890–896.

61. Smitz J, Picton H, Platteau P, et al. Principal findings from a multicenter trial investigating the safety of follicular-fluid meiosis-activating sterol for in vitro maturation of human cumulus-enclosed oocytes. *Fertil Steril* 2007; **87**: 949–964.

62. Papanikolaou EG, Platteau P, Albano C, et al. Immature oocyte in-vitro maturation: clinical aspects. *Reprod Biomed Online* 2005; **10**: 587–592.

63. Nogueira D, Cortvrindt R, Eveaerdt B, Smitz J. Effects of long-term in vitro exposure to phosphodiesterase type-3 inhibitors on follicle and oocyte development. *Reproduction* 2005; **130**: 177–186.

64. Picton HM, Harris SE, Muruvi W, Chambers EL. The in vitro growth and maturation of follicles. *Reprod Rev* 2008; **136**: 703–715.

65. Sadeu JC, Cortvrindt R, Ron-El R, Kasterstein E, Smitz J. Morphological and ultrastructural evaluation of cultured frozen-thawed human fetal ovarian tissue. *Fertil Steril* 2006; **85**: 1130–1141.

66. Sadeu JC, Mazoyer C, Smitz J. Human follicle culture in vitro In: Rizk B, Garcia-Velasco J, Sallam H, Makrigiannakis A, eds. *Infertility and Assisted Reproduction*. Cambridge, UK: Cambridge University Press, 2008; 25–38.

67. Amorim CA, Van Langendonckt A, David A, Dolmans MM, Donnez J. Survival of human pre-antral follicles after cryopreservation of ovarian tissue, follicular isolation and in vitro culture in a calcium alginate matrix. *Hum Reprod* 2009; **24**: 92–99.

68. Telfer EE, McLaughlin M, Ding C, Thong KJ. A two-step serum-free culture system supports development of human oocytes from primordial follicles in the presence of activin. *Hum Reprod* 2008; **23**: 1151–1158.

69. West ER, Xu M, Woodruff TK, Shea LD. Physical properties of alginate hydrogels and their effects on in vitro follicle development. *Biomaterials* 2007; **28**: 4439–4448.

70. West-Farrell ER, Xu M, Gromberg MA, et al. The mouse follicle microenvironment regulates antrum formation and steroid production: alternations in gene expression profiles. *Biol Reprod* 2009; **80**: 432–439.

71. Xu M, Kreeger PK, Shea LD, Woodruff TK. Tissue-engineered follicles produce live, fertile offspring. *Tissue Eng* 2006; **12**: 2739–2746.

72. Xu M, West E, Shea LD, Woodruff TK. Identification of a stage-specific permissive in vitro culture environment for follicle growth and oocyte development. *Biol Reprod* 2006; **75**: 916–923.

73. Silber S, Kagawa N, Kuwayama M, Gosden R. Duration of fertility after fresh and frozen ovary transplantation. *Fertil Steril* 2010; **94**: 2191–2196.

74. Donnez J, Silber S, Andersen CY, et al. Children born after ovarian transplantation. A review of 13 live births. *Ann Med* 2011; **43**: 437–450.

Chapter

13 Prenatal diagnosis after assisted reproductive technology

Ido Ben-Ami and Ron Maymon

Introduction

Over the last three decades, prenatal screening for Down's syndrome (DS) has become an integrated part of antenatal care in most developed countries. In the second trimester, the most common markers are maternal serum human chorionic gonadotrophin (hCG) or its free β-subunit (Fβ-hCG), alpha-fetoprotein (AFP), and unconjugated estriol (uE_3). Large studies using combinations of hCG or Fβ-hCG and either or both of the other markers have confirmed model predictions that about two thirds of DS-affected pregnancies can be detected with a false positive rate (FPR) of about 5% [1,2]. The most recent addition to the second-trimester serum markers has been inhibin-A, which is found at higher levels in affected pregnancies [3,4]. This combination of markers (the "quadruple test") allows the detection of about 75% of DS-affected pregnancies with a FPR of approximately 5% if gestational age is based on an ultrasound scan [5].

It is presently accepted that ultrasound can identify and measure subcutaneous fluid collections between the soft tissue covering the fetal spine and the overlying skin during the late first trimester [6–8]. The thickness of this hypoechoic ultrasonographic feature, defined as nuchal translucency (NT), is associated with chromosomal abnormalities [6–8], cardiac and other structural defects [9], as well as an increased risk of spontaneous abortion [10]. In the first trimester, the combination of maternal serum pregnancy-associated placental protein-A (PAPP-A) and Fβ-hCG can achieve a detection rate of approximately 60% with a FPR of about 5% [11].

Combining NT with these first-trimester biochemical serum markers resulted in a combined screening test [6]. It has been reported that such a combination may allow about an 85% DS detection rate with a 5% FPR [12–14], a significant improvement of other DS screening tests. Later, a model of an integrated screening for DS was proposed, which was based on the combination of first-trimester NT measurement and serum PAPP-A levels with second-trimester AFP, β-hCG, E_3, and inhibin. The integrated test could allow a 90% DS detection rate for a 1% FPR [4].

Another sonographic marker that can be used both in the first and second trimester in order to improve the prediction of DS is nasal bone (NB) evaluation. Cicero and colleagues [15] found that absence of the NB during first-trimester sonography was associated with trisomy 21 (Figure 13.1). The authors estimated that if NB assessment were combined with maternal age and NT measurement, 93% of DS cases would be detected at a 5% FPR and that 85% of cases would still be detected if the FPR were set at 1%. In subsequent studies, the same investigators found that an absent NB was also associated with trisomy 18, trisomy 13, and monosomy X [16]. These data suggest that in high-risk pregnancies, NB assessment is a sensitive and highly specific marker and could be a useful adjunct to NT and serum biochemistry [17].

In addition to increased NT and absent NB, chromosomal abnormalities are associated with a pattern of characteristic sonographic findings in the first trimester. Trisomy 21 was found to be associated with a reverse flow pattern in the ductus venosus (Figure 13.2), tricuspid regurgitation, and maxillary hypoplasia [18]. Although first-trimester sonographic markers are potentially the best, some concerns have arisen about their clinical application. Pitfalls may be due to the inability to examine the markers, incorrect assessment, or incorrect interpretation of the findings [18].

It is well known that the maternal serum concentrations of placental and fetal proteins may be affected

Pregnancy After Assisted Reproductive Technology, ed. Eric R. M. Jauniaux and Botros R. M. B. Rizk. Published by Cambridge University Press.

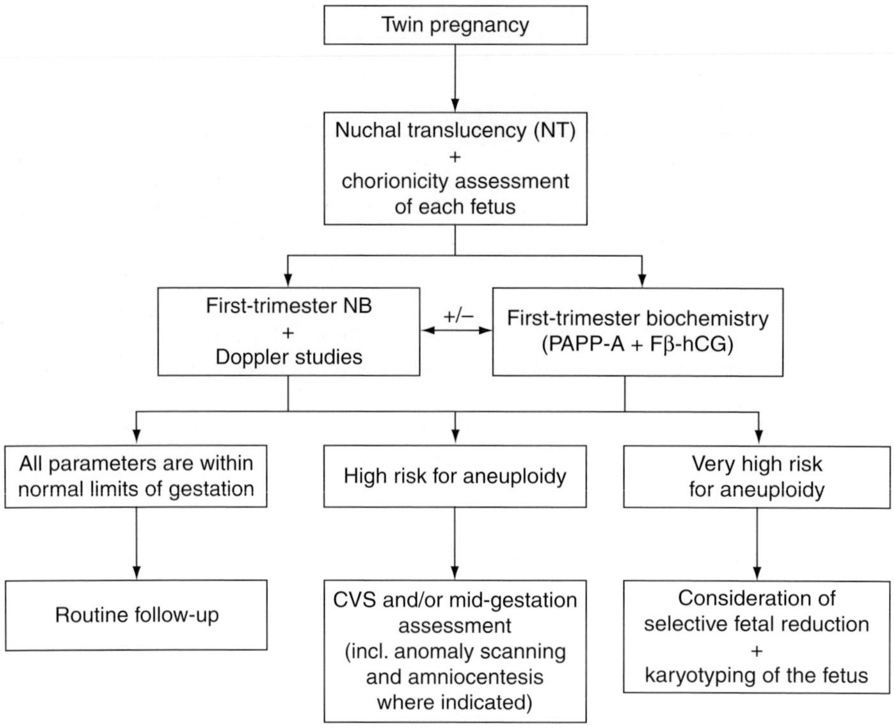

Figure 13.1. Flow chart of first-trimester screening for chromosomal abnormalities in a twin pregnancy. Selective fetal reduction could be postponed until after a detailed anomaly scan (around 13–14 weeks' gestation). Chorionic villous sampling is reserved for high-risk cases for chromosomal aberrations or carriers of a single gene disorder or balanced translocation.

NB, nasal bone; PAPP-A, pregnancy-associated placental protein-A; Fβ-hCG, free β-subunit of human chorionic gonadotrophin; CVS, chorionic villous sampling.

by various conditions, such as diabetes mellitus, maternal smoking, multiple gestation, ethnic subgroups, and wrong dates [1]. Therefore, adjustment criteria were introduced to correct the FPR and the detection rate (DR), thus providing a more accurate patient-specific calculated risk [1].

Over the past decade, the wide use of various assisted reproductive technologies (ARTs) has risen dramatically. Women who conceived following ART have thus far received the same antenatal screening approach as those who conceived spontaneously [19]. This policy would appear to be inadequate as women who conceived following ART treatment are generally older than are women with spontaneously conceived pregnancies, and are therefore more likely to be carrying a child affected by a chromosomal disorder (primarily trisomy 21) [20,21]. Fetuses conceived after intracytoplasmic spermatozoon injection (ICSI) are also known to have an increased risk of chromosomal aberrations [22–25]. In addition, these women may suffer from various underlying metabolic, endocrinological, or genetic diseases, for which ART has been indicated in the first place [19]. Taken together, these factors may lead to overuse of invasive cytogenetic testing, and thus may contribute to the 20% amniocentesis rate in pregnant women who conceived with ART [26]. Besides the risk of miscarriage following an invasive procedure, high-risk results are associated with emotional sequelae as they raise the anxiety level throughout the process of counseling, invasive procedure, and until a reassuring result is received.

Furthermore, ART has led to a high prevalence of twin pregnancies and a higher order of multiple gestations, which even further complicate the antenatal screening algorithm. Therefore, the importance of accurate noninvasive prenatal screening in this population is even higher than in spontaneous pregnancies.

This chapter aims to explore the challenging issue of antenatal DS screening in pregnancies resulting from ART (singletons, twins, and high-order multiple gestations). The implication and the management in the attempt to achieve the best evaluation of DS risk for every type of gestation will be discussed.

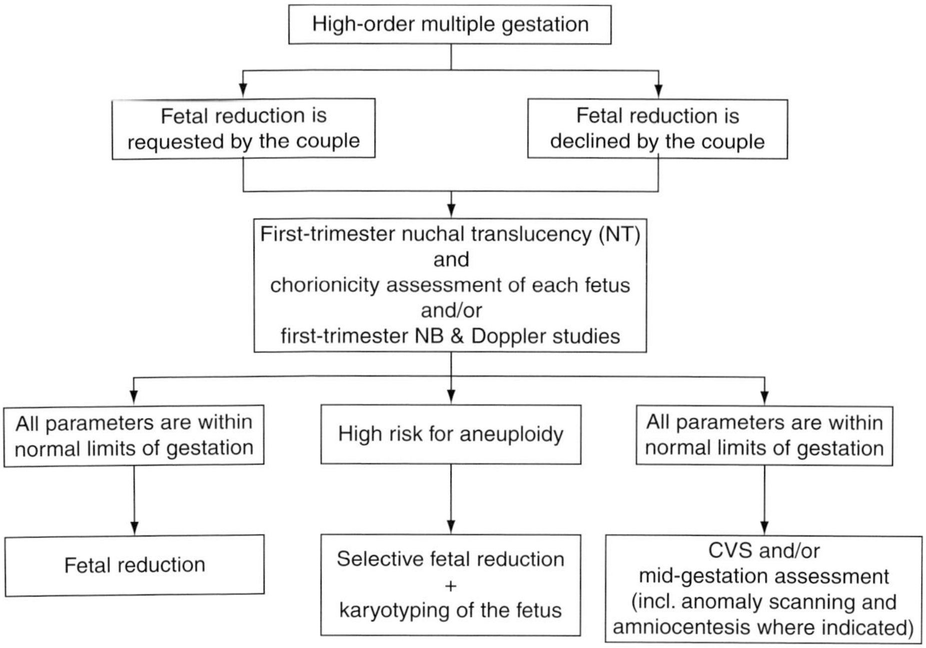

Figure 13.2. Flow chart of first-trimester screening for chromosomal abnormalities in a high-order multiple gestation. Fetal reduction could be postponed until after a detailed anomaly scan (around 13–14 weeks' gestation). Chorionic villous sampling is reserved for only high-risk cases for chromosomal aberrations or carriers of a single gene disorder or balanced translocation.
NB, nasal bone; CVS, chorionic villous sampling.

Singleton pregnancies

In ART pregnancies, the gestational age can be calculated from the oocyte retrieval; nevertheless, an "artificial menstrual dating" is constructed by calculating the oocyte retrieval minus two weeks or embryo transfer minus 16 days to convert the menstrual dating. This date is then considered the basis for further gestational age calculation.

Second-trimester screening

Chronologically, second-trimester serum screening was introduced first and thus more experience has been gained with it. There are conflicting data in the literature surrounding maternal serum triple marker screening analyte levels and the DS FPR in pregnancies conceived through ART (Table 13.1). Several studies have found insignificant changes in maternal serum hCG concentrations in pregnancies achieved by ART treatment compared with naturally conceived pregnancies. Other authors, however, have found higher hCG concentrations in pregnancies resulting from ART compared with spontaneous pregnancies (overall range: 0.88–1.53 multiples of the mean (MoM), Table 13.1) [27–38].

High hCG levels may be explained partly by a greater number of corpora lutea [30], by undiagnosed multiple early implantation sites, or by progesterone supplementation, which increases placental hCG production [39]. Nevertheless, it is unlikely that most of these proteins will remain in the maternal circulation for as long as four months when the biochemical screening is performed [29,40]. Alternatively, it may represent placentation failure that could result in changes in the trophoblast function and thus hCG production [38].

Women who conceived after oocyte donation represent a unique clinical model, as these women lack a corpus luteum and no induction of ovulation could have been carried out [19]. Unlike what occurs in self-oocyte in vitro fertilization (IVF), where multiple corpora lutea may produce very high concentrations of progesterone, in oocyte donation pregnancies the progesterone is exclusively derived from a therapeutic source. Hence, the changes in the second-trimester serum markers can be attributed almost entirely to changes in the feto-placental unit metabolism.

Table 13.1. The biochemistry serum screening profile in pregnancies achieved by assisted reproductive technology

ART	Number of cases	AFP MoM	uE_3 MoM	hCG MoM	Reference
IVF	67	0.89	NR	1.23	[29]
IVF	41	1.02	NR	1.52	[28]
IVF	327	0.98	0.92	0.93	[27]
IVF	69	0.95	0.9	1.22	[30]
IVF	42	0.88	NR	1.15	[41]
IVF	151	0.99	0.94	1.14	[31]
IVF	70	1.13	0.98	1.31	[33]
IVF	46	1.04	1.11	1.38	[32]
IVF	71	1.13	0.94	1.12	[34]
IVF	58	0.95	NR	1.19	[35]
IVF	96	0.98	NR	1.2	[38]
IVF	970	0.97	0.9	1.1	[36]
IVF	88	0.99	1.12	1.12	[37]
OI	1,632	1.02	0.92	1.09	[27]
OI+IUI	43	0.76	NR	1.09	[43]
ICSI	23	0.76	NR	0.88	[41]
ICSI	48	1.22	NR	1.53	[38]
ICSI	545	0.95	1	1.01	[36]
OD	37	1.45	0.97	1.32	[32]

ART, assisted reproductive technology; AFP, α-fetoprotein; uE_3, unconjugated estriol; hCG, human chorionic gonadotrophin; MoM , multiples of the mean; IVF, in vitro fertilization; OI, ovulation induction; IUI, intrauterine insemination; ICSI, intracytoplasmic spermatozoon injection; OD, oocyte donation; NR, not recorded.

A comparison of maternal serum screening results between 37 oocyte donation and 46 self-oocyte IVF-conceived singletons of similarly aged women revealed a similar daily pattern of first-trimester serum β-hCG in both groups. Importantly, these maternal serum hCG concentrations were found to be higher when compared to spontaneous pregnancies from the same population (1.38 and 1.32 median MoM for IVF and oocyte donation, respectively, in comparison with 0.99 median MoM from the same reference laboratory; Table 13.1). Because neither chromosomal abnormalities nor fetal or neonatal deaths were recorded in either group, it was concluded that the high maternal serum hCG concentrations may be a marker for other adverse obstetric outcomes rather than indicating a higher risk for a DS fetus [32].

The effect of ART on AFP and uE_3 levels is also controversial (Table 13.1). Several studies have demonstrated decreased levels of maternal serum AFP and uE_3 in IVF-conceived pregnancies [29–31,36,41], while others found insignificant changes in their concentrations compared with naturally conceived pregnancies [28,33,37]. Interestingly, pregnancies resulting from oocyte donation showed 45% increase in AFP concentrations, which could not be explained by the age-related 4.4% per 10-year increment of serum AFP concentrations [32]. Likewise, the median levels of both AFP and uE_3 were found to be significantly higher in women using a donor ovum versus those using their own ovum, although it was concluded that these changes are not large enough to warrant correction of AFP and uE_3 [27]. A comparison between two groups of unstimulated assisted-conception pregnancies, that is, own-oocyte frozen embryos (own-FET) versus oocyte-donated embryos, revealed that the oocyte-donated group had only significantly increased AFP concentrations compared to the own-FET group (1.38 versus 0.99 median MoM, respectively, $P = 0.002$) [42]. In contrast, pregnancies conceived by intrauterine insemination (IUI) often present with lower maternal serum AFP than naturally conceived pregnancies [43].

The data concerning maternal serum inhibin levels in ART pregnancies are limited. Wald et al. [31] found that the median serum inhibin levels in 39 singleton pregnancies conceived by IVF were not significantly different from 195 controls. In contrast, our group [44] found that the median serum inhibin levels of 170 ART singleton pregnancies were significantly higher as compared to 4334 spontaneous singletons (1.11 MoM versus 0.99 MoM, respectively, $P < 0.001$).

Following correction for gestational age by means of the dating scan and for maternal age at conception, it was concluded that the high second-trimester FPR in the IVF patients is mainly attributed to factors that are directly associated with the pregnancy itself. These findings support the concept that such pregnancies may have a primary underlying pathology. This may result from various unknown metabolic disturbances in the feto-placental unit to placental-related obstetric complications [29]. Indeed, IVF pregnancies were found to be associated with a higher incidence of low birth weight and premature delivery compared with spontaneous conception [45,46]. These complications are typically predicted and characterized by high maternal serum hCG and AFP [47].

First-trimester screening

Theoretically, first-trimester screening should be directly influenced by ART, particularly by the hormonal treatments and the presence of multiple corpora lutea. Moreover, the effect of ART is likely to persist throughout the first trimester of gestation. Thus, one would expect that serum marker changes induced by this treatment would be more marked during the first trimester and mainly be reflected by high maternal serum hCG and low PAPP-A levels [19].

In fact, the effect of ART on first-trimester screening is also controversial (Table 13.2). Most studies of first-trimester screening report decreased PAPP-A levels in IVF pregnancies with unaltered levels of Fβ-hCG [45–50]. However, other authors found decreased PAPP-A levels and increased Fβ-hCG levels [51,52] or decreased Fβ-hCG levels [48,49], and some show no changes in maternal serum values in IVF pregnancies [50–52]. In ICSI pregnancies, a decrease in PAPP-A levels has been reported with unaltered levels of Fβ-hCG [47–49,51,53]. One study reported increased levels of Fβ-hCG [53] and other studies have found no changes in maternal serum values in ICSI pregnancies [51,54].

The lower PAPP-A concentrations (range: 0.71–1.13 median MoM; Table 13.2) might be attributed to early testing in the ART group or might be secondary to early metabolic impairment of the feto-placental unit [55]. Lower PAPP-A and Fβ-hCG concentrations at 10 to 14 weeks of gestation were also reported to be associated with the subsequent development of various pregnancy complications [55].

In contrast to the fluctuating maternal serum results, NT measurements are found to be more consistent. Indeed, NT thickness does not seem to be affected by ART in most studies [50,53,56,57]. However, some studies have found an increased NT thickness in IVF or ICSI pregnancies [46,58] or a decreased NT thickness [58].

Initial data suggest that NB status is independent of serum biochemistry. Although absent NB is associated with increased NT thickness, these ultrasound findings can be combined as long as the calculation of DS risk takes this association into account. Therefore, adding NB assessment to measurements of NT and maternal serum markers has the potential to improve accuracy of risk assessment, and the inclusion of NB likelihood ratios to risk estimates is statistically valid. In a prospective study of a high-risk population with a median maternal age of 35 years assessed by NT, NB, and biochemistry, it was estimated that 93.6% of DS cases would be detected at a FPR of 5% [59]. Although these data are promising, they reflect the experience of highly specialized and high-risk centers and are not generalizable to less-experienced centers [17].

Sequential screening

The effect of ART on integrated (first- and second-trimester) screening was assessed in a group that underwent a serial nondisclosure integrated DS screening test. The study protocol included first-trimester combined NT, Fβ-hCG, and PAPP-A

Table 13.2. The biochemistry serum screening profile in pregnancies achieved by assisted reproductive technology

ART	Number of cases	PAPP-A MoM	Fβ-hCG MoM	NT MoM	Reference
IVF	220	1.0	1.21	0.97	[56]
ICSI	30	0.86	1.09	1.00	[56]
OD	161	1.04	0.96	0.96	[56]
IVF	47	1.02	1.14	0.97	[50]
OI	63	0.89	1.02	1.08	[50]
IVF	71	0.96	1.16	1.16	[34]
IVF	203	0.76	0.94	0.94	[49]
ICSI	192	0.71	1.04	0.98	[49]
IVF	47	1.06	0.83	NR	[51]
ICSI	222	1.13	1.13	NR	[51]
OI	97	1.26	0.98	NR	[51]
IVF	277	0.94	1.13	1.03	[52]
OI	323	0.91	1.06	1.02	[52]
IUI	247	0.98	1.08	0.97	[52]
OD	56	1.00	1.22	0.96	[52]
IVF	92	0.83	0.87	NR	[48]
ICSI	57	0.7	0.82	NR	[48]
IVF	32	0.79	0.84	1.1	[54]
ICSI	42	0.96	1.13	1.02	[54]
IVF	512	0.78	0.96	1.5	[58]
ICSI	396	0.79	0.98	1.6	[58]

ART, assisted reproductive technology; PAPP-A, pregnancy-associated placental protein-A; Fβ-hCG, free β-subunit of human chorionic gonadotrophin; NT, nuchal translucency; MoM, multiples of the mean; IVF, in vitro fertilization; ICSI, intracytoplasmic spermatozoon injection; OD, oocyte donation; OI, ovulation induction; IUI, intrauterine insemination; NR, not recorded.

testing. The second-trimester triple serum screening included AFP, intact hCG, and uE_3. After excluding aneuploidies, miscarriages, anatomical anomalies, and cases with incomplete follow-up, the serum samples of normal cases were assessed and correlated. Nuchal translucency measurement was not significantly changed in either group. However, the IVF group had lower PAPP-A levels and higher AFP. Both groups had similar rates of first-trimester FPR, but the IVF group had a significantly higher mid-gestation FPR rate (10% versus 5%; P=0.029). This has contributed to amniocentesis uptake rates of 15% and 13% for the IVF and natural conception pregnancies, respectively. It was concluded that ART singleton patients should be screened either by the integrated first- and second-trimester screening tests or the use of NT alone [34].

A later report from the same group assessed the profile of markers that constitute the integrated test, measuring its FPR among a preselected group of unaffected IVF pregnancies. These results were compared with the reference laboratory values that reflect the general obstetric population, which underwent the same investigative protocol. The IVF group had significantly lower PAPP-A levels (0.78 versus 1.03; t-test, P<0.05) and higher NT (1.14 versus 1.01, P<0.05) values, respectively. All the other markers were similar for both groups. On the basis of the integrated test, a higher rate of IVF pregnancies were defined as being screen-positive (6.1% versus 3.7%), although the values did not reach a level of statistical significance [57].

It is postulated that DS screening in ART pregnancies is associated with a higher FPR. To decrease the magnitude of such uncertain experience, it is advised to use better screening modalities, such as the combined or integrated tests [39]. In practice, pregnancies achieved by ART receive obstetric care from very early in the first trimester. Therefore, it may be advantageous to offer them NT as the initial DS screening method. In high-risk cases, if there is an experienced sonographer, addition of other sonographic markers, such as NB and Doppler flow studies, might enhance the detection rate. In centers that still conduct the triple test, when the NT screening is negative, it would be reasonable to subsequently offer the second-trimester serum testing, producing a combined risk assessment. The likelihood ratio (LR) should be applied from the NT screen to the risk from the serum screen or vice versa. One should be able to work out either one or both of the ratios from the reports if they include the age-specific risk (AR) and the final risk (FR) expressed as odds, using the formula : LR=FR/AR [19]. These calculations assume that the NT measurement was performed using the Fetal Medicine Foundation protocol [6].

Twin pregnancies

Twin pregnancies are becoming more frequent in most developed countries due to the increased use of ART and advanced maternal age (see Chapter 8). The combined effect results in older women having a greater chance of conceiving twins [60]. These pregnancies present numerous diagnostic and management challenges from conception to delivery. They may be at a higher risk for chromosomal abnormality [61] as well as for structural defects [62]. The methods currently widely used for DS screening in twins include maternal age, mid-gestation maternal serum screening, and first-trimester NT measurements (with or without serum markers). Screening of twin pregnancies is considered to be extremely difficult because of the clinical, technical, and ethical challenges posed for diagnosis and clinical management of such pregnancies [61,63], with some centers not offering DS screening in twin pregnancies [62,63].

Second-trimester screening

As serum screening was introduced before the other methods, there is more experience with it worldwide. It is now accepted, however, that DS serum screening is of limited value in twin pregnancies [61,64]. For example, modeling predicts that in 30-year-old women, second-trimester AFP, uE_3, Fβ-hCG, and inhibin with a 1 in 250 term cutoff risk will detect just one quarter of affected twin pregnancies compared with two thirds in singletons, albeit with fewer false positives. The reason for the poorer results is that in twins that are discordant for DS, feto-placental products from the unaffected fetus can mask the abnormal levels produced by the affected fetus [61]. Furthermore, while a pregnancy at high risk may be identified, serum biochemistry results will not be able to pinpoint which twin is affected [63].

It is well established that all the serum markers used in DS screening are increased about two-fold, on average, in twins. The interpretation of screening tests in twins is similar to that in singletons, in that a DS risk is estimated from the maternal age and overlapping marker distributions. For DS twin pregnancies, the average level although increased is not doubled and can be calculated from the averages in DS and unaffected singletons [61]. Despite these limitations, centers still offer mid-gestation serum screening for twin pregnancies, either because of a limited capacity for first-trimester screening or due to women booking late for prenatal care.

Two studies that compared DS screening tests in unaffected IVF and spontaneous twin pregnancies used this screening method [65,66]. In the former, the authors showed Fβ-hCG levels to be 20% higher in IVF twin pregnancies compared to spontaneously conceived ones (2.20 MoM and 1.83 MoM, respectively). This difference was of only marginal statistical significance (P=0.08). No difference was observed in AFP MoM levels between the two twin groups. The authors concluded that because of the increased FPR in this population, these issues should be discussed when offering the mid-gestation DS screening test in IVF twin pregnancies [65]. In the second study, there was no significant difference in the mean MoM value of the triple serum analytes, although the ART cases had the highest hCG levels [66]. Possible reasons for the higher hCG levels may be either the medication associated with ART, advanced maternal age, or placentation failure in IVF gestation [65].

There is only limited data regarding serum inhibin levels in ART pregnancies. Our group [44] found that there was no statistically significant difference between the median serum inhibin levels of 37 ART twin pregnancies and 50 spontaneous twin pregnancies (1.98 and 2.18 MoM, respectively, P=0.62).

First-trimester screening

A cornerstone in first-trimester evaluation in twins is an accurate determination of the chorionicity [67]. Ultrasound, using single or composite parameters, has enabled the determination of chorionicity in the majority of cases. Determination of chorionicity becomes increasingly difficult with advancing gestational age and high-resolution first-trimester or early second-trimester (10–14 weeks) abdominal or transvaginal sonography has been shown to offer the highest specificity and sensitivity in diagnosing chorionicity [68].

The "lambda" sign (also known as the "twin peak" sign) refers to the triangular projection of tissue extending up to the base of the inter-twin membrane in dichorionic placentation. This term represents the echodense chorionic villi between the two layers of chorion at its origin from the placenta. As the pregnancy advances into the second and third trimesters, regression of the chorion frondosum to form the chorion laeve means that the twin peak sign cannot be reliably used to determine chorionicity. Traditionally, the membrane "take-off" in a monochorionic gestation has been described with the "T" sign, where the membrane approaches the placenta at around a 90 degree angle [68].

Although one may expect that the majority of ART twins are dichorionic, an increased incidence of monozygotic twining is reported in these pregnancies [69]. One theory behind this observation is minor trauma to the blastocyst during the process of ART [69]. Early detection of monochorionic twins has major implications for pregnancy management especially if invasive karyotyping or selective fetal reduction is later indicated.

An initial study which looked at the influence of chorionicity on first-trimester biochemical marker levels concluded that there was no statistically significant difference between marker levels in monochorionic and dichorionic twins – despite there being the suggestion of lower values of PAPP-A levels in the former case [70]. Subsequent small studies have confirmed no difference in marker levels between mono- and dichorionic twins [71,72]. Later on, it was demonstrated that first-trimester screening in twin pregnancies requires adjustment of the calculated MoM to account for the presence of two fetuses. For Fβ-hCG, this should be by dividing the observed corrected MoM by 2.023. For PAPP-A two different factors are required: 2.192 in dichorionic twins and 1.788 in monochorionic twins [73].

First-trimester NT measurements in twin pregnancies are not affected by the problems encountered in serum screening. Indeed, in a study of 60 unaffected twins that sequentially underwent both first-trimester NT and mid-gestation triple serum screening, the screen positive rate was found to be much lower using NT measurements alone than mid-gestation serum levels (5% versus 15%). Thus, in twins, serum screening may lead to an 18% amniocentesis rate in this group [74]. This has serious perinatal consequences because the fetal loss related to amniocentesis is more than double in twins compared to matched singletons [75]. Because NT screening is fetus specific, it is regarded as the method of choice for both spontaneous and ART twin pregnancies (Figures 13.3–13.7) [19]. This is supported by the observation that NT in DS fetuses was found to be similar to that found in affected singletons [7].

The common fetus-specific method of calculating DS risk in twins assumes that the NT measurements in the two fetuses are independent and this is now known to be incorrect. A series of 181 unaffected twins from Denmark reported a correlation coefficient of 0.34 between the pairs of NTs, expressed in log MoMs for crown–rump length (CRL). A similar substantial degree of correlation was found both in the 31 monochorionic twins, with a correlation coefficient of 0.40, and in the 150 dichorionic twins, with a correlation coefficient of 0.32 [72]. Similarly, a recent study reported a correlation coefficient of 0.43 in 246 dichorionic twins with euploid fetuses [76]. Therefore, the DS risk in an individual fetus is dependent on both the specific NT and that of the co-twin.

Recently, our group estimated the DS detection rate for NT screening in twins when fetus-specific risk allows for between-fetus NT correlation. The correlation coefficient in unaffected pregnancies was 0.43 (P<0.0001) and estimated to be 0.23 and 0.11 in discordant and concordant twins. At 12 weeks of gestation, the model-predicted detection rate for a 3% FPR was 68% when between-fetus correlation is not taken into account,

(a) (b)

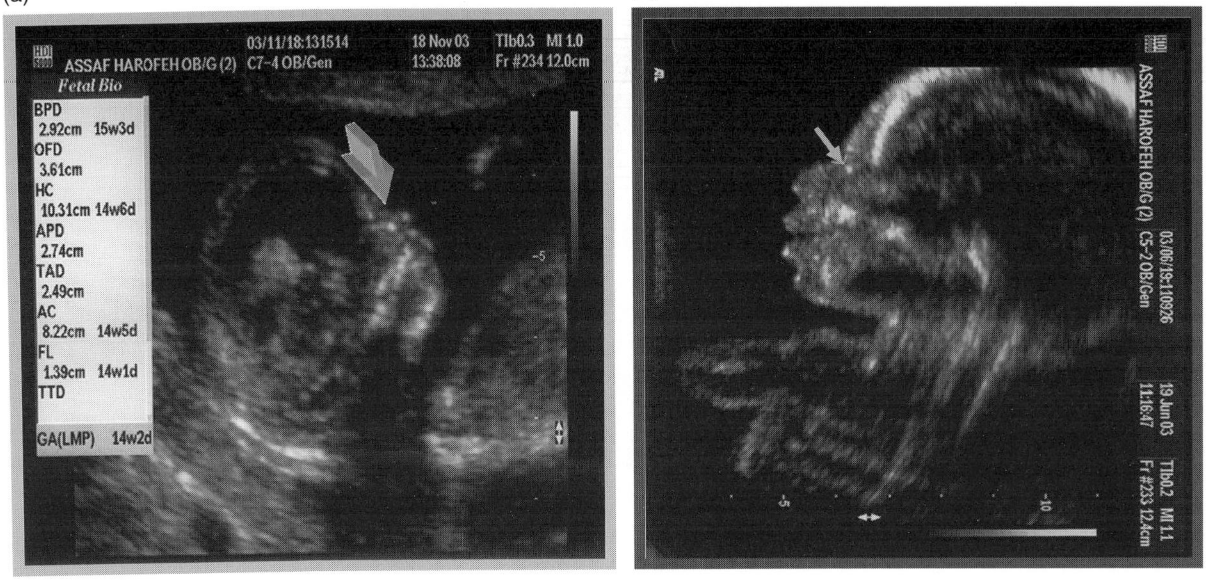

Figure 13.3. Midsagittal scan of the fetal head and thorax, (a): 14 weeks and (b): mid-gestation. Note the hypoplastic nasal bone (arrow heads) of each of the two Down's syndrome fetuses.

(a) (b)

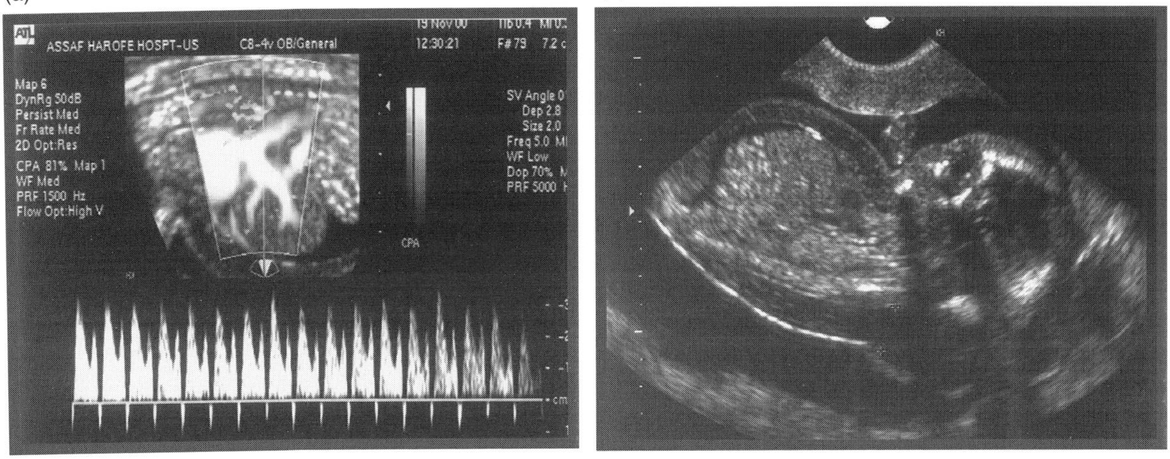

Figure 13.4. (a): color Doppler flow of a hydropic fetus. Note the intense intrahepatic flow, the enlarged ductus venosus, with a persistent A wave indicating a reversed flow; (b): transvaginal scan of the same fetus (note the ascites and the increased nuchal translucency)

increasing to 73% when it was applied. Similarly, for other false-positive rates and gestational weeks there was a predicted 4%–6% increase in detection. We concluded that using a fetus-specific DS risk algorithm leads to a worthwhile increase in detection [77].

In multiple pregnancies, the maternal age-specific DS risks, meaning that at least one fetus is affected, is no higher in twins than in singletons [61]. Caution is needed when interpreting the maternal age background risk in cases of oocyte donation. In this case, the age of the donor should be used for the DS risk calculation. Within this context, it is vital to define a prior risk for each fetus, which is half the age-specific risk as that in a singleton [78].

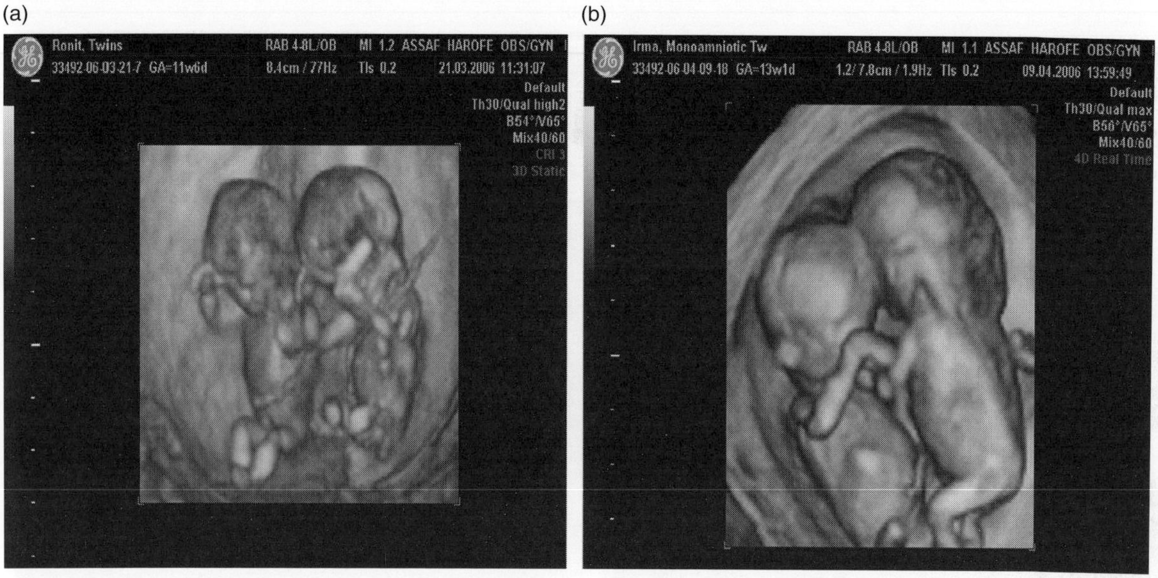

Figure 13.5. (a): three-dimensional ultrasound image of a bichorionic twin pregnancy. Note the thin nuchal translucency in the right-hand fetus; (b): three-dimensional ultrasound image of monoamniotic twins. One fetus is embracing the other. Note the increased nuchal translucency of the posterior fetus.

Excluding one report, which demonstrated a significantly lower NT (0.88 MoM) in IVF twins [54], most studies found no difference in the median of NT measurements (mm) and mean (MoM) NT among ART twins compared to spontaneous twins [26,79]. The IVF group had a lower FPR by a combination of first-trimester NT and maternal age (6.5% compared to 10% and 13% for the controlled ovarian hyperstimulation and spontaneous twins, respectively), but this value did not reach a level of statistical significance.

There are only limited data available on the use of NB evaluation for DS risk assessment in multiple gestations. In a retrospective study it was shown that the addition of NB to NT, PAPP-A, and Fβ-hCG increased the DS DR from 79% to 89% at a 5% screen-positive rate. It was concluded that in twins first-trimester screening with NB is valuable [80].

Combined nuchal translucency and serum markers

As in singleton pregnancies, combining the NT results with the serum markers in twin pregnancies is likely to yield a better screening performance than that obtained using either NT or serum markers alone [59,63]. In twin pregnancies, however, interpreting all the results of these markers is more difficult because the serum biochemistry concentration relates to the pregnancy while each NT measurement is fetus specific. Therefore, the combination of serum and NT measurements results in the calculation of a pregnancy-specific estimation.

Assuming that first- and second-trimester serum analytes are not correlated and that the levels of serum markers are twice that expected in singletons [1,61,81], the models of combining the LR of NT in MoMs and serum biochemistry of each co-twin can be applied as they are in singletons. The larger of the two CRLs should be used to estimate the overall gestational age for use in determining the MoMs. The overall DS risk can be calculated from the sum of the two individual NT LRs multiplied by the biochemistry LR [66].

In a study which examined the effect of IVF on first-trimester serum markers and NT in 30 twins (16 IVF and 14 ICSI), no difference was found in the levels of Fβ-hCG and PAPP-A between the study and the control cases [54]. Another group has suggested combining the individual fetal NT with the results of serum markers, thereby obtaining the entire pregnancy-specific "pseudorisk" [78]. According to this model, for a 5% FPR NT alone, first-trimester combined NT and serum biochemistry as well as the integrated tests will yield a 69%, 72%, and 80% detection rate, respectively. Similar first-trimester screening results were reported

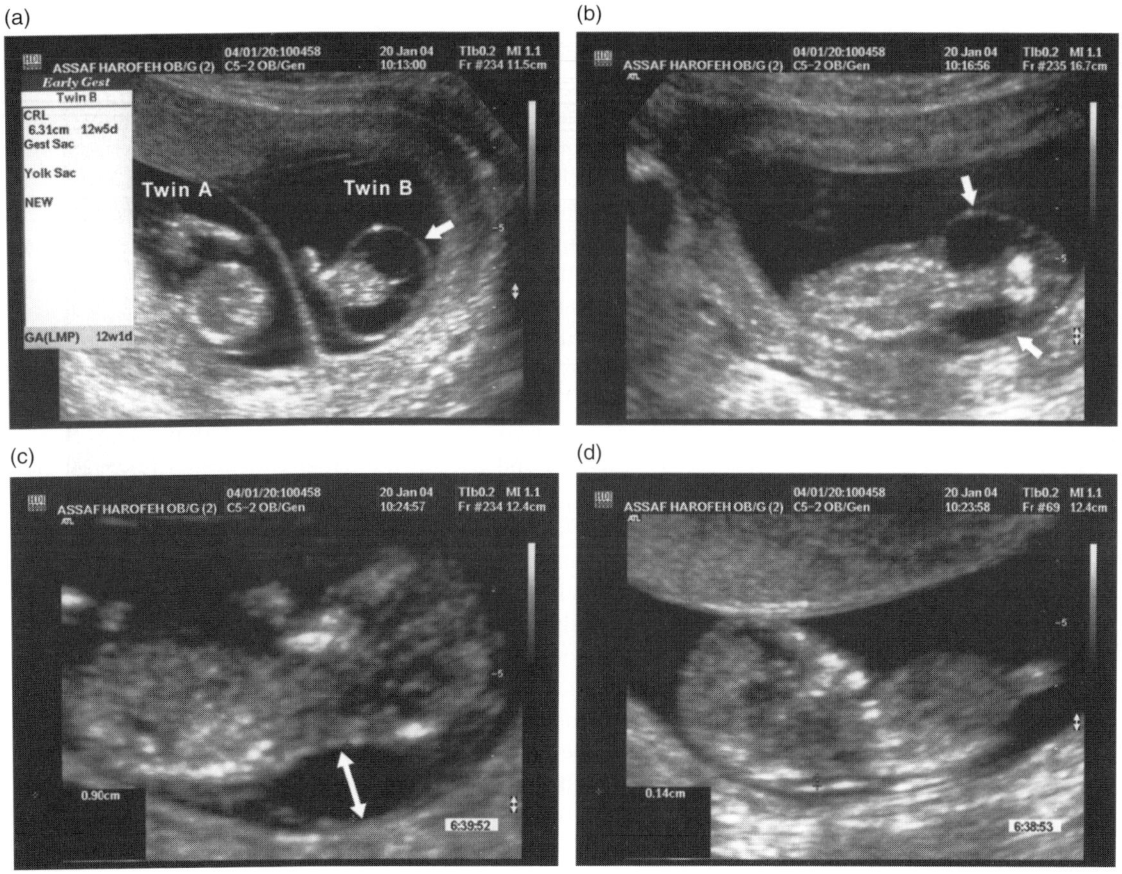

Figure 13.6. Montage plate of a bichorionic twin pregnancy (a). Twin B has an enlarged nuchal translucency ((b) and (c)), and twin A has a normal nuchal translucency (d).

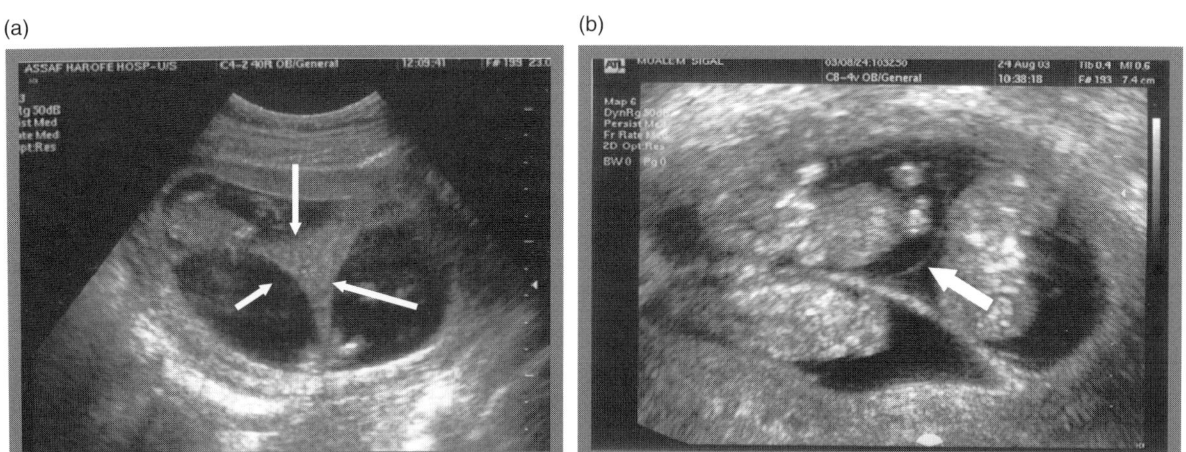

Figure 13.7. (a): transabdominal scan of a trichorionic triplet pregnancy. Note the three "peak signs" of the thick placenta at its insertion onto the chorionic plate; (b): transvaginal scan of a triplet pregnancy. In one gestational sac there is a monochorionic twin with a thin membrane forming the "T" sign.

by another group [60]. However, in contrast to second-trimester screening, chorionicity had no impact on the first-trimester serum biochemical marker levels in twin pregnancies [70]. In a later study, Spencer and Nicolaides [63] reported their experience for DS screening in the first trimester of 230 twin pregnancies (21% conceived by ART), using the combination of maternal serum biochemistry and NT: 9.2% of these pregnancies were found to be screen positive, similar to our current NT screening results. Therefore, adding first-trimester maternal serum biochemistry to NT may improve the detection rate by about 5%–6%. However, when invasive testing is indicated, NT alone is the screening modality women should be counseled to choose, as ultrasound is the best means of specifically locating the affected co-twin [63].

To the best of our knowledge, only one study has reported mid-gestation Fβ-hCG levels to be 20% higher in IVF twin pregnancies compared to spontaneously conceived ones. This difference was of marginal statistical significance only [65]. Another small series found high levels of hCG and uE_3 among ART twins, which was not statistically significant [66].

Mid-gestation serum screening alone is of limited value in ART-achieved twin pregnancies, and in view of the impressive progress recently achieved using early ultrasound, it should be abandoned. The benefits of an algorithm that combines NT and serum biochemistry are that it may increase the detection rates to the level of singletons, and may even reduce the FPR. Because those women receive careful prenatal care from early in their pregnancies, it seems reasonable to offer them ultrasound screening with NT measurement. Presently, it is the best available modality and a highly efficient screening method for multiple pregnancies. The valuable information obtained early in gestation, including chorionicity determination, can contribute to overall management if either fetal reduction is planned or the data are used as a screening modality for other structural anomalies associated with increased NT (see Figure 13.3).

High-order multiple pregnancies

The artificial production of large numbers of high-order multiple gestations was followed by an urgent need to screen for DS among these pregnancies and the subsequent recognition of the complexity of such procedures.

Serum screening

Triplet pregnancies are primarily iatrogenic conceptions following successful infertility therapy [82]. In such a selected population, serum screening is not widely applicable, although studies have been published [81]. Furthermore, the use of fetal reduction, which parallels the widespread use of assisted conception [82,83], further complicates the screening algorithm, mainly because elevated mid-gestation maternal serum AFP levels are present after first-trimester fetal reduction. Grau and coworkers [84] reviewed maternal serum and amniotic fluid levels of AFP from 40 women who underwent fetal reduction at approximately 12 weeks of gestation. Respectively, 95% and 25% of the patients who had mid-gestation AFP measured in maternal serum and amniotic fluid had elevated values. Fortunately, none of those abnormal levels were associated with neural tube defects, although two structural defects were detected by other means. The difference between serum and amniotic fluid AFP was attributed to either one or several mechanisms: all pregnancies were reduced to twins and one to triplets, and it is not uncommon to find elevated maternal serum AFP in such pregnancies. Alternatively, fetal AFP could have been released from the dead fetuses because of their having undergone autholysis [85]. In such circumstances, the transport of AFP across fetal membranes and the placenta may be enhanced by the remaining live co-twin(s) [84]. Lynch and Berkowitz [85] reported similar findings and concluded that mid-gestation maternal serum AFP is always elevated after multifetal pregnancy reduction and thus is not necessarily indicative of fetal defects. In contrast, Groutz et al. [86] found elevated AFP maternal serum in only two of the 28 studied cases, both having adverse perinatal outcomes; that is, severe preeclampsia in one and exomphalos in the other.

Several groups [86–88] studied the effect of first-trimester fetal reduction on the triple test results (AFP; uE_3, and hCG), and confirmed the elevation of maternal serum AFP. Rotmensch et al. [89] reported mid-gestation triple serum screening results from 27 high-order multiple gestations reduced to twins. About 90% of women exhibited maternal serum AFP levels >2 MoM, but only one of the newborns had structural anomalies. In their experience, this marker did not correlate with either the number of reduced fetuses or adverse obstetric outcome. In this study, however, the mean hCG and uE_3 serum levels were also slightly increased (1.22±0.49 MoM; 1.15±0.31 MoM, respectively). Although previous studies found that both hCG and uE_3 were not altered [87,88], the effect of first-trimester reduction on DS screening efficacy remains undetermined [86–89], and amniocentesis is not indicated in those cases. Moreover, ultrasonography for evaluation of fetal anatomy should be considered mainly because maternal serum AFP cannot be used in these patients to screen for fetal abnormalities [85]. Finally, it was found that following multifetal reduction to twin pregnancies, the maternal serum levels of inhibin A decrease to the level of twin pregnancies during the second trimester. It was concluded that inhibin A may be used effectively as a marker for DS screening in cases of twin pregnancy following multifetal reduction [90].

Ultrasound screening

Because NT is perceived as a valuable marker for detecting fetal abnormalities and complications, its importance is clear-cut for multiple pregnancies in which biochemical screening is of limited value. In twin pregnancies, first-trimester ultrasound screening for chromosomal abnormalities is both reliable and feasible [91].

Our group assessed pregnant patients who conceived following assisted reproduction and were carrying three or more fetuses [92]. Each fetus was ultrasonographically assessed by measuring the CRL and NT thickness using a published protocol [6,7].

Twenty-four pregnant patients, initially carrying 79 fetuses aged between 10 and 14 weeks of gestation, were compared with consecutively matched, singleton controls [92]. Nuchal translucency measurements were feasible for both study and control fetuses, which exhibited similar NT measurements for the 5th, 50th, and 95th percentiles. In addition, mean NT thicknesses (mm or MoMs) were similar for both groups (1.41±0.41 mm and 1.35±0.39 mm, respectively, and 0.87±0.23 MoM and 0.83±0.25 MoM, respectively). No instances of chromosomal abnormalities were detected in either group, and of those infants who had no karyotyping, no traits were observed postnatally that warranted a chromosomal analysis. As there is no other effective screening modality for these pregnancies, it is reasonable to recommend NT measurement for antenatal screening services for higher-order multiple gestations [19,92]. Moreover, contrary to others who have reported obtaining an NT thickness only in about 83% of the assessed singletons [11], we succeeded in measuring it in all of our cases [92].

We believe our observations [92] validate the using of NT measurements originally obtained in singletons [6,7] and twins [91,93,94] among higher-order multiple gestations. Furthermore, this sonographic screening method provides additional data for the identification of an abnormal fetus, thus lowering the complications of leaving an abnormal one after the reduction [95].

Screening before multifetal pregnancy reduction

A critical problem of high-order multiple gestation management protocols is fetal reduction. Most authorities agree that reducing multifetal pregnancies to twins improves pregnancy and perinatal outcome [82]. Moreover, this possibility offers an alternative, aside from terminating the entire pregnancy, to those women carrying either a higher number of fetuses than desired or an affected one [83].

Fetal reduction is commonly carried out at the end of the first trimester through a transabdominal intrathoracic introduction of a fine needle under ultrasound guidance and injection of concentrated potassium chloride solution [82,95]. While agreement exists [82, 95] as to the number of fetuses to be left (twin pregnancies having the best outcome) [96], the choice as to which fetuses to terminate is governed by a number of variables. Thus, before feticide, a careful ultrasonographic assessment of the entire pregnancy is recommended to determine the actual number of living fetuses, their location, the placentation for monochorionic twins (Figure 13.7) [97], presence of visible fetal anomalies, or fetal discordancy [83,98], as well as slower fetal heart rate [99]. Those parameters may indicate an anomaly or poor prognosis for the survival of that fetus [98,99]. Additionally, it seems important to offer pre-procedure, noninvasive genetic testing and a careful scanning, especially for those patients with a significantly increased risk of karyotypic abnormalities by virtue of their age [95].

Berkowitz et al. [95] have reported that among 200 patients who underwent fetal reduction, six of the remaining fetuses had either anatomical [6] or chromosomal [11] abnormalities. Based on this observation, pre-procedure genetic counseling and careful scanning was proposed, especially for those patients with an increased risk of karyotype abnormalities [95]. To overcome such problems, first-trimester ultrasound screening using NT measurement appears to be the best option. In this respect, first-trimester ultrasound screening using NT measurements seems to be a most promising option.

Lipitz et al. [100] recommend performance of fetal reduction in triplets at 13–14 weeks' gestation rather than 11–12 weeks; as this allows a more detailed anomaly scan at a slightly more advanced gestational age. According to their experience, pregnancy loss was similar (about 4%) in either group. They concluded that screening before fetal reduction at 13–14 weeks' should include NT measurement and ruling out relative intrauterine growth restriction and structural anomalies. At this gestational age, the gender of the fetus can also be determined, a factor which may be of clinical importance for families at risk for chromosomal X-linked disorders [47]. In triplet pregnancies, such an early detailed fetal anomaly scan requires a very experienced sonographer and a modern ultrasound machine with high resolution.

Because the transvaginal sonography provides a better image of the lower fetus, combined transvaginal and transabdominal scans may be required [15]. With such high scanning performance, it seems reasonable to consider additional sonographic markers or fetal biometric measurements such as the fetal NB, flow velocity patterns in the ductus venosus, tricuspid regurgitation, and maxillary hypoplasia at the time of an NT scan [101]. Additional studies are needed to determine the most efficient screening combination by means of ultrasound for the subgroup of high-order multiple gestation.

Brambati and colleagues [102] and Eddleman and coworkers [103] reported performing CVS before multifetal pregnancy reduction. The message from these two studies is that in high-risk groups for chromosomal aneuploidy, CVS should be offered before embryo reduction is employed. Eddleman et al. [103] further supported their management protocol by stating that "rarely, there is a visible anomaly or a smaller than expected crown-rump length that influences the decision about which fetus to remove." According to their report, however, CVS procedures alone were associated with 1.2% sampling errors, which is actually the primary risk for aneuploidy in this group.

Although pre-reduction CVS has its advantages, primarily in older patients, the following disadvantages hinder the widespread use of this practice: the risk of abortion; the objective difficulty in carrying out villocentesis in multiple pregnancies; the difficulty in identifying ill fetuses to be eliminated within a few days of taking the sample; and the higher stress level in patients caused by the two invasive procedures carried out within a few days of each other [104].

It is our contention to suggest the following approach, which includes NT measurement as part of pre-procedure noninvasive genetic testing, before any embryo reduction. This is followed by reducing the one exhibiting the highest risk, once such a fetus is detected, and thereby lowering the probability of leaving an affected fetus after the procedure [95]. Using this policy, we encountered a triplet pregnancy in which one fetus exhibited an NT of 3 mm (>95th percentile for CRL [105]). The other two fetuses had NTs within the normal limit for gestation [105]. Before reducing that fetus and by using the same fine needle, a few milliliters of amniotic fluid were aspirated for chromosomal analysis. This test revealed a fetus affected with trisomy 13. Mid-gestation amniocentesis performed later confirmed a euploid karyotype of the remaining fetuses. A similar experience was reported by Monni et al. [104].

Our current policy [92,105] is:

(i) Routine examination of fetal NT and determination of chorionicity before any multifetal pregnancy reduction. Examination of NB, flow velocity patterns in the ductus venosus, tricuspid regurgitation, and maxillary hypoplasia is reserved for high-risk cases. Patients could be offered the choice to postpone the reduction to around 14 weeks after a detailed anomaly scan.
(ii) Reduction and karyotyping of the high-risk one and/or the malformed fetus.
(iii) Performance of mid-gestation amniocentesis, where indicated.

The performance of genetic amniocentesis after multifetal pregnancy reduction does not increase the risk of pregnancy loss over that observed in association with reduction itself [106]. We think that CVS should be reserved only for highly selected instances, including parents with balance translocations or who are carriers of a single gene disorder for which prenatal diagnosis is available.

Conclusion

Women who progress to a multifetal pregnancy after assisted conception are naturally wary of any invasive prenatal diagnostic procedure. As they receive careful antenatal care from the start of their pregnancies, and because their serum markers are less discriminative for chromosomal screening, it seems reasonable to offer them ultrasound assessment including NT measurement, which presently is the only available and highly efficient screening method. This valuable information can contribute to overall management if fetal reduction is planned and as a screening modality for other structural anomalies associated with increased NT (Figure 13.4).

References

1. Wald NJ, Kennard A, Hackshaw A, McGuire A. Antenatal screening for Down's syndrome. *J Med Screen* 1997; **4**: 181–246.
2. Cuckle H. Antenatal screening for Down's syndrome. *Lancet* 1998; **352**: 1144–1145.
3. Van Lith JM, Pratt JJ, Beekhuis JR, Mantingh A. Second-trimester maternal serum immunoreactive inhibin as a marker for fetal Down's syndrome. *Prenat Diagn* 1992; **12**: 801–806.
4. Wald NJ, Watt HC, Hackshaw AK. Integrated screening for Down's syndrome on the basis of tests performed during the first and second trimesters. *N Engl J Med* 1999; **341**: 461–467.
5. Wald NJ, Huttly WJ, Hackshaw AK. Antenatal screening for Down's syndrome with the quadruple test. *Lancet* 2003; **361**: 835–836.
6. Snijders RJ, Noble P, Sebire N, Souka A, Nicolaides KH. UK multicentre project on assessment of risk of trisomy 21 by maternal age and fetal nuchal-translucency thickness at 10–14 weeks of gestation. Fetal Medicine Foundation First Trimester Screening Group. *Lancet* 1998; **352**: 343–346.
7. Pandya PP, Snijders RJ, Johnson SP, De Lourdes Brizot M, Nicolaides KH. Screening for fetal trisomies by maternal age and fetal nuchal translucency thickness at 10 to 14 weeks of gestation. *Br J Obstet Gynaecol* 1995; **102**: 957–962.
8. Szabo J, Gellen J. Nuchal fluid accumulation in trisomy-21 detected by vaginosonography in first trimester. *Lancet* 1990; **336**: 1133.
9. Reynders CS, Pauker S, Benacerraf BR. First trimester isolated fetal nuchal lucency: significance and outcome. *J Ultrasound Med* 1997; **16**: 101–105.
10. Fukada Y, Yasumizu T, Takizawa M, Amemiya A, Hoshi K. The prognosis of fetuses with transient nuchal translucency in the first and early second trimester. *Acta Obstet Gynecol Scand* 1997; **76**: 913–916.
11. Haddow JE, Palomaki GE, Knight GJ, et al. Screening of maternal serum for fetal Down's syndrome in the first trimester. *N Engl J Med* 1998; **338**: 955–961.
12. Spencer K, Souter V, Tul N, Snijders R, Nicolaides KH. A screening program for trisomy 21 at 10–14 weeks using fetal nuchal translucency, maternal serum free beta-human chorionic gonadotropin and pregnancy-associated plasma protein-A. *Ultrasound Obstet Gynecol* 1999; **13**: 231–237.
13. De Biasio P, Siccardi M, Volpe G, et al. First-trimester screening for Down syndrome using nuchal translucency measurement with free beta-hCG and PAPP-A between 10 and 13 weeks of pregnancy – the combined test. *Prenat Diagn* 1999; **19**: 360–363.
14. de Graaf IM, Pajkrt E, Bilardo CM, et al. Early pregnancy screening for fetal aneuploidy with serum markers and nuchal translucency. *Prenat Diagn* 1999; **19**: 458–462.
15. Cicero S, Curcio P, Papageorghiou A, Sonek J, Nicolaides K. Absence of nasal bone in fetuses with trisomy 21 at 10–14 weeks of gestation: an observational study. *Lancet* 2001; **358**: 1665–1667.
16. Cicero S, Rembouskos G, Vandecruys H, Hogg M, Nicolaides KH. Likelihood ratio for trisomy 21 in fetuses with absent nasal bone at the 10–14-week scan. *Ultrasound Obstet Gynecol* 2004; **23**: 218–223.
17. Rosen T, D'Alton ME, Platt LD, et al. First-trimester ultrasound assessment of the nasal bone to screen for aneuploidy. *Obstet Gynecol* 2007; **110**: 399–404.
18. Borrell A. Promises and pitfalls of first trimester sonographic markers in the detection of fetal aneuploidy. *Prenat Diagn* 2009; **29**: 62–68.
19. Maymon R, Jauniaux E. Down's syndrome screening in pregnancies after assisted reproductive techniques: an update. *Reprod Biomed Online* 2002; **4**: 285–293.
20. Geipel A, Gembruch U, Ludwig M, et al. Genetic sonography as the preferred option of prenatal diagnosis in patients with pregnancies following intracytoplasmic sperm injection. *Hum Reprod* 1999; **14**: 2629–2634.
21. Pinborg A, Loft A, Rasmussen S, et al. Neonatal outcome in a Danish national cohort of 3438 IVF/ICSI and 10,362 non-IVF/ICSI twins born between 1995 and 2000. *Hum Reprod* 2004; **19**: 435–441.
22. Gjerris AC, Loft A, Pinborg A, Christiansen M, Tabor A. Prenatal testing among women pregnant after assisted reproductive techniques in Denmark 1995–2000: a national cohort study. *Hum Reprod* 2008; **23**: 1545–1552.

23. Aboulghar H, Aboulghar M, Mansour R, et al. A prospective controlled study of karyotyping for 430 consecutive babies conceived through intracytoplasmic sperm injection. *Fertil Steril* 2001; **76**: 249–253.

24. Bonduelle M, Van Assche E, Joris H, et al. Prenatal testing in ICSI pregnancies: incidence of chromosomal anomalies in 1586 karyotypes and relation to sperm parameters. *Hum Reprod* 2002; **17**: 2600–2614.

25. Jozwiak EA, Ulug U, Mesut A, Erden HF, Bahçeci M. Prenatal karyotypes of fetuses conceived by intracytoplasmic sperm injection. *Fertil Steril* 2004; **82**: 628–633.

26. Maymon R, Dreazen E, Rozinsky S, et al. Comparison of nuchal translucency measurement and mid-gestation serum screening in assisted reproduction versus naturally conceived singleton pregnancies. *Prenat Diagn* 1999; **19**: 1007–1011.

27. Barkai G, Goldman B, Ries L, et al. Down's syndrome screening marker levels following assisted reproduction. *Prenat Diagn* 1996; **16**: 1111–1114.

28. Heinonen S, Ryynänen M, Kirkinen P, Hippeläinen M, Saarikoski S. Effect of in vitro fertilization on human chorionic gonadotropin serum concentrations and Down's syndrome screening. *Fertil Steril* 1996; **66**: 398–403.

29. Ribbert LS, Kornman LH, De Wolf BT, et al. Maternal serum screening for fetal Down syndrome in IVF pregnancies. *Prenat Diagn* 1996; **16**: 35–38.

30. Frishman GN, Canick JA, Hogan JW, et al. Serum triple-marker screening in in vitro fertilization and naturally conceived pregnancies. *Obstet Gynecol* 1997; **90**: 98–101.

31. Wald NJ, White N, Morris JK, Huttly WJ, Canick JA. Serum markers for Down's syndrome in women who have had in vitro fertilisation: implications for antenatal screening. *Br J Obstet Gynaecol* 1999; **106**: 1304–1306.

32. Maymon R, Shulman A. Comparison of triple serum screening and pregnancy outcome in oocyte donation versus IVF pregnancies. *Hum Reprod* 2001; **16**: 691–695.

33. Bar-Hava I, Yitzhak M, Krissi H, et al. Triple-test screening in in vitro fertilization pregnancies. *J Assist Reprod Genet* 2001; **18**: 226–229.

34. Maymon R, Shulman A. Serial first- and second-trimester Down's syndrome screening tests among IVF-versus naturally-conceived singletons. *Hum Reprod* 2002; **17**: 1081–1085.

35. Raty R, Virtanen A, Koskinen P, et al. Serum free beta-HCG and alpha-fetoprotein levels in IVF, ICSI and frozen embryo transfer pregnancies in maternal mid-trimester serum screening for Down's syndrome. *Hum Reprod* 2002; **17**: 481–484.

36. Muller F, Dreux S, Lemeur A, et al. Medically assisted reproduction and second-trimester maternal serum marker screening for Down syndrome. *Prenat Diagn* 2003; **23**: 1073–1076.

37. Rice JD, McIntosh SF,Halstead AC. Second-trimester maternal serum screening for Down syndrome in in vitro fertilization pregnancies. *Prenat Diagn* 2005; **25**: 234–238.

38. Perheentupa A, Ruokonen A, Tuomivaara L, Ryynänen M, Martikainen H. Maternal serum beta-HCG and alpha-fetoprotein concentrations in singleton pregnancies following assisted reproduction. *Hum Reprod* 2002; **17**: 794–797.

39. Weisz B, Rodeck C.H. An update on antenatal screening for Down's syndrome and specific implications for assisted reproduction pregnancies. *Hum Reprod Update* 2006; **12**: 513–518.

40. Marrs R, Kletzky OA, Howard WF, Mishell DR Jr. Disappearance of human chorionic gonadotropin and resumption of ovulation following abortion. *Am J Obstet Gynecol* 1979; **135**: 731–736.

41. Lam YH, Yeung WS, Tang MH, et al. Maternal serum alpha-fetoprotein and human chorionic gonadotrophin in pregnancies conceived after intracytoplasmic sperm injection and conventional in-vitro fertilization. *Hum Reprod* 1999; **14**: 2120–2123.

42. Shulman A, Maymon R. Mid-gestation Down syndrome screening test and pregnancy outcome among unstimulated assisted-conception pregnancies. *Prenat Diagn* 2003; **23**: 625–628.

43. Hsu TY, Ou CY, Hsu JJ, et al. Maternal serum screening for Down syndrome in pregnancies conceived by intra-uterine insemination. *Prenat Diagn* 1999; **19**: 1012–1014.

44. Maymon R, Cuckle H,Herman A. Maternal serum inhibin levels in twin and singleton pregnancies conceived by assisted reproduction. *Hum Reprod* 2006; **21**: 1305–1308.

45. Jackson RA, Gibson KA, Wu YW, Croughan MS. Perinatal outcomes in singletons following in vitro fertilization: a meta-analysis. *Obstet Gynecol* 2004; **103**: 551–563.

46. Kalra SK, Molinaro TA. The association of in vitro fertilization and perinatal morbidity. *Semin Reprod Med* 2008; **26**: 423–435.

47. Ogle R, Jauniaux E, Pahal GS, et al. Serum screening for Down syndrome and adverse pregnancy outcomes: a case-controlled study. *Prenat Diagn* 2000; **20**: 96–99.

48. Hui W, Lam YH, Tang MH, et al. Maternal serum pregnancy-associated plasma protein-A and free beta-human chorionic gonadotrophin in pregnancies conceived with fresh and frozen-thawed embryos from

in vitro fertilization and intracytoplasmic sperm injection. *Prenat Diagn* 2005; **25**: 390–393.

49. Engels MA, Kooij M, Schats R, et al. First-trimester serum marker distribution in singleton pregnancies conceived with assisted reproduction. *Prenat Diagn* 2010; **30**: 372–377.
50. Wojdemann KR, Larsen SO, Shalmi A, et al. First trimester screening for Down syndrome and assisted reproduction: no basis for concern. *Prenat Diagn* 2001; **21**: 563–565.
51. Bellver J, Lara C, Soares SR, et al. First trimester biochemical screening for Down's syndrome in singleton pregnancies conceived by assisted reproduction. *Hum Reprod* 2005; **20**: 2623–2627.
52. Lambert-Messerlian G Dugoff L, Vidaver J, et al. First- and second-trimester Down syndrome screening markers in pregnancies achieved through assisted reproductive technologies (ART): a FASTER trial study. *Prenat Diagn* 2006; **26**: 672–678.
53. Ghisoni L, Ferrazzi E, Castagna C, et al. Prenatal diagnosis after ART success: the role of early combined screening tests in counselling pregnant patients. *Placenta* 2003; **24**: S99–S103.
54. Orlandi F, Rossi C, Allegra A, et al. First trimester screening with free beta-hCG, PAPP-A and nuchal translucency in pregnancies conceived with assisted reproduction. *Prenat Diagn* 2002; **22**: 718–721.
55. Ong CY, Liao AW, Spencer K, Munim S, Nicolaides KH. First trimester maternal serum free beta human chorionic gonadotrophin and pregnancy associated plasma protein A as predictors of pregnancy complications. *BJOG* 2000; **107**: 1265–1270.
56. Liao AW, Heath V, Kametas N, Spencer K, Nicolaides KH. First-trimester screening for trisomy 21 in singleton pregnancies achieved by assisted reproduction. *Hum Reprod* 2001; **16**: 1501–1504.
57. Maymon R, Shulman A. Integrated first- and second-trimester Down syndrome screening test among unaffected IVF pregnancies. *Prenat Diagn* 2004; **24**: 125–129.
58. Gjerris AC, Loft A, Pinborg A, Christiansen M, Tabor A. First-trimester screening markers are altered in pregnancies conceived after IVF/ICSI. *Ultrasound Obstet Gynecol* 2009; **33**: 8–17.
59. Cicero S, Avgidou K, Rembouskos G, Kagan KO, Nicolaides KH. Nasal bone in first-trimester screening for trisomy 21. *Am J Obstet Gynecol* 2006; **195**: 109–114.
60. Spencer K. Screening for trisomy 21 in twin pregnancies in the first trimester using free beta-hCG and PAPP-A, combined with fetal nuchal translucency thickness. *Prenat Diagn* 2000; **20**: 91–95.
61. Cuckle H. Down's syndrome screening in twins. *J Med Screen* 1998; **5**: 3–4.
62. Doyle PE, Beral V, Botting B, Wale CJ. Congenital malformations in twins in England and Wales. *J Epidemiol Community Health* 1991; **45**: 43–48.
63. Spencer K, Nicolaides KH. Screening for trisomy 21 in twins using first trimester ultrasound and maternal serum biochemistry in a one-stop clinic: a review of three years experience. *BJOG* 2003; **110**: 276–280.
64. Wald N, Cuckle H, Wu TS, George L. Maternal serum unconjugated oestriol and human chorionic gonadotrophin levels in twin pregnancies: implications for screening for Down's syndrome. *Br J Obstet Gynaecol* 1991; **98**: 905–908.
65. Raty R, Virtanen A, Koskinen P, et al. Maternal midtrimester serum AFP and free beta-hCG levels in in vitro fertilization twin pregnancies. *Prenat Diagn* 2000; **20**: 221–223.
66. Maymon R, Neeman O, Shulman A, Rosen H, Herman A. Current concepts of Down syndrome screening tests in assisted reproduction twin pregnancies: another double trouble. *Prenat Diagn* 2005; **25**: 746–750.
67. Sepulveda W. Chorionicity determination in twin pregnancies: double trouble. *Ultrasound Obstet Gynecol* 1997; **10**: 79–81.
68. Shetty A, Smith A. The sonographic diagnosis of chorionicity. *Prenat Diagn* 2005; **25**: 735–739.
69. Wenstrom KD, Syrop CH, Hammitt DG, Van Voorhis BJ. Increased risk of monochorionic twinning associated with assisted reproduction. *Fertil Steril* 1993; **60**: 510–514.
70. Spencer K. Screening for trisomy 21 in twin pregnancies in the first trimester: does chorionicity impact on maternal serum free beta-hCG or PAPP-A levels? *Prenat Diagn* 2001; **21**: 715–717.
71. Gonce A, Borrell A, Fortuny A, et al. First-trimester screening for trisomy 21 in twin pregnancy: does the addition of biochemistry make an improvement? *Prenat Diagn* 2005; **25**: 1156–1161.
72. Wojdemann KR, Larsen SO, Shalmi AC, et al. Nuchal translucency measurements are highly correlated in both mono- and dichorionic twin pairs. *Prenat Diagn* 2006; **26**: 218–220.
73. Spencer K, Kagan KO,Nicolaides KH. Screening for trisomy 21 in twin pregnancies in the first trimester: an update of the impact of chorionicity on maternal serum markers. *Prenat Diagn* 2008; **28**: 49–52.
74. Maymon R, Dreazen E, Rozinsky S, et al. Comparison of nuchal translucency measurement and second-trimester triple serum screening in twin versus singleton pregnancies. *Prenat Diagn* 1999; **19**: 727–731.

75. Kidd SA, Lancaster PA, Anderson JC, et al. A cohort study of pregnancy outcome after amniocentesis in twin pregnancy. *Paediatr Perinat Epidemiol* 1997; **11**: 200–213.

76. Cuckle H, Maymon R. Down syndrome risk calculation for a twin fetus taking account of the nuchal translucency in the co-twin. *Prenat Diagn* 2010; **30**: 827–833.

77. Maymon R, Rosen H, Baruchin O, Herman A, Cuckle H. Model predicted Down syndrome detection rates for nuchal translucency screening in twin pregnancies. *Prenat Diagn* 2011; **31**:426–429.

78. Wald NJ, Rish S,Hackshaw AK. Combining nuchal translucency and serum markers in prenatal screening for Down syndrome in twin pregnancies. *Prenat Diagn* 2003; **23**: 588–592.

79. Maymon R, Jauniaux E, Holmes A, et al. Nuchal translucency measurement and pregnancy outcome after assisted conception versus spontaneously conceived twins. *Hum Reprod* 2001; **16**: 1999–2004.

80. Cleary-Goldman J, Rebarber A, Krantz D, Hallahan T, Saltzman D. First-trimester screening with nasal bone in twins. *Am J Obstet Gynecol* 2008; **199**: 283. e1–e3.

81. Spencer K, Salonen R,Muller F. Down's syndrome screening in multiple pregnancies using alpha-fetoprotein and free beta hCG. *Prenat Diagn* 1994; **14**: 537–542.

82. Berkowitz RL, Lynch L, Stone J, Alvarez M. The current status of multifetal pregnancy reduction. *Am J Obstet Gynecol* 1996; **174**: 1265–1272.

83. Maymon R, Herman A, Shulman A, et al. First trimester embryo reduction: a medical solution to an iatrogenic problem. *Hum Reprod* 1995; **10**: 668–673.

84. Grau P, Robinson L, Tabsh K, Crandall BF. Elevated maternal serum alpha-fetoprotein and amniotic fluid alpha-fetoprotein after multifetal pregnancy reduction. *Obstet Gynecol* 1990; **76**: 1042–1045.

85. Lynch L, Berkowitz RL. Maternal serum alpha-fetoprotein and coagulation profiles after multifetal pregnancy reduction. *Am J Obstet Gynecol* 1993; **169**: 987–990.

86. Groutz A, Amit A, Yaron Y, et al. Second-trimester maternal serum alpha-fetoprotein, human chorionic gonadotropin, and unconjugated oestriol after early transvaginal multifetal pregnancy reduction. *Prenat Diagn* 1996; **16**: 723–727.

87. Shulman L, Phillips O. Re: second-trimester maternal serum alpha-fetoprotein, human chorionic gonadotropin, and unconjugated oestriol after early transvaginal multifetal pregnancy reduction. *Prenat Diagn* 1997; **17**: 488–490.

88. Shulman L, Phillips O, Cervetti TA. Maternal serum analyte levels after first-trimester multifetal pregnancy reduction. *Am J Obstet Gynecol* 1996; **174**: 1072–1074.

89. Rotmensch S, Celentano C, Shalev J, *et al.* Midtrimester maternal serum screening after multifetal pregnancy reduction in pregnancies conceived by in vitro fertilization. *J Assist Reprod Genet* 1999; **16**: 8–12.

90. Chen HJ, Huang LW, Lin YH, *et al.* Midtrimester maternal serum inhibin A levels after multifetal pregnancy reduction. *Prenat Diagn* 2007; **27**: 431–434.

91. Pandya PP, Hilbert F, Snijders RJ, Nicolaides KH. Nuchal translucency thickness and crown-rump length in twin pregnancies with chromosomally abnormal fetuses. *J Ultrasound Med* 1995. **14**: 565–568.

92. Maymon R, Dreazen E, Tovbin Y, et al. The feasibility of nuchal translucency measurement in higher order multiple gestations achieved by assisted reproduction. *Hum Reprod* 1999; **14**: 2102–2105.

93. Sebire NJ, Snijders RJ, Hughes K, Sepulveda W, Nicolaides KH. Screening for trisomy 21 in twin pregnancies by maternal age and fetal nuchal translucency thickness at 10–14 weeks of gestation. *Br J Obstet Gynaecol* 1996; **103**: 999–1003.

94. Sebire NJ, Souka A, Skentou H, Geerts L, Nicolaides KH. Early prediction of severe twin-to-twin transfusion syndrome. *Hum Reprod* 2000; **15**: 2008–2010.

95. Berkowitz RL, Lynch L, Lapinski R, Bergh P. First-trimester transabdominal multifetal pregnancy reduction: a report of two hundred completed cases. *Am J Obstet Gynecol* 1993; **169**: 17–21.

96. Evans MI, Berkowitz RL, Wapner RJ, et al. Improvement in outcomes of multifetal pregnancy reduction with increased experience. *Am J Obstet Gynecol* 2001; **184**: 97–103.

97. Sepulveda W, Sebire NJ, Odibo A, Psarra A, Nicolaides KH. Prenatal determination of chorionicity in triplet pregnancy by ultrasonographic examination of the ipsilon zone. *Obstet Gynecol* 1996; **88**: 855–858.

98. Dickey R, Olar TT, Taylor SN, et al. Incidence and significance of unequal gestational sac diameter or embryo crown-rump length in twin pregnancy. *Hum Reprod* 1992; **7**: 1170–1172.

99. Achiron R, Tadmor O,Mashiach S. Heart rate as a predictor of first-trimester spontaneous abortion after ultrasound-proven viability. *Obstet Gynecol* 1991; **78**: 330–334.

100. Lipitz S, Shulman A, Achiron R, Zalel Y, Seidman DS. A comparative study of multifetal pregnancy reduction from triplets to twins in the first versus early second trimesters after detailed fetal screening. *Ultrasound Obstet Gynecol* 2001; **18**: 35–38.

101. Cuckle HS. Growing complexity in the choice of Down's syndrome screening policy. *Ultrasound Obstet Gynecol* 2002; **19**: 323–326.

102. Brambati B, Tului L, Baldi M, Guercilena S. Genetic analysis prior to selective fetal reduction in multiple pregnancy: technical aspects and clinical outcome. *Hum Reprod* 1995; **10**: 818–825.

103. Eddleman KA, Stone JL, Lynch L, Berkowitz RL. Chorionic villus sampling before multifetal pregnancy reduction. *Am J Obstet Gynecol* 2000; **183**: 1078–1081.

104. Monni G, *et al.* Importance of nuchal translucency measurement in multifetal pregnancy reduction. *Ultrasound Obstet Gynecol*, 1999. **13**(5): 377–8.

105. Maymon R, Herman A. Multifetal pregnancy reduction. *Am J Obstet Gynecol* 2001;**185**: 772–774.

106. Selam B, Torok O, Lembet A, *et al.* Genetic amniocentesis after multifetal pregnancy reduction. *Am J Obstet Gynecol* 1999; **180**: 226–230.

Chapter 14

Children born after assisted reproductive technology

Alastair G. Sutcliffe and Tajinder Singhrao

Introduction

The birth of the first in vitro fertilization (IVF) baby Louise Brown on the July 25, 1978 hallmarked an era of change for infertile couples and would-be parents [1]. In 1992, the first successful results of intracytoplasmic spermatozoon injection (ICSI) treatment were published, as was the first successful report of preimplantation genetic diagnosis (PGD) using human embryos [2,3]. Assisted reproductive technology (ART) has since provided the opportunity for a successful pregnancy and birth of a healthy child/children for infertile parents, single parents, and parents concerned about passing on genetically inherited diseases. Within the U.K., the Human Fertilisation and Embryology Authority (HFEA) maintains registry data, providing limited information on children born following ART from 1991 to the present day. Over 12 000 babies are born within the U.K. every year as a direct result of ART [4].

With limited knowledge of the immediate, short-, and long-term outcomes for children born following ART, there are concerns regarding the future of the "ART generation." The social, physical, and reproductive health implications for the child born as a direct result of ART were completely unknown at the outset and have been both debated and, to some degree, identified alongside clarification of issues regarding legal parental responsibility, disclosure of ART, and genetic tracing/testing.

Many national IVF registers did not exist at the beginning of human ART. European data (EIM) have been collected since 1999 by the European Society of Human Reproduction and Embryology (ESHRE) and U.K. data have been collected since 1991. Long-term follow-up data have therefore been a constant limitation for assessment of the health of children born after ART. Many studies have previously focused on assessment of short-term outcomes in babies and young children [5,6]. By definition, studies of ART children are prospective and longitudinal. Small sample sizes, self-reporting, and poor follow-up rates have been a stumbling block and contribute to the pitfalls in interpreting results from some early studies and conclusions extrapolated from them. The ability to differentiate childhood and adolescent morbidity resulting directly from ART versus the underlying parental infertility itself or another independent factor as the primary cause also provides a potential confounding factor within a study design and remains problematic [7].

Antenatal and perinatal complications

Iatrogenic multiple pregnancies pose the greatest risk of obstetric complications and adverse long-term outcomes associated with ART. Multiple and high-order pregnancies correlate directly with the number of embryos transferred per cycle, thus making it a modifiable risk factor [8].

Multiple pregnancy increases the risk of spontaneous abortion, preterm delivery, low birth weight, perinatal mortality, and cerebral palsy (see Chapter 8). Currently within the U.K., a live birth rate of 24.1% per ART cycle is seen. Just under a quarter of these (23.2%) are multiple births (HFEA, 2008) [5], compared with 30% in the U.S. and 21% in Europe (2002–4005 data) [9]. Current restrictions on maximum numbers of embryo transfers per IVF cycle have reduced the number of triplet or high-order births, but twin births are still common [8]. They remain the worst undesirable health outcome from

Pregnancy After Assisted Reproductive Technology, ed. Eric R. M. Jauniaux and Botros R. M. B. Rizk. Published by Cambridge University Press.

ART worldwide, and there is some progress to be made before this becomes a thing of the past. Guidelines published by the British Fertility Society and Association of Clinical Embryologists in 2008 encourage clinics within the U.K. to provide elective single embryo transfer (eSET). Other countries such as Sweden have mandated this practice. As pediatricians, we call for the same practice worldwide.

Across the world, there is much variation in legislation, funding, and uptake of eSET. Sweden has the highest overall rates (69.4%, 2005); legislation enforces the use of single embryo ART unless there are exceptional circumstances [9]. Randomized Swedish data have demonstrated a statistically significant reduction ($P<0.001$) in multiple pregnancy rates with eSET (0.8%) when compared with double embryo transfers (DET) (33.1%) [8]. Updated figures for 2007 have shown a stable live birth rate in patients receiving eSET up to the age of 40 years [10]. In contrast, in 2007 only 2.8% of ART cycles were eSET in the U.S. Australia and New Zealand (56.9%, 2006), Belgium (48%, 2005), and Finland (49.7%, 2005) also have high rates of eSET uptake. Legislation in New Zealand outlines the first-line use of eSET if a patient is 35 years of age or younger, and the first two attempts are publicly funded. Patients in Belgium are allowed six publicly funded cycles, with eSET mandatory for the first cycle if the woman is younger than 36 years old [9]. Twin pregnancies have since decreased from 19% to 3% in Belgium, without a reduction in the overall pregnancy rate [11]. Guidelines produced from the Canadian Fertility and Andrology Society and the Society of Obstetricians and Gynaecologists of Canada suggest eSET for women 35 years and younger for their first or second cycle, and those who are 36 or 37 years of age with a good prognosis [9].

A recent meta-analysis performed by McLernon et al., comparing the outcomes of single and double embryo transfers, confirmed that two eSET IVF cycles (one fresh and one frozen) were needed to achieve similar pregnancy rates to those observed in one DET IVF cycle (38% and 42%, respectively). However, eSET significantly lowered the risk of preterm birth (OR 0.33, 95% CI: 0.20–0.55) and delivery of a low birth weight baby independent of embryo quality, patient age (up to 36 years), and previous duration of infertility. Multiple birth rates were much lower and similar to naturally conceived spontaneous pregnancies (1% versus 32%). While authors advocate the use of eSET, they acknowledge that DET may still be the treatment of choice in an older patient, where live birth rates after IVF cycles are much lower despite multiple embryo transfer [12].

The concept of eSET may be unacceptable to parents who may perceive the risk of a multiple pregnancy associated with DET as an increased chance of completing their family with a single treatment and pregnancy, a desire to have twins, a successful pregnancy (versus a failed cycle), and as a generally positive short-term outcome of ART [12]. The need for multiple cycles may also increase the emotional burden for parents. Evidence has shown that economic factors such as public funding can also influence the desirability of eSET for a patient. Kjellberg et al. assessed maternal and pediatric costs per delivery from birth up to six months of eSET and DET in Sweden and found eSET to be more cost-effective than DET. They provide an argument that eSET is more financially viable for couples seeking ART, where demand exceeds fixed financial supply [13]. This may also have an implication for some countries reluctant to increase eSET due to concern regarding lower birth rates per cycle and anticipated fiscal difficulties.

Despite the established association of preterm birth, low birth weight, and increased perinatal mortality for multiple pregnancies, there remains an increased baseline risk for singleton births following ART compared with singletons born from natural conception.

The association that ART may increase perinatal mortality for singletons was first identified in 1985. A meta-analysis performed on early and more recent data by Helmerhorst et al. confirmed a positive association between very preterm births of less than 32 weeks (RR 3.27, 95% CI: 2.05–3.28), preterm births (RR 2.04, 95% CI: 1.82–0.32), very low birth weight of less than 1500 g (RR 3.00, 95% CI: 2.04–7.36), low birth weight of less than 2500 g (RR 1.40, 95% CI: 1.11–5.71), small for gestational age (RR 1.54, 95% CI: 1.41–4.66), admission to a neonatal ICU (RR 1.27, 95% CI: 1.11–6.40), and perinatal mortality (RR 1.68, 95% CI: 1.12–1.55), when compared with matched non-ART controls. Non-matched study results showed a similar trend [14].

These trends demonstrate a significantly raised risk of perinatal morbidity for singleton ART pregnancies and have been echoed with strong reinforcement in other meta-analyses. Jackson et al. found very similar odds ratios (ORs) for all the previously given parameters when performing a random-effects meta-analysis, excluding very preterm delivery (not assessed) [15]. McGovern et al. assessed the risk of preterm babies resulting from IVF and gamete intra-Fallopian transfer and found the relative risk (RR) of preterm delivery to be almost double that seen in naturally conceived singleton pregnancies (RR 1.98, 95% CI: 1.72–7.22). The risk of very preterm delivery was increased further (RR 2.49, 95% CI: 0.87–6.21) [16].

The increased risk of perinatal morbidity and mortality observed following ART is attributable in some part to underlying infertility itself, which is regarded as an independent risk factor. This link has been confirmed in numerous studies. A Danish cohort study assessing time to a singleton pregnancy in females who were planning pregnancy found a positive correlation between increasing length of time to pregnancy (less than six months, one to 12 months, and greater than 12 months) and the associated RR of a preterm delivery, independent of infertility treatment. They concluded that patients with clinical subfertility or infertility are more prone to preterm delivery [17]. A study conducted in Sweden found that women with a history of infertility of one year or greater had a higher mean age, lower parity, more stillbirths, and a higher than average rate of low birth weight children and preterm deliveries when compared with women without a history of infertility [18]. A case-control study by Draper et al., investigating the separate contribution of ART and infertility to perinatal mortality, found that infertility independently increased perinatal mortality (OR 2.9, 95% CI: 1.04–8.5), with over half of cases associated with preterm delivery. Multiple and singleton births were included in this data [19].

The role of IVF techniques themselves may also be implicated in producing adverse perinatal outcomes. Wang et al. assessed IVF and gamete intra-Fallopian transfer (GIFT) techniques for association with perinatal outcome. They found a higher incidence of low and very low birth weight babies (OR 1.76, 95% CI: 1.32–8.25 and OR 1.61, 95% CI: 1.02–5.46, respectively) when ART was compared with the normal obstetric population (see Table 14.1) [20].

Table 14.1. Perinatal complications

Multiple pregnancy is the largest contributory factor to obstetric complications and perinatal morbidity and is predominantly iatrogenic in the context of ART.
High-order pregnancy is the most undesirable health outcome from ART worldwide, associated with higher rates of preterm birth, low birth weight, and increased perinatal mortality.
Multiple and high-order pregnancies correlate directly with the number of embryos transferred per cycle and can be reduced by elective single embryo transfer.
Double embryo transfer may be appropriate in older patients where live birth rates after IVF cycles are much lower.
Infertility is thought to be an independent risk factor for increased perinatal morbidity and mortality following ART.
Singleton ART pregnancies also have an increased risk of perinatal morbidity. Infertility itself may account for this.

Congenital anomalies, imprinting disorders, and neurodevelopment

Much attention has been drawn to the risk of malformations and congenital anomalies following ART. According to ESHRE, the total risk for all children of a birth defect is 3% (April, 2009), based on European and Nordic registry data [21]. The effects of standard IVF, micromanipulation techniques, embryo culture conditions, and spermatozoon selection in patients with an underlying genetic predilection for infertility have been much debated. Does this increase the risk of genetic, epigenetic, and aberrant congenital malformation? Current expert thinking estimates that the risk of major malformations after IVF and ICSI is raised by about 1.1–3.5-fold, with no significant difference observed between standard IVF and ICSI [5].

In 1987 Lancaster raised concern about the association of ART and congenital malformations when he reported an increased number of neural tube defects and transposition of the great arteries in children born after ART [22]. Many studies have since attempted to address this important issue; however, results have proved inconsistent and can be attributed to the difficulties encountered in interpretation of studies including study design and power, sample size, retrospective self-reported data collection of anomalies, and time to pregnancy in case-control studies (also acknowledged by the HFEA). Some early studies were not designed to answer questions relating to birth defects, confounded by the relatively low prevalence, low numbers of ART, disparities of the definition of major malformations, and the time and type of clinical assessment of malformations identified. Not all studies take into account genetic screening, spontaneous and induced abortion, and the rates of chromosomal abnormalities or major malformations within these populations.

Hansen et al. performed the first systematic review and fixed-effect meta-analysis addressing major malformation risk after ART in an attempt to substantiate this link. The meta-analysis revealed a 30%–40% increased risk of all birth defects when compared with spontaneous conceptions, with a changing "number needed to harm" rate (the number of children needed to be conceived by ART for one additional child to be born with a birth defect), depending on the prevalence of a disorder within a population [23].

A meta-analysis performed by Rimm et al. aiming to estimate the risk of major malformations in IVF and ICSI found a statistically significant increase in ART versus natural conception (OR 1.29, 95% CI: 1.01–1.67). No statistically significant difference was noted between IVF and ICSI. They acknowledged that all studies included lacked a control group consisting of infertile patients spontaneously conceiving and that this may bias the results alongside the inability to separate procedure-associated risk from other factors [24].

Most recently, Reefhuis et al. conducted a case-control study using data from the U.S. National Birth Defects Society for singletons born after ART. They found strong associations of ART with septal heart defects (adjusted OR 2.1, 95% CI: 1.4–1.0), cleft lip with or without cleft palate (adjusted OR 2.4, 95% CI: 1.5–2.1), esophageal atresia (adjusted OR 4.5, 95% CI: 1.1–90.5), and anorectal atresia (adjusted OR 3.7, 95% CI: 1.9–5.1) [25]. Critical correspondence subsequently published by Rimm et al. highlighted a lack of a control group consisting of subfertile couples and that, due to large numerical discrepancies in maternal age groups between the ART and non-ART groups (13% versus 55% of 35 years or older, respectively), age stratification may have been more appropriate. They postulated that risks identified may have been overstated due to the statistical methods used, and that other factors with a currently unknown extent may well contribute to an overall increase in major malformations seen in the ART group [26].

Difficulties in obtaining a proper control group consisting of subfertile or infertile couples who conceive naturally has been addressed in one longitudinal study by Zhu et al., who sought a link between time to pregnancy and prevalence of congenital malformations in fertile patients, infertile patients who had conceived naturally, and those who conceived using ART (national Danish birth cohort data). Infertility was defined as twelve months or more duration before pregnancy was achieved, and prevalence of congenital malformations ascertained from hospital discharge diagnoses. They found that infertile couples who conceived irrespective of ART treatment had a higher prevalence of congenital neurological, gastrointestinal, and musculoskeletal malformations (hazard ratio 1.20, 95% CI: 1.21–3.57 for infertile couples and natural conception cases, and 1.39, 95% CI: 1.21–3.57 for infertile couples using ART). The prevalence increased with increasing time to pregnancy. However, an increased prevalence of genital organ malformations (hazard ratio 2.32, 95% CI: 1.24–4.35), chromosomal abnormalities, and other malformations was seen among the ART group when compared with infertile patients and natural conception cases. Although the study was not powered to assess the prevalence of particular malformations, penoscrotal and perineal hypospadias were higher in singletons born after ART. The prevalence of balanic and penile hypospadias was unchanged. They concluded that hormonal treatments associated with ART may be responsible for genital malformations, but they also identified an association with infertility [27].

Lie et al. performed a meta-analysis looking at the risk of birth defects of ICSI compared with standard IVF, and found a weakly positive association (RR 1.12, 95% CI: 0.91–7.28; P=0.12). They did not find significantly raised risks for cardiovascular defects, musculoskeletal defects, hypospadias, neural tube defects, or oral clefts, and concluded that there was not a significant difference of major malformations between standard IVF and ICSI. They did note, however, the ambiguity of the term major malformation, which encompasses an anatomical defect that needs treatment or possible functional implications. Without a clear definition, this precludes a lack of general consensus of such regarded conditions within the analyzed studies. They also acknowledged under-reporting of prenatal diagnoses and induced abortions may have introduced bias into their results [28].

Again an argument exists that age at conception and infertility itself play a role in a positive association between ART and an increased risk of spontaneous and genetic major malformations. Currently, 35.1% of women seeking ART within the UK are more than 37 years of age [5]. While this may reflect a desire to conceive at a later age, it may also mirror a period of unrecognized subfertility for affected couples who, by definition, will have been trying to conceive for at least one year without achieving success. Ghazi et al. observed, when investigating delivery outcome in infertile patients, that the rate of major malformations may have been increased in patients with a history of four or more years of infertility [18].

This has also been acknowledged by ESHRE in their position statement on birth defects in IVF children. They acknowledge the need for continuous monitoring, stating that: "*Children from couples who get pregnant after ART like IVF/ICSI have a 40–50% increased risk for a birth defect. A similar increased risk has been reported for subfertile couples who get pregnant spontaneously after a prolonged time period. This increased risk seems thus mainly to be due to parental characteristics from the infertility status and not the treatment given*" [21].

Assisted reproductive technology has also been implicated in the production of epigenetic malformations and recognized syndromes. These changes occur most commonly via alteration in the normal methylation pattern of DNA or histone protein modification rather than through DNA damage itself. The resulting effect is abnormal silencing of one allele in inherited autosomal genes that are usually expressed together. Allele dysfunction associated with imprinting is parent-specific [29,30].

A valid link may exist between ART and the predisposition to an imprinting disorder. Spermatozoa are known to complete imprinting processes earlier in development than oocytes, which undergo re-methylation processes immediately prior to or post-ovulation. Ovarian hyperstimulation and oocyte retrieval, alongside culture conditions, may therefore alter subsequent normal reconstitution of methylated genes. Interestingly, almost all human genetic phenotypes seen after ART occur via hypomethylation of the affected maternal allele [29].

Currently, ten human phenotypes resulting from imprinting disorders have been identified, with particular interest directed toward the relationship of ART and Angelman syndrome (AS) and Beckwith–Wiedemann syndrome (BWS). Angelman syndrome has an approximate prevalence of 1 in 12 000 individuals. Children with AS suffer with severe intellectual disability, speech impairment, ataxia, seizures, and microcephaly. Beckwith–Wiedermann syndrome affects 1 in 13 700 children. Patients may suffer with pre- and postnatal overgrowth, neonatal hypoglycemia, exomphalos, macroglossia, and hemihyperplasia. Children who suffer with BWS are at increased risk of developing embryonal tumors [29,30].

Manipalviratn et al. conducted a review on data and consolidated clinical cases of AS and BWS reported after ART. They observed increased prevalence rates for BWS in ART children in an American registry (4.6% ART population prevalence versus 0.76% in the general population); a similar prevalence has been noted in France (4% versus 1.3%) and the Netherlands (5.6% versus 0.92%). Regional U.K. data have also shown a positive trend (4% versus 1.2% and 2.9% versus 0.8%, respectively), with a recent two-center study demonstrating a prevalence of 1 in 1524 ART-associated cases compared with a general population prevalence of 1 in 13 700 children. Australian case-control data noted a BWS prevalence of 1 in 4000 ART children, compared with 1 in 35 580 live births. Danish and Swedish cohort data have not shown a relationship of BWS with ART. More than 60 BWS patients born after ART and ovulation induction have been identified worldwide. Of the ART patients who underwent genetic mutation identification in the nine studies identified, 90%–100% were born with the same epigenetic mutation: hypomethylation of the affected maternal allele. Epigenetic changes are thought to normally account for only 50%–60% of sporadic BWS cases [29].

There have been fewer identified AS cases associated with ART than with BWS. Three genetic mechanisms are known to be responsible in producing the AS phenotype, accounting for the majority of cases. Less than 5% of cases are attributed to an imprinting defect (approximately 1 in 300 000 births). When looking at existing data for AS children born after ART, Manipalviratn et al. found that five children out of a total of seven reported IVF and ICSI cases resulted from an epimutation [29]. Amor and Halliday also reviewed existing literature on AS and imprinting disorders. They calculated that, should an association between ART and AS with an imprinting defect as the etiologic factor be a truly non-random event, this would be expected to occur in one per 20 million births [30]. There does appear to be a non-random association of epimutations causing AS with ART. This relationship may of course be multifactorial. Other potential risk factors may be overshadowed by the concerns relating to ART techniques and imprinting disorders. Infertility itself has been implicated.

Angelman syndrome resulting from imprinting defects has been seen in children born to subfertile parents who did not undergo fertility treatment. The role played by ovulation induction is also not clear [30].

Confirmation of a true relationship between ART in general and imprinting syndromes is limited by the rarity of these disorders. Large multicenter studies may never have sufficient power to answer this question. The question that mild cases of BWS may be under-reported within the general population, and that a higher prevalence within ART populations is thus a reflection of increased medical scrutiny of these children has also been raised previously. Ultimately these diseases still remain rare whether they are seen within ART or non-ART populations [29].

Concerns exist regarding the extent, if any, of neurodevelopmental morbidity and persistent neurological impairment associated directly with ART techniques. Questions have been raised relating to the potential association of ART with adverse neurodevelopmental outcome in infancy, cerebral palsy, epilepsy, and longer-term neurological sequelae that may only manifest or become identifiable in adolescence.

A systematic review conducted by Middleburg et al. assessed ART outcomes of neuromotor development, cognition, speech and language, and behavior. Most studies included data for children born after conventional IVF, ICSI, and cryopreservation at infancy and school age. Registry-based studies analyzed showed no increased risk of severe cognitive impairment, mental retardation, and speech and language, behavior, and neuromotor disorders correlating with the results of larger methodologically sound and controlled original studies. They highlight the lack of neurodevelopmental data after infancy, and therefore a potential underestimation or even underdiagnosis of minor neurodevelopmental disorders that may become apparent with longer follow-up, such as fine manipulative disability or dyslexia [31].

A European study assessing the cognitive and motor development of five-year-old children born after ART found no significant difference in those children born after IVF or ICSI when compared to naturally conceived controls. The ART children included from all centers were Caucasian, born from a singleton pregnancy after 32 weeks' gestation, and first- or second-born, with a native language of the country where they were assessed. Verbal IQ, performance IQ, and a combination of these scores (full scale IQ) were assessed using the Wechsler preschool and primary scale of intelligence (revised), and McCarthy scales of children's abilities: motor scale. The authors observed that after adjustment for demographic variables, ART children with mothers within the 34–35-year age category scored lower than children born from natural conception, although this difference was relative and corresponded to less than one IQ point between groups. They also observed that maternal education appeared to influence outcome in performance scale subsets (block design subset and object assembly) and verbal scale subsets, concluding that maternal age and education may play a role in the cognitive development of ART children [32].

Belva et al. used a Belgian ICSI cohort aged eight years, and compared medical and neurological outcomes with spontaneously conceived controls. The ICSI children included were singletons and born at term. No significant difference in neurological assessment was found within this group [33]. Leunens et al. took this work forward and assessed the cognitive and motor development of a Belgian cohort of ICSI children, at the ages of eight and, two years later, at 10 years. Comparatively, no significant difference was noted between ICSI children and controls at eight or 10 years for motor, manual, and ball skills. Total, verbal, and performance intelligence scores were also similar to those of controls [34].

One study has assessed the educational ability of adolescents post-ART. Wagenaar et al. assessed 233 8- to 18-year-old children born after IVF with the same number of naturally conceived controls born to parents with fertility problems. No differences in school functioning: education level, general cognitive ability, school performance, rates of learning, or developmental disorders were found. The authors concluded that children and adolescents born after IVF do not seem to suffer educational difficulties resulting from ART treatment [35].

To date, outcomes have not reliably or consistently shown any difference between children born after ART and natural conception for neurological development from birth to adolescence. Studies discussed here, however, have been based largely on singleton pregnancies and babies born after 32 weeks' gestation with a normal birth weight. Information relating to adolescent cognitive and neurological development is sparse. The full extent of adverse ART-influenced neurological outcomes in adolescents is yet to be comprehensively evaluated.

Concerns regarding cerebral palsy and a possible link to ART have been extensively investigated; registry-based data have contributed significantly to current thinking. Neurological and psychiatric diagnoses have been linked to ART registers in Scandinavian countries, allowing for statistical risk calculation estimates for adverse neurological and psychiatric outcomes after ART.

Literature on this subject is summarized succinctly by Middelburg et al., who included key studies from registry-based cohorts in their systematic review. In vitro fertilization has previously been identified as an independent risk factor for cerebral palsy. However, risks appear to be mainly attributable to a higher rate of multiple pregnancy and increased risk of preterm delivery and low birth weight with ART rather than to ART itself [31]. The possibility of intrauterine death of a single foetus during a twin pregnancy may influence the neurological outcome of the surviving twin. This potential link has been investigated by Pinborg et al., who identified that 10% of singleton children born after IVF originated from twin pregnancies. Spontaneous abortion of a single fetus was found to increase the risk of cerebral palsy (OR 1.9, 95% CI: 0.5–7.2) in the surviving sibling, with increased risks of low birth weight and preterm birth also noted (see Table 14.2). A positive correlation between neurological sequelae and lengthened duration of pregnancy at the time of spontaneous abortion was observed [36]. Of course, an argument again exists around the true role of infertility itself in the multifactorial causes of cerebral palsy within ART cohorts.

Table 14.2. Congenital anomalies, imprinting disorders, and neurodevelopment

There is a 30% increased risk of spontaneous and/or genetic major malformation in babies born to couples undergoing ART.
ESHRE advise that this increased risk seems mainly attributable to subfertility and infertility rather than a direct result of ART treatment.
A link may exist between imprinting disorders and ART, in particular Beckwith–Wiedemann syndrome and Angelman syndrome. Increased prevalence of these disorders caused by epigenetic mutation has been observed in ART cohorts in many different countries.
No difference between children born after ART and natural conception for intellectual development from birth to adolescence has been identified.
Higher rates of cerebral palsy are seen with ART, predominantly due to higher rates of multiple pregnancy, preterm delivery, and low birth weight.

Long-term health implications

Assessment of other aspects of physical well-being after ART such as childhood cancer, subsequent infertility, and general health have been approached using different methods of assessment. These have included hospitalization rates and health resource use.

Leslie et al. performed the first study looking at health resource use and hospitalization rates after IVF, in a small Australian study assessing primigravid mothers and their children from 30 weeks' antenatal gestation to one year of age. They confirmed previous findings that babies born after IVF were more likely to be admitted to neonatal intensive care units. They did not observe a discrepancy in medical problems or overutilization of health resources; however, the IVF cohort used was unusual in that no difference in preterm birth, low birth weight, or congenital abnormalities was noted between them and the control group [37].

A large retrospective Swedish study used hospital discharge data linked to the births registry, identifying all hospital admissions for IVF and non-IVF children between 1981–1997. Analysis in children up to the age of 14 years was undertaken. Neonatal admission observed was three times higher in the IVF cohort, with hospital admission in children born after ART being consistently higher until six years of age (OR 1.1–2.3). Increased ORs for admission with cerebral palsy (OR 1.7), epilepsy (OR 1.5), asthma (OR 1.4), and infections (OR 1.4) were observed in the IVF group, perhaps reflecting long-term neurological and respiratory sequelae resulting from preterm birth. Admission for congenital malformation was also raised (OR 1.8) as was cancer; however, rates did not appear to be raised within the IVF cohort. Increased hospitalization, especially in the neonatal period, may be attributable to increased rates of preterm birth and subsequent morbidity following IVF for both singletons and multiples. Interestingly, the increased baseline risk after the neonatal period, corrected after adjustment for time to pregnancy, perhaps implicates parental anxiety as a contributing factor. The average number of days spent in hospital for IVF children was 9.5 versus 3.6 for non-IVF cohorts. Hospitalization rates between IVF and non-IVF twins were similar [38].

Childhood cancers are devastating, life-changing, and potentially life-shortening for any patient unfortunate to receive an oncological diagnosis. It is not surprising that concerns regarding the incidence of cancer after ART are still being investigated. Hypotheses include hormonal ovarian hyperstimulation and in vitro embryo culture and manipulation as potential stages of the ART process where genetic expression may be altered, resulting in a predisposition to malignancy. Interestingly, suggested links also implicate epigenetic changes as a causative factor.

A meta-analysis performed by Raimondi et al. reviewed key literature relating to IVF and childhood cancer from cohort studies performed in Europe, Scandinavia, Australia, the U.S., and Brazil. A standardized incidence ratio was used to assess the relationship between IVF and cancer, calculated using expected numbers and actual observed cases. Although individual study outcomes varied, the meta-analysis failed to identify a link between ART and childhood cancer. They acknowledge that they were unable to adjust analysis for follow-up length, and advocate pooled analysis of data for further investigation [39].

A study assessing the childhood cancer risk in a large Danish cohort following drug-induced ovulation stimulation compared rates with childhood cancer incidence in the Danish population. The overall standardized incidence ratio (SIR) of childhood cancer post-ART was calculated as 1.14 (95% CI: 0.1–8.5). No association between early childhood tumors and non-hematopoietic malignancies was identified. An increased risk of hematopoietic cancer in childhood and later in life was observed, but this was not statistically significant. Authors concluded that results were reassuring; however, they also identified the need for an adequately powered study to investigate the relationship between ovulation-inducing drugs and childhood malignancy [40].

Again, initial studies attempting to substantiate a possible link have been plagued with pitfalls such as poor or variable follow-up rates, small sample size, and a lack of comparison with non-ART incidence rates within a given population. Worldwide pooled analysis is currently being undertaken by Felix et al., who produced an interim report in 2009, outlining the difficulties encountered with analysis of existing cohort data. At the time of publication, the authors felt that, worldwide, data collection after ART in its current form was sufficiently deficient to address the relationship between ART and cancer. Efforts to counteract this include expansion of cohort children, registry linkage for ART offspring diagnosed with cancer, and co-variate stratification including infertility, socioeconomic status, and hormonal stimulation [41].

At present it appears that there is reassuringly little evidence to support a link between childhood cancer and ART. Stand-alone studies suggesting that a link exists have used small cohorts and have failed to demonstrate a consensus for particular cancer subtypes implicated. It is reassuring that an observed or repeated anecdotal association has not been identified. However, the fact remains that currently there is a paucity of long-term large cohort data without adequate long-term follow-up. Without further information, a true association cannot be substantiated or refuted.

The impact of ART on reproductive ability is yet to be fully investigated, with concerns centered around ICSI treatment. Within the U.K., ICSI comprises 46% of all IVF treatment (HFEA, 2008), and has bypassed donor insemination in terms of live birth rate while also offering the chance to conceive a child genetically related to both parents [5]. Although providing a solution to male factor subfertility, it seems that this is not enough to halt the cause-and-effect pattern of inherited male infertility, primarily resulting from the presence of underlying Y chromosome genetic abnormalities within spermatozoa from affected males, and subsequent inheritance of these male sex chromosomal aberrations by male ICSI offspring. In fact, ICSI may facilitate inheritance of male infertility that initially occurred de novo within the prospective father.

It has been documented previously that chromosomal abnormalities within couples undergoing ICSI are higher than the baseline rates observed within the general population, with many affecting sex chromosomes, particularly in males. Recognized Y chromosome abnormalities in males undergoing infertility treatment include numerical sex chromosome aberrations, such as Klinefelter's syndrome (47XXY), unbalanced and balanced translocations, and microdeletions [42,43].

Numerical sex chromosome aberrations are not directly inherited by offspring. Translocations may not be inherited at all, inherited in their balanced form, or in an unbalanced form. Patients with inherited balanced translocations are healthy but infertile, whereas an unbalanced translocation may result in spontaneous abortion. Congenital malformations and significant neurodevelopmental impairment are associated with unbalanced translocations when the outcome of pregnancy is a living child [42].

Microdeletions hold particular significance for fertility outcomes in ART offspring. They are genetic aberrations that usually occur spontaneously and result in infertility. Three independent, large loci for spermatogenesis have been identified on the long arm of the Y chromosome, and it is thought that microdeletions occurring within these regions are responsible for 10%–15% of cases of azoospermia and oligospermia. It has previously been demonstrated that ICSI treatment allows transfer of microdeletions from father to son, iatrogenically transforming a de novo condition into an inherited disorder [42,43].

Autosomal genetic aberrations may also affect fertility outcomes indirectly. Cystic fibrosis (CF) mutations are common in Caucasians and have an association with congenital bilateral absence or atrophy of the vas deferens, an inadvertent complication causing unexpected infertility on a background of significant health morbidity in children born with CF after ART [43].

The ability to transfer male factor infertility from parent to child via ICSI is a hugely significant finding and poses, for prospective parents and clinicians, the dilemma of deliberating the extra medical and psychological impact this may have on a male child, alongside the ethical considerations requiring serious forethought. In relation to microdeletions identified prior to treatment, disclosure of fertility treatment would be needed to explain infertility in male progeny. Of course, ICSI may hold the solution to the problem for these affected males, but also allows us to continue a cycle reliant on ART to produce another generation with knowledge that this group of ART offspring will have increased health morbidity manifesting as infertility as a direct result of ICSI treatment. Concerns exist as to whether these microdeletions could lengthen in males affected after ART as generations increase, resulting in a more severe and perhaps treatment-resistant male infertility. These concerns have yet to be substantiated [43]. Alternative treatments available for this group include donor insemination, PGD, and gender selection.

Genetic testing and counseling has consistently been advocated for ICSI candidates with azoospermia and severe oligospermia, although no universally accepted method exists in practice. Attempts to identify Y chromosome microdeletions may be confounded by the presence of small microdeletions, as these may not be identified using conventional karyotyping [42,43]. Given the higher incidence of genetic aberrations in parents undergoing ICSI and the potential consequences of autosomal and sex chromosome aberrations imposed on resulting progeny, it seems that karyotyping in the least may allow for anticipation of reproductive impairment and general long-term health of a child.

Of course, complex interplay exists between the effects of infertility, ART, and health outcomes. The manifestations of long-term cardiovascular morbidity may not be seen until adulthood and middle-age. Low birth weight has been consistently demonstrated on a global scale to have an independent association with coronary heart disease, stroke, hypertension, and non-insulin dependent diabetes in adult life, a phenomenon thought to be due to developmental plasticity in utero, more commonly referred to as the Barker hypothesis [44].

Emotional well-being of children born after ART has not been forgotten among the considerations and identification of physical outcomes. Factors potentially affecting social and psychological development include parenting issues, non-disclosure of ART, disclosure to the child/adolescent on the proviso that this is contained within the family and thus becomes a "family secret," and manifest family discord resulting from any of the aforementioned factors. Assisted reproductive treatment itself has been implicated as a stress-inducing factor that may adversely affect adaptation to parenthood, therefore influencing the relationship between parent and child [5].

Childhood and adolescent studies addressing the impact of ART on inter-family relationships and social and emotional development have not shown any convincing or reproducible relationship between adverse psychosocial outcomes and ART. A large European study assessing socioemotional development in five-year-old children born after ICSI and IVF found no negative difference on family function and emotional well-being. They observed ICSI mothers to have a higher level of commitment to parenting and reported fewer feelings of hostility toward their offspring at a statistically significant level [45]. A recent review of existing literature examining the psychological outcome after IVF found no difference in children up to the age of eight years. The authors acknowledge that psychosocial function needed further assessment in children aged more than eight years, having identified indications of behavioral problems and socioemotional problems from some studies examined [46]. Wagenaar et al. performed a study looking at behavior and socioemotional functioning of Dutch 9- to 18-year-olds born after IVF, as perceived by parents and teachers. Overall, no difference was found when compared with matched controls, although a trend toward internalization and withdrawn behavior was noted in IVF children. Results were not reproduced when this study was repeated in 2011 [47,48]. Colpin and Bossaert performed a small study assessing parenting and psychosocial adjustment on families with ART children aged two years, and reassessed the cohort when the children were between 15 and 16 years old. The IVF group included IVF teenagers who were privy to their parents IVF treatment and a subset of children who were not. They found no significant differences in parenting of adolescents or psychosocial adjustment in IVF children compared with controls, nor in informed IVF teenagers versus those oblivious to their mode of conception (see Table 14.3) [49].

Table 14.3. Long-term health implications

No reproducible association between childhood cancer and ART has been identified. Efforts to improve data collection are ongoing in preparation for worldwide pooled analysis.
Male infertility may be influenced by ICSI treatment. ICSI may allow a sporadic Y chromosome microdeletion causing infertility in a father to be transferred to a son, which would not occur through natural conception.
ART children born at a low birth weight have an increased risk of coronary heart disease, stroke, hypertension, and non-insulin dependent diabetes in adult life, but this happens in all such births.
The needs and rights of the child should be considered prior to treatment and considered with equal weighting to those of the couple having treatment.
ART does not appear to have a negative psychosocial impact on children and adolescents.
Disclosure of treatment allows the ART child access to information regarding biological parents or siblings for genetic and marital purposes. This also allows discussion of important health issues such as inherited infertility.
The psychological aspect of ART and disclosure, and family and sexual relationships in later life, especially in those who may be infertile themselves, is also an important aspect not to be forgotten.
We do not know the effect that ART may impose on adult health. Adult cancer risk, fertility patterns, cardiovascular morbidity, susceptibility to systemic illness, and life expectancy is not known and, to some extent, yet to be observed.

Ethical considerations

A spectrum of moral and ethical considerations exists as a minefield when navigating through the subject of ART. It begins with the initial decision to treat infertility of two adults, progressing to include the multidimensional challenges that subsequent children, adolescents, and adult offspring may face as a direct result of ART.

Sutcliffe et al. noted concerns that children in our society do not receive the consideration they ought [5]. Does ART allow precedence of the rights of the would-be parent to overshadow those of the resulting child/children? Assisted reproductive technology complicates parentage in the first instance by discrepancies in embryo transfer numbers per cycle as an iatrogenically created issue. The strongest association of adverse outcome with ART is caused by multiple pregnancy; therefore, beneficence toward the child would perhaps dictate that all women under the age of 37 years should undergo eSET in order to minimize the risk of low birth weight, prematurity, and cerebral palsy.

Assisted reproductive technology also produces a dilemma regarding disclosure of treatment to offspring. When is the right time to divulge this information; how will it be regarded; and what does the parent expect the child to do with it? Of course, parents may translate infertility into feelings of inadequacy and this may also affect disclosure. As discussed previously, if ART treatment is disclosed on the understanding that this is to be kept a "family secret," this may hold psychological consequences for the child. Disclosing this information may also inadvertently involve or affect other family members. It may implicate others also suffering from subfertility or infertility. In cases of embryo donation and donor insemination, it may reveal the existence of a biological parent or half-siblings previously unknown to that child/adolescent. Those born from ART after 2005 in the U.K. can obtain information about their genetic relatives via HFEA, after the age of 18 years, should they wish [50]. Siblings may be conceived naturally or by ART and this may alter self-perception and induce feelings of competition, inferiority, jealousy, and resentment toward them. It must therefore not be forgotten that long-term effects of ART also include effects on family dynamics and relationships.

Sexual and marital relationships are not unaffected by ART. There exists the possibility of unfortunate and inadvertent incest in offspring born after donor insemination and embryo donation. In 2008, British adolescents aged 18 years and those contemplating marriage from 16 years old were given the right to contact HFEA to find out whether they were conceived by ART and whether they are related to their future life partner, in an attempt to minimize this risk [50]. Disclosure of ART treatment allows the opportunity to increase awareness and acknowledgment of this issue, providing an argument that ART allows non-disclosing parents to put their own rights before the rights of their offspring.

Parents may not be the only persons who may compromise the rights of the child. The example of iatrogenic ICSI-related inheritance of Y chromosome microdeletions demonstrates that clinicians may encourage and indirectly support this. Although microdeletion testing and chromosome analysis is undertaken in males with severe oligospermia and azoospermia, options include proceeding with ICSI if a microdeletion or other abnormality is found. We do not know what psychological effect that inherited iatrogenic infertility will have on male children born after ICSI, and the relationships that they form. Are we feeding a biological "greed" by proceeding with ICSI in these circumstances? This does not come without a significant physical cost for male offspring and may not be recognized as non-maleficence from this perspective. Acknowledgment of this, alongside feelings toward disclosure of ART and infertility of offspring in the early stages of treatment requires serious forethought, counsel, and may never be completely achieved by those who desire to be biological parents to their child.

As clinicians, do we have the right to decide that infertility will be acceptable to an individual who has not been born on their behalf? In the case of eSET and DET, are we accepting the adverse physical health outcomes of multiple pregnancy as acceptable? One must question whether we are correctly adhering to the Hippocratic oath from this position. Could it be that we are responsible for permanently overriding and subsequently trivializing the reproductive rights of the child? These are important issues to consider.

Over the last three decades IVF has evolved from a scientific breakthrough into ART – encompassing reliable reproductive techniques with worldwide success. The outcomes of IVF and ICSI have been scrutinized constantly, in order to identify any unacceptable health risk to ART children and adolescents. Studies aiming to assess a link (or absence thereof) between ART and childhood outcomes are continuously improving in study method, design, and population numbers. Linked registry data will also allow health trends to be observed on a wider scale and investigated over a lifetime. Of course, this should lead to a more accurate understanding of the short- and long-term health risks associated with ART. Pursuing definitive answers will be difficult for rare associations such as imprinting disorders, but important nonetheless. Ultimately, the needs and the rights of the child must be considered prior to treatment and put before those of the prospective parents.

Louise Brown will be celebrating her 34th birthday in 2012. One aspect of paramount importance to ART is the absolute limitation of time. We do not have any experience of what middle- and older age holds for ART-born adults who were once infants, children, and adolescents. We also have little appreciation of the impact childhood morbidity may play in longer-term health outcomes. The Barker hypothesis implicates developmental plasticity as a predisposing factor for diabetes and cardiovascular morbidity in later life in low birth weight babies [44]. Whether ART will have an additional effect remains to be determined. Adult cancer risk, fertility patterns, susceptibility to systemic illness, and life expectancy are unknown. The psychological aspect of ART and disclosure, family and sexual relationships in later life, especially in those who may be infertile themselves, is also an important aspect not to be forgotten. Future prospective studies on longer-term health outcomes will hopefully hold some of these answers (see Table 14.4).

Conclusion

Multiple pregnancies as a result of double or multiple embryo transfer remains the biggest factor for adverse perinatal outcome including preterm delivery and low birth weight. This may also result in chronic lifelong health morbidity as cerebral palsy or manifest as cardiovascular disease, diabetes, or stroke in adult life. There is an increased baseline risk of preterm delivery, perinatal mortality, and congenital anomalies estimated at 30% by ESHRE after ART. This is thought to be related to underlying subfertility or infertility. Rare epigenetic syndromes including Angelman syndrome and Beckwith–Wiedemann syndrome may have an association with ART. Imprinting aberrations as the underlying genetic malformation have been noted in higher proportions after ART than observed in the general population. As these syndromes are rare, an established link may never be statistically proven.

Neurodevelopmental differences have not been demonstrated in ART children when compared with naturally conceived controls. Most of the existing evidence relates to singleton children born after 32 weeks' gestation. The increased risk of cerebral palsy after ART is attributable to preterm birth and low birth weight. The main modifiable risk factor for this is multiple embryo transfer.

To date, there has been no reproducible link or trend observing increased childhood cancer rates following ART around the world. Infertility may be inherited via ICSI treatment in cases where sporadic Y-chromosome microdeletions resulting in azoospermia or oligospermia are treated by this method. Psychosocial development from childhood and into adolescence is not demonstrably different to those born by natural conception.

Ethical considerations must include the rights of the child, with special regard to disclosure, fertility, relationships, and the possible existence/desire to explore biological family links.

References

1. Steptoe PC, Edwards RG. Birth after the reimplantation of a human embryo. *Lancet* 1978; **2**: 366.
2. Palermo G, Joris H, Devroey P, Van Steirteghem AC. Pregnancies after intracytoplasmic injection of single spermatozoon into an oocyte. *Lancet* 1992; **340**: 17–18.
3. Handyside AH, Lesko JG, Tarin JJ, Winston RM, Hughes MR. Birth of a normal girl after in vitro fertilisation and preimplantation diagnostic testing for cystic fibrosis. *N Engl J Med* 1992; **327**: 905–909.
4. Human Fertilisation and Embryology Authority. *Fertility Facts and Figures 2008*. (Available at: http://www.hfea.gov.uk/104.html) [Accessed January 23, 2011.]
5. Sutcliffe AG, Ludwig M. Outcome of assisted reproduction. *Lancet* 2007; **370**: 351–359.
6. Steel AJ, Sutcliffe A. Long-term health implications for children conceived by IVF/ICSI. *Hum Fertil* 2009; **12**: 21–27.
7. Buck Louis GM, Schisterman EF, Dukic VM, Schieve LA. Research hurdles complicating the analysis of infertility treatment and child health. *Hum Reprod* 2005; **20**: 12–18.
8. Karlstrom PO, Bergh C. Reducing the number of embryos transferred in Sweden–impact on delivery and multiple birth rates. *Hum Reprod* 2007; **22**: 2202–2207.
9. Maheshwari A, Griffiths S, Bhattacharya S. Global variations in the uptake of single embryo transfer. *Hum Reprod Update* 2011; **17**: 107–120.
10. Thurin A, Hausken J, Hillensjo T, et al. Elective single-embryo transfer versus double-embryo transfer in in vitro fertilisation. *N Engl J Med* 2004; **351**: 2392–2402.
11. Gordts S, Campo R, Puttemans P, et al. Belgian legislation and the effect of elective single embryo transfer on IVF outcome. *Reprod Biomed Online* 2005; **10**: 436–441.
12. McLernon DJ, Harrild K, Bergh C, et al. Clinical effectiveness of elective single versus double embryo transfer: meta analysis of individual patient data from randomised trials. *BMJ* 2010; **341**: c6945.
13. Kjellberg AT, Carlsson P, Bergh C. Randomised single versus double embryo transfer: obstetric and paediatric outcome and a cost-effectiveness analysis. *Hum Reprod* 2006; **21**: 210–216.
14. Helmerhorst FM, Perquin DAM, Donker D, Keirse MJ. Perinatal outcome of singletons and twins after assisted conception: a systematic review of controlled studies. *BMJ* 2004; **328**: 261.
15. Jackson RA, Gibson KA, Wu Y, Croughan MS. Perinatal outcomes in singletons following in vitro fertilisation: a meta analysis. *Obstet Gynaecol* 2004; **103**: 551–563.
16. McGovern PG, Llorens AJ, Skurnick JH, Weiss G, Goldsmith LT. Increased risk of preterm birth in singleton pregnancies resulting from in vitro fertilisation–embryo transfer or gamete intrafallopian transfer: a meta analysis. *Fertil Steril* 2004; **82**: 1514–1520.

17. Henriksen TB, Baird DD, Olsen J, et al. Time to pregnancy and preterm delivery. *Obstet Gynecol* 1997; **89**: 594–599.

18. Ghazi HA, Spielberger C, Kallen B. Delivery outcome after infertility–a registry study. *Fertil Steril* 1991; **55**: 726–732.

19. Draper ES, Kurinczuk JJ, Abrams KR, Clarke M. Assessment of separate contributions to perinatal mortality of infertility history and treatment: a case control analysis. *Lancet* 1999; **353**: 1746–1749.

20. Wang JX, Clark AM, Kirby CA, et al. The obstetric outcome of singleton pregnancies following in vitro fertilisation/gamete intra-fallopian transfer. *Hum Reprod* 1994; **9**: 141–146.

21. ESHRE position statement: Birth defects in IVF children 2009. European society of human reproduction and embryology. (Available at: http://www.eshre.eu/ESHRE/English/Guidelines-Legal/ESHRE-Position-Papers/page.aspx/942) [Accessed January 18, 2011.]

22. Lancaster PA. Congenital malformations after in-vitro fertilisation. *Lancet* 1987; **2**: 1392–1393.

23. Hansen M, Bower C, Milne E, de Klerk N, Kurinczuk JJ. Assisted reproductive technologies and the risk of birth defects–a systematic review. *Hum Reprod* 2005; **20**: 328–338.

24. Rimm AA, Katayama AC, Diaz M, Katayama KP. A meta-analysis of controlled studies comparing major malformation rates in IVF and ICSI infants with naturally conceived children. *J Assist Reprod Genet* 2004; **21**: 437–443.

25. Reefhuis J, Honein MA, Schieve LA, et al. Assisted reproductive technology and major structural birth defects in the United States. *Hum Reprod* 2009; **2**: 360–366.

26. Rimm AA, Katayama AC, Katayama P. Letters to the editor: ART and major structural birth defects in the United States. *Hum Reprod* 2009; **24**: 1765–1771.

27. Zhu JL, Basso O, Obel C, Bille C, Olsen J. Infertility, infertility treatment and congenital malformations: Danish national birth cohort. *BMJ* 2006; **333**: 679.

28. Lie RT, Lyngstadaas A, Orstavik KH, et al. Birth defects in children conceived by ICSI compared with children conceived by other IVF methods: a meta analysis. *Int J Epidemiol* 2005; **34**: 696–701.

29. Manipalviratn S, DeCherney A, Segars J. Imprinting disorders and assisted reproductive technology. *Fertil Steril* 2009; **91**: 305–315.

30. Amor DJ, Halliday J. A review of known imprinting syndromes and their association with assisted reproduction technologies. *Hum Reprod* 2008; **23**: 2826–2834.

31. Middleburg KJ, Heineman MJ, Bos AF, Hadders-Algra M. Neuromotor, cognitive, language and behavioural outcome in children born following IVF or ICSI–a systematic review. *Hum Reprod Update* 2008; **14**: 219–231.

32. Ponjaert-Kristoffersen I, Bonduelle M, Barnes J, et al. International collaborative study of intracytoplasmic sperm injection-conceived, in vitro fertilisation-conceived, and naturally conceived 5 year old child outcomes: cognitive and motor assessments. *Pediatrics* 2005; **115**: e283–e289.

33. Belva F, Henriet S, Liebaers I, et al. Medical outcome of 8 year old singleton ICSI children (born > or 32 weeks' gestation) and a spontaneously conceived comparison group. *Hum Reprod* 2007; **22**: 506–515.

34. Leunens L, Celestin-Westreich S, Bonduelle M, Liebaers I, Ponjaert-Kristoffersen I. Follow-up of cognitive and motor development of 10 year old singleton children born after ICSI compared with spontaneously conceived children. *Hum Reprod* 2008; **23**: 105–111.

35. Wagenaar K, Ceelen M, Van Weissenbruch MM, et al. School functioning in 8 to 18 year old children born after in vitro fertilisation. *Eur J Paediatr* 2008; **167**: 1289–1295.

36. Pinborg A, Lidegaard O, La Cour Freiesleben N, Andersen AN. Consequences of vanishing twins in IVF/ICSI pregnancies. *Hum Reprod* 2005; **20**: 2821–2829.

37. Leslie GI, Gibson FL, McMahon C, Tennant C, Saunders DM. Infants conceived using in-vitro fertilisation do not over-utilise health care resources after the neonatal period. *Hum Reprod* 1998; **13**: 2055–2059.

38. Ericson A, Nygren KG, Olausson PO, Kallen B. Hospital care utilisation of infants born after IVF. *Hum Reprod* 2002; **17**: 929–932.

39. Raimondi S, Pedotti P, Taioli E. Meta-analysis of cancer incidence in children born after assisted reproductive technologies. *Br J Cancer* 2005; **93**: 1053–1056.

40. Brinton LA, Kruger Kjaer S, Thomsen BL, et al. Childhood tumor risk after treatment with ovulation-stimulating drugs. *Fertil Steril* 2004; **81**: 1083–1091.

41. Felix AS, Bruinsma F, Klemetti R, et al. International pooled analysis of cancer incidence in children after assisted reproductive technologies: interim report. *Future Oncol* 2009; **5**: 901–906.

42. Aittomaki K, Wennerholm UB, Bergh C, et al. Safety issues in assisted reproduction technology: should ICSI patients have genetic testing before treatment? A practical proposition to help patient information. *Hum Reprod* 2004; **19**: 472–476.

43. Kurinczuk JJ. Safety issues in assisted reproduction technology. From theory to reality–just what are the data telling us about ICSI offspring health and future fertility and should we be concerned? *Hum Reprod* 2003; **18**: 925–931.

44. Barker DJ. The developmental origins of adult disease. *J Am Coll Nutr* 2004; **23**: 588S–595S.

45. Barnes J, Sutcliffe AG, Kristoffersen I, et al. The influence of assisted reproduction on family functioning and children's socio-emotional development: results from a European study. *Hum Reprod* 2004;**19**: 1480–1487.

46. Wagenaar K, Huisman J, Cohen-Kettenis PT, Delemarre-van de Waal HA. An overview of studies on early development, cognition and psychosocial well-being in children born after in vitro fertilisation. *J Dev Behav Paediatr* 2008; **29**: 219–230.

47. Wagenaar K, Van Weissenbruch MM, Knol DL, *et al.* Behaviour and socioemotional functioning in 9–18-year old children born after in vitro fertilisation. *Fertil Steril* 2009; **92**: 1907–1914.

48. Wagenaar K, Van Weissenbruch MM, Van Keeuwen FE, et al. Self-reported behavioural and socioemotional functioning of 11- to 18- year old adolescents conceived by in vitro fertilisation. *Fertil Steril* 2011; **95**: 611–616.

49. Colpin H, Bossaert G. Adolescents conceived by IVF: parenting and psychosocial adjustment. *Hum Reprod* 2008; **23**: 2724–2730.

50. Human Fertility and Embryology Authority. *Information for Donor Conceived People 2011.* (Available at: http://www.hfea.gov.uk/5526.html) [Accessed January 30, 2011.]

Chapter 15

Ethical and legal perspectives of assisted reproductive technology pregnancies

Françoise Shenfield

Introduction

For over three decades now, the term assisted reproduction (ART) has been associated with procedures that have enthralled the public, both challenging and participating with the modern and post-modern societal evolution of the family, and also preyed on widespread fantasies. Ethically speaking, the issues have been many, as the possibility of seeing a human embryo outside its natural environment led to much debate about the status of this entity. However, this chapter will concentrate on aspects that directly relate to the children born from ART. Assisted reproduction is seen in the large sense, not confined to in vitro fertilization (IVF) and related techniques like ovum donation, surrogacy, and preimplantation genetic diagnosis (PGD), but also including simpler techniques of spermatozoon donation and posthumous inseminations. One may argue that of all relevant issues, using the simple ethical tools of balancing the patient's autonomy, doing as much good and as little harm as possible (in ethical terms, the beneficence and non-maleficence calculus), and the respect of justice, the issue of multiple pregnancy stands out in its frequency, severity, and the possible negative consequences for both the gestating woman and her offspring. It may also be the consequence of simple ovulation induction, and will be discussed as it forms the most frequent complication of ART internationally.

At the onset of IVF, which revolutionized fertility treatments, society's interest and concern about the human embryo were very vocal. All over Europe, the inevitable consequence was that legislation ensued to provide a regulatory framework and the watchdog deemed necessary to reassure all stakeholders. In the U.K., the Human Fertilisation and Embryology (HFE) Act [1] was passed by Parliament in 1990, and many other countries passed specific laws regulating embryo research and often access to treatment, while U.S. jurisdictions vary between states and usually are less comprehensive. Furthermore, many laws were revised, completed, or amended in order to clarify the legal status of scientific advances like somatic cell nuclear transfer, or to keep up with social changes. In the U.K., this led to the new HFE Act in 2008 [2]. The initial French "bioethics laws" of 1994, revised in 2004, right now are going through the French Parliament for possible modifications concerning the anonymity of gametes, and allowing some embryo research under conditions rather than forbidding it with exceptions – a welcome progress a few months after the attribution of the Nobel Prize for medicine to R. G. Edwards last autumn. These laws are more or less restrictive, like the Italian law of 2005 [3], which forbids any gamete donations and embryo cryopreservation. However, a third phase has recently evolved, that of judicial challenge. Indeed, this happened recently for two of the strictest European legislations. First, in Italy, where statutory replacement of all oocytes fertilized in IVF (with a maximum of three) was subjected to successful judicial challenge. The practice was wisely declared inappropriate by the Supreme Court, invoking clinical judgment and the prime interest of the health of the future mother and her offspring, and leading to a positive trend to reduction in the number of multiple pregnancies [4]. Second, an interesting event is that Germany, where legislation that very symbolically mentions protection of the embryo in its title, has forbidden PGD since 1990, and is considering some amendments after a Berlin court decided not to sanction a team that successfully performed this to avoid the birth of a very sick child [5].

Pregnancy After Assisted Reproductive Technology, ed. Eric R. M. Jauniaux and Botros R. M. B. Rizk. Published by Cambridge University Press.

Such decisions emphasize the fact that the welfare of the most vulnerable party, the future child, may be the essential ethical issue that trumps all others, as this represents the very core of and reason for the specialty of infertility treatment. Indeed in the U.K., the HFE Act actually requires the practitioners of ART to consider the "welfare of the child born as a result of the treatment, and of any other child which may be affected by the birth." The Act also set up the Human Fertilisation and Embryology Authority (HFEA) in order to regulate human embryo research and licence centers, as well as fertility treatments involving the creation of embryos outside the body (i.e., IVF) or donated ova and spermatozoa (e.g., donor insemination (DI)). What was new at the time of writing this chapter, is the possibility that HFEA will be abolished and some regulatory duties concerning safe standards and safety would be devoluted to other existing bodies while statutory duties, of course, must continue.

It is, however, impossible to cover all related subjects, from the preimplantation embryo to the future child, the internationally varied legal background, and their ethical implications, in just one chapter. Thus, the focus will definitively be on the offspring. We will not discuss embryo research, even though the legal status of this preimplantation entity [6] has been at the core of the ART ethical debate and of much legal discourse for at least 30 years since the first successful IVF. We will discuss "third-party" reproduction involving gamete donations or surrogacy, and the infrequent but emotionally laden field of posthumous reproduction, PGD and the selection of the embryo to lead to the birth of a healthy child or a savior sibling, and the prevention of multiple pregnancy, all matters that more directly influence the status and well-being of ART offspring. We will also discuss social gender selection and the currently much-debated field of cross-border reproductive care (CBRC), the former having an eternal dimension raising perennial concerns of non-discrimination, and the latter symptomatic of what patients may do when they either wish to avoid their own restrictive legislation, like in Italy where all gamete donations are now forbidden (re Law 4) [3], or when there is difficulty of access to specific groups or techniques. The interaction between ethics and law is unavoidable, and legislation is not necessarily ethical although ideally it aspires to be [7]; therefore, the two subjects are discussed in symbiosis.

Indeed the subject of filiation, who is the legal parent of an ART conceived child, and the discussion of some problems that may arise consequently to the severance from biological links in some techniques, illustrate this symbiosis well. Filiation is generally described as having three components: legal, biological, and affective/psychosociological. The psychological component is both sensitive and complex, evoking as it does many of the most awe-inspiring subjects within the human psyche, the begetting of life, sexuality (or its denial through many of the methods of assisted reproduction), and death (as in the use of gametes after the death of the provider). Certainly, we may be reassured on this score as, in fact, several psychological studies over the years have confirmed the feeling many clinicians have had that such children, most desired from well before conception, are objectively doing very well with their intended parents, who have had a complex and often lengthy path before they achieve their goal and assume this most wanted parental responsibility [8].

Access to assisted reproductive technologies, justice, and barriers

Before going into the specific aspects of ART, however, it must be made clear that a major ethical issue is still at stake, that of fair access to ART with its variability both in Europe, as witnessed by the European IVF monitoring data on behalf of the European Society of Human Reproduction and Embryology (ESHRE) [9], and even more acutely worldwide [10] from low to high resource countries. A just and equitable healthcare system should provide fairly for the needs of the patients, with equity of access at a national level, and this naturally should also apply to fertility treatments [11]. Indeed, much of the value of international comparisons resides in the possibility of contrasting the different ways in which similar circumstances, in this case the treatments of infertility, are viewed by different societies. The disparities of access, because of lack of homogeneous national funding or the legal exclusion of specific treatments, are major reasons for CBRC, for instance, an international phenomenon that is now receiving intense exposure and where data have started to gather [12], highlighting the unfairness of access to fertility treatments worldwide, which will be discussed last.

At the international level, there are many countries where most ART treatments are in the private sector with no state subsidy, leading to inequity because of parental means, both in high resource areas like the

U.S., countries in transition like India or China, or even more strikingly in low resource countries [10].

In addition, at the national level there are many ways where access can be limited by the providers of ART treatment. Apart from the well-known phenomenon of postcode lottery in the U.K., a new phenomenon must be highlighted, that of the extra barriers put in the path of many patients. The ethical conundrum resides in the fact that they are sometimes clinically appropriate, but may also be used again merely as a disguised way of restricting access to treatment and of rationing. In the general debate about personal responsibility for health, the importance of lifestyle factors, which may adversely affect fertility, has been the matter of much discussion, and led the ESHRE ethics and law taskforce to discuss the fairness of imposing further delays on infertile couples as conditions to treatment, looking at obesity, smoking, and alcohol consumption [13]. Indeed, fertility doctors have a double responsibility to the patient(s) and to the future child, or as stated in the U.K. statutory, a "welfare of the child" consideration [1,2].

The ethical analysis [14] of the "welfare of the child" states that treatment should be refused only if there is a risk of serious harm to the future child, although the profession also has a duty to reduce reproductive risks. Thus, the question is whether it is justifiable to (strictly) implement conditions to starting ART when lifestyle changes are advisable for better efficiency, or to protect the future offspring. Thus, discussing lifestyle changes and their imposition as the key to access to treatments, we concluded [13] that treatment may be conditional to lifestyle changes if there is indeed strong evidence that without this there was a risk of serious harm to the child, or that the treatment became disproportional in terms of cost-effectiveness or obstetric risks. There are major differences when one considers smoking, obesity, or alcohol dependency, the last having the most serious potential danger for the future child with a possible fetal alcohol syndrome. Here the taskforce states that "in view of the risks for the future child, fertility doctors should refuse treatment to women used to more than moderate drinking who are not willing or able to minimize their alcohol consumption."

Another factor to consider, more common with smoking and obesity, is treatment efficiency, especially when such treatment comes from the "common purse." Indeed "the primary issue here is to what extent fertility doctors should insist on prior lifestyle modification by the woman (and her partner) that may either preempt the need for medical assistance or else lead to a greater effectiveness and/or a reduction of reproductive risks." With regard to obesity and smoking, "the available data seem to suggest that treating women with severe or morbid obesity would require special justification," and evidence suggests that "a positive reproductive effect of weight loss and smoking cessation can reasonably be assumed." We might thus "insist that a serious effort at achieving [tackling such issues] must be made before treatment can be considered," but the most important concern is to a possible time-delay for women whose ovarian reserve is threatened by their age; it would be unfair not to offer a chance of treatment if postponement means that delays would seriously impair the chance for women approaching the end of their fertile period. This essential point also highlights the duty-of-care and responsibility of the clinician to his/her patient, and the moral dilemma encountered with state-imposed funding limits. Furthermore, if (fertility doctors) "mak[e] assisted reproduction conditional on lifestyle modification or efforts to that effect, [they] should support their patients in achieving the intended results." Here duty-of-care is the essential ethical issue as well as a legal one, and the core of the patient/doctor relationship in general.

Ethical issues in third-party reproduction: gamete donations and surrogacy

There are also specific ethical issues, present since the beginning of available ART techniques, which are still the subject of current discussion, such as the fair compensation of gamete donors and surrogates, their anonymity or lack thereof, as well as who is allowed to donate gametes to whom (if at all). They will now be discussed, as they epitomize much of the varied approaches to third-party reproduction, reflecting often different societal and cultural values.

Thus, two main issues surround gamete donations: the traditional and more recently questioned anonymity of the donors of the gamete(s)/embryos, which must be put in the context of the sense of identity of the offspring in relation to that of his/her intended (or psychosocial) parent(s), and access to his/her origins. The other issue is older still, but often rekindled, especially when donation becomes relatively scarce: should donors be (highly) compensated for their donation, what is fair compensation, and when does it become disproportionate and akin to payment?

At the first examination, the issue of payment for donation (a contradiction in terms) may not appear to be as important for the future child's welfare as the question of the donor's anonymity [15]. One should consider, however, that the issue of buying gametes, offering disproportionate compensation for gametes' donors or to surrogates, is also very much value laden, as it teases out the limits of how much any society wishes to put a price on everything, at the expense of ignoring an important value, that of solidarity.

Indeed it seems obvious, at least from a semantic point of view, that a gift should be free. Furthermore, the fact is that if society intends to pay gamete donors, the term "donation" itself should be changed to "sale" of gametes and embryos [16]. However, in most countries where gamete donation is used as a means of solving infertility problems, those who recruit the donors have difficulties in matching the supply to the demand, especially in the case of oocytes and embryos. Thus, it has been argued that pragmatism should prevail in a scarce-supply environment and that some type of financial inducement might not be forbidden. In the U.K., this must of course be within the frame of English law, which states that ""no money or other kind of benefit shall be given or received in respect of any supply of gametes or embryos unless authorized by directions" [2]. The notion of gifting is also enshrined in French law among others, while in Spain the amount of the usual compensation to ovum donors (€900) is larger than that allowed in the U.K. (up to £750). Interestingly, however, sharing of ova is allowed in the U.K., and this means a large reduction of IVF fees in the private sector, which still performs about two thirds of IVF cycles and most ovum donations. All this, however, must fit within the EU tissue directive, which stresses that human "products" must not be the matter of financial transactions [17].

Similarly, variations of compensation for surrogacy with its contractual basis in the U.S. – while it is either forbidden or strictly regulated in some European countries – also highlight this difficulty concerning proportionate compensation, in order not to entice and possibly abuse poorer women to take a risk on behalf of the intended parents. The issues are complicated by the fact that all parties share a responsibility to the surrogate, with attention to minimization of risk for her, and the necessity to respect her fundamental autonomy during the pregnancy. Indeed, to ensure minimal risk, one may recommend single embryo transfer for surrogate pregnancy [18].

In both surrogacy and gamete donations, openness by the parents toward the child about its mode of conception is advisable, but the years' long debate on anonymity in gamete donations epitomizes the polarization of different positions, and highlights the meaning of "origins," including genetic origins. Several legislations, such as from Sweden or the U.K., require mandatory enrolment of donors ready to reveal their identity to the offspring on their majority, and several others stick to anonymity as a principle, like Spain, or France where the discussion has been rekindled during the current parliamentary debate concerning the revision of ART legislation. A fair compromise seems to be that of the double-gate approach [19], which leaves parents to decide what kind of donors, who never have legal parental responsibility, to use for their offspring.

Similar societal differences in approach are seen when one considers whether to allow ART access to single women, men, or same-gender couples, which necessarily implies gamete donations and/or surrogacy. This is forbidden in French law, where "assisted reproduction treatments are solely to be used for a couple's parenting project" and "the man and woman which constitute this couple (must be) of a reproductive age," thus excluding same-gender couples, while in the U.K. they can now have their name as co-parent on a birth certificate of an ART child, since the HFE Act 2008 was made compatible with non-discriminatory, previous legislation. Indeed, the follow-up of children, issue of insemination, for lesbian couples has been extensively studied, showing no adverse effect [20] in spite of the rare cases that get press exposure [21].

Finally, all these cases may seem relatively straight forward compared to posthumous reproduction [22]. The keys are that there should be support from the surviving family of the widow, and especially the availability of prior written consent, as otherwise there is the possibility that decisions are taken that do not conform to the deceased person's wishes. This means that, in the absence of such specific advanced directives, including most cases of accidental persistent vegetative state or sudden death, as was raised recently in the U.S. [23], no action to obtain reproductive material can be performed and no use can be made of the gametes or embryos. Indeed, the presence of cryo-stored gametes or embryos shows that a parental project existed but it does not demonstrate after his/her death that the deceased accepted the continuation of the project. A parental project further means that only the partner of the deceased, not potential grandparents, should be allowed their use, and the easiest solution is to have written prior consent with legal effect. Again there is little evidence about the effect on future children, but it is recommended that family support for this project should be available to the surviving partner.

Preimplantation genetic diagnosis, uses, and abuses

When a child is planned, most intended parents wish for a healthy child, and to avoid serious disability at birth, accept the routine antenatal screening offered to women in many countries without prejudice of the sometimes difficult decision to be taken if an anomaly is discovered. Thus, in general, the ethical dilemmas of PGD are not dissimilar to those encountered in antenatal screening. Preimplantation genetic diagnosis is the ultimate step in antenatal screening, retrogressing from diagnosis on the fetus in utero to the embryo in vitro, and may be called "pregravid diagnosis," as indeed the mother-to-be is not pregnant until a fertilized embryo (after PGD or not) has been replaced and implanted in utero following the necessary IVF.

The eugenics debate has long been used in this field, as it has been argued that some couples would demand, after preimplantation diagnosis, the assurance of a "perfect" baby, although in practice couples voice their wish for "normality" rather than "perfection," and this often after having the personal experience of genetic disease [24]. But is the basic philosophy of preconception and preimplantation diagnosis akin to eugenics, in that it selects gametes or embryos? Although concerns that "a more and more restrictive definition of normality and humanity would ensue from a wide application of PGD" [25] must be at least considered, the fact that eugenics actually means the imposition of a policy on a specific population indicates that this term of eugenic practice does not apply to PGD, where the gamete providers, an informed couple, seek and give informed consent to a complex procedure that applies to them and no one else, case by case.

Late-onset disorders

This same casuistic analysis remains the best argument against this historically tainted terminology of eugenics, and also applies when PGD is performed to avoid a late-onset serious disease or its predisposition. Although few voices have opposed its use to prevent the birth of a newborn with retinoblastoma, the case for avoiding late-onset disease, like hereditary forms of breast cancer, is much more controversial. Furthermore, although the absolute risk figures for women carrying BRCA1/2 are relatively high, preventive measures like mastectomy exist. Thus, it is a double dilemma whether it is ethically acceptable to test and select embryos because of an increased risk – instead of a certainty – of developing a particular, grave disease especially if it is later in life, rather than one affecting a baby or a young child with a high degree of certainty.

In such cases, it is essential to take into account the severity of the familial illness and the effects on the quality of life of the future offspring, even though it may be almost impossible to assess objectively. Thus, subjective assessment is used, and the technique may be offered in cases of a disastrous family history, and with appropriate genetic and implication counseling. The sword of Damocles hanging on such families with a choice between possible death in early adulthood or maiming surgery is enough to warrant this on compassionate grounds [26].

Another concern is that the imperfection in predicting the development of the disease forces us to accept that a number of embryos will be discarded that will not develop the disease. The discarding of potentially healthy embryos is indeed a specific ethical dilemma, pertaining to PGD in general, when the disease is sex linked, or of variable penetration. The embryos rejected for transfer may not be donated to other infertile couples in view of the possible risk to the offspring (unknown as yet from the embryo biopsy), although they may be given for research with the consent of both gamete providers.

Savior sibling

Another specific dilemma concerns the use of PGD to select an embryo that is human leukocyte antigen (HLA) compatible for a sick sibling, for whom all other treatments have been ineffective. This example of PGD for HLA matching is a paradigm in the discussion that is at the heart of this book, the children of

ART, and the welfare of the future child. The main argument against this kind of request is the possible instrumentalization of the future child, infringing the Kantian categorical imperative to "act so that you treat humanity, whether in your own person or in that of another, always as an end and never as a means only."

Two U.K. cases actually illustrate this very core issue, the possible "use" of one human being "merely" for the sake of another. The Hashmis wished to conceive an embryo both free from the disease, and matching their son, seriously ill with thalassemia, hoping for compatible cord blood stem cells as a cure at the delivery of the sibling. The Whitakers' sick child suffered from Diamond–Blackfan anemia, a disease that is mostly non-genetic, and thus the future planned child was not at risk of this condition and would arguably be planned "merely to save the older sibling" and PGD not used to primarily exclude a serious genetic disease (as well as to plan a "savior sibling"), as in the case of thalassemia. After much public debate, and a successful PGD in Chicago for the Whitakers, resulting in the birth of a savior sibling, the HFEA, which had refused their request on Kantian grounds, stated the following year that further similar cases would be licensed in the U.K., thus accepting the danger to the life of the existing sibling as a sufficiently compelling reason. In fact, even from the point of view of the future child, it may be seen as beneficial to be able to save its sibling as a matter of solidarity, and seems acceptable if the future child's operation involves minimal risk (e.g., cord blood or bone marrow donation). This is now positively enshrined in the new HFE Act [2].

Another concern is which motive is acceptable for the selection of embryos. Here the "postnatal" test is useful, as it states that it is ethically acceptable to create a child that can be used for a certain goal if it is acceptable to use an existing child for the same goal while, of course, parents' self-interest is not acceptable [27]. This very matter led to a lot of attention when hearing impaired couples wished to have embryos selected with the same impairment and took part very vocally in the public debate prior to the vote of the revised UK legislation. This has also been strictly and clearly forbidden, another symbolic confirmation that the "welfare of the future child" trumps other important values such as the respect of the intended patients' autonomy. This theme is indeed recurrent in all ethical debates in ART, as our responsibility to the most vulnerable party, the offspring, is generally considered to weigh heavily in an ethical calculus with many strands, some of which may be contradictory.

But the "promotion of informed reproductive decisions" [28] is indeed caring and sensitive terminology to qualify this pregravid diagnosis, a complex task where a multidisciplinary approach, including counseling, is essential [27]. Let us not forget, however, that the danger at the societal level is that those opting out will be portrayed as irresponsible and be stigmatized.

Social gender selection

Finally, the advent of PGD and the possibility of pregravid diagnosis to families affected by an X-linked disorder rekindled the question of gender selection for social reasons. The matter of gender social selection is not novel in historical terms: baby girls have been left exposed on the hillside to die from time immemorial, and female and adolescent children submitted to negative discrimination in health and education systems of old in many societies. But the availability of technology, whether low key (spermatozoon selection) or complex and intensive (PGD), has rendered the efficacy of gender selection more accurate and therefore less innocuous than the old mythology of having sex at a certain time, or ingesting a special regime at conception in order to achieve the desired effect. Although some propose a compromise with the possibility of family balancing, which means never accepting social "sexing" for the first child but always for a child of another gender to the first born [29], tolerating this "balancing" would imply that families with same-gender children may be somewhat unbalanced, a negative qualification by comparison with the supposedly ideal boy and girl balanced family.

Worldwide, the practice of gender selection is more often to favor the birth of a son rather than a daughter. In fact, gender discrimination is common worldwide, and can have many guises and rationalizations. Some arguments trying to justify gender selection as a reproductive choice are worse than others. For instance, the known imbalance of genders already existing in some societies has led to comments that this would lead to an increased "value" of females, a demeaning attitude for whichever gender becomes thus of scarcity value. This terminology of the market place reduces further the status of women (in practice, rather than men) to mere chattels.

The obvious imbalance of gender rationing observed in areas of India [30] and China [31] is one extreme piece of evidence of its occurrence, where it is known to result mostly from the use of prenatal ultrasound gender diagnosis followed by termination of pregnancy (TOP)[32] rather than from PGD. Nevertheless, it has been argued that PGD –discarding an embryo for being of the wrong gender – is a lesser evil than TOP, as the fetus is even nearer achieving its potential (at least its legal) personhood, and itself more serious than spermatozoon sorting.

However, one must state that moral appraisal of such a grave issue does not depend on the method used. Discrimination is wrong at whatever level, whether after birth, during fetal life, or at the pregravid state. We would like to adhere to the strict view here, holding that any kind of selection, called balancing or not, is inherently sexist, and is likely to reinforce sexist attitudes already too prevalent in most societies.

Without pointing out the obvious (a child knowing of the method used for his/her conception may have the feeling of "being conditionally wanted" and/or feel even more intense pressure than usual in her/his society to fulfil a gender stereotype in behavior, profession, and private life), and without raising the specter of eugenics and the worn slippery slopes' warning, one may also feel that children would benefit from being born in a society where acceptance rather than rejection of any difference (of phenotype, gender, or disabilities) is the norm. Regardless of personal or cultural motivations, the message that gender selection for non-medical reasons (including balancing) sends to the broader society and the world at large is the suboptimal worth of women. The stakes are too high to allow any compromise until equality of opportunity (lack of discrimination) between the genders is shown to be really implemented as demanded by Human Rights declarations [33].

International concerns in assisted reproductive technology

Here we discuss the consequences of the most common complication worldwide, multiple pregnancy, and a phenomenon that has always existed for people with means, crossing national borders to obtain a treatment not available at home, but which is spreading thanks to low-cost travel.

Avoiding multiple pregnancy

The dangers of multiple pregnancies are well documented and is the subject of Chapter 8. These dangers exist for the future mother and for the children-to-be, due mainly to the complications of intrauterine growth retardation, preterm delivery, and their long-term consequences. In ART, this iatrogenic event is the physician's responsibility, not to cause unnecessary harm. In addition, there may be conflict between the reproductive autonomy of the patients, especially when they are submitted to financial pressure, and the professional autonomy of the physician, particularly in the decision about the number of embryos to be transferred and the decision to perform multifetal pregnancy reduction (MFPR). For all these reasons, it seems obvious that prevention is preferable to submitting patients to difficult decisions when they are carrying a much-wanted pregnancy. Indeed, regardless of the information provided before the treatment, people will still generally view MFPR as an emotional upheaval [34].

Furthermore, the high number of multiple pregnancies after ART is not only a personal issue but also a public health one; the issue of justice and equitable access to ART is another major component of the preventive aspect, as several studies have correlated better public funding and access to ART with lesser rates of multiple pregnancies. Thus, "public funding should give patients a reasonable chance of achieving a healthy singleton birth," and in order to give a clear message to all stakeholders, "multiple pregnancies should not be reported as a success, but as a complication of MAR, and separately to the singleton pregnancy rate".

Finally, we have evidence that another kind of pressure may occur when couples cross national borders to seek fertility treatment, the relatively newly quantified phenomenon of CBRC [12]; a multiple pregnancy of high order conceived after CBRC is less likely to be reduced than if conceived at home, as shown for pregnant women consulting at UCLH fetal medicine unit over a ten-year period [35].

Cross-border reproductive care

Intended parents go abroad for treatment because of law evasion when the law excludes them as a particular population group, or when the technique is either forbidden per se (surrogacy or gamete donations), or when there are access limitations at home (long waiting lists). They may also seek better quality of care or cheaper treatment abroad, especially after previous failure at home. The fact that health professionals prefer this term to the more derogatory terminology of "tourism" means to emphasize that most patients who cross borders in search of reproductive treatment do this because they must and not by choice, or for fun as one would for a holiday [36]. The ethical and legal issues of CBRC were considered by the ESHRE task-force for ethics and law [36], and again the relevance of equitable access to ART treatments for all citizens was highlighted [11]. One might also consider extending "the portability of health insurance (at least for treatment that is not prohibited in the home country) to reproductive health; install a system of accreditation in order to guarantee that all patients get safe and effective treatment wherever they go; promote awareness and information campaigns by the government, patients and professional organizations to warn its citizens for possible dangers of cross-border reproductive care and finally ensure that all professional parties, referring agents as well as doctors/teams caring abroad are aware of their responsibilities and relevant ethical guidance."

As clinicians, we know that many colleagues are involved in CBRC, and unlike some politicians or media in the press, hold no a priori prejudice against this common phenomenon, as it clearly enhances our patients' autonomy to be able to choose treatment abroad. Law evasion is not necessarily wrong per se; "there may be good reasons for people to violate national law," which are not necessarily immoral, such as escaping the total ban on gamete donations in Italy, or that of oocytes donation in Germany.

Clinicians can advise patients to make sure the chosen center abroad follows good clinical practice [37], especially with a limit of a maximum of two embryos transferred bar exceptional circumstances linked to their age. It is also important to get into more detailed ethical discussions about the lack of pressure on oocyte donors or surrogates they might require, mostly linked to disproportionate compensation. Indeed, the recently published good practice guide for clinicians and clinics (GPG) [38] articulates guidance around six principles: equity, quality, safety, evidence-based care, patient involvement, and redress for respective patients, donors and surrogates, the future child, and professionals. For instance, defining that "quality . . . implies that patients are not subjected to unnecessary procedures," and stressing that "for surrogates, single embryo transfer is the only available option" represent one aspect of the beneficence/non-maleficence (doing as much good and as little harm as possible) balance; additionally, giving patients information about success rates, encouraging colleagues to communicate before and after treatment, enhancing patients' autonomy as well as safety; and last but not least, the repeatedly mentioning minimization of multiple pregnancy protect the welfare of the future child.

Conclusion

After over four million babies have been born worldwide, one might argue that it is time IVF was seen as routine, and was perhaps less rather than more regulated. In spite of all the ethical dilemmas discussed in this chapter, a true libertarian would argue that society and the professions involved are interfering with the autonomy of the future parents, informed consenting adults, by restricting their choice to have several embryos replaced, or to have oocyte donation at a very advanced age, for instance. However, if the notion of responsibility is as dear to us personally and to society as it is to Hans Jonas, who made it the key to his ethical theory by citing as a paradigm the case of parents toward their children and future generations [39], we can find in this a common thread, which is included in the British legislation as an injunction, "to take into account the welfare of the child when offering licenced fertility treatment." This "responsibility principle" [39], together with concerns about (mostly women's) exploitation, with a purely "market" approach to surrogacy or ovum donation, for instance [40], make the common ground to the different dilemmas outlined and also transcend national borders. Indeed, when women are subjected to disproportionate financial enticement to "donate," it makes a mockery of their informed consent, as the pressure induced by low income is hard to resist.

Finally, the interests of future generations include the difficult dilemma presented by the need for surveillance of children resulting from the new techniques. This may give answers about the risk and possible long-term consequences of the newer procedures like PGD, but it is always important to respect the confidentiality and privacy of the parents and avoid stigmatization of the children. This, in the end, may only be achieved by a sensitive approach to the solidarity between the present and future generations. Both at the personal and societal level, nationally and internationally, the interests of the child-to-be (the aim desired in assisted conception, and a vulnerable future party to protect) must be the most important concern. To act responsibly is an ethical imperative.

References

1. HFE Act, 1990. (Available at: http://www.dh.gov.uk/en/.../Legislation/Actsandbills/DH)
2. HFE Act, 2008. (Available at: http://www.dh.gov.uk/en/.../Legislation/Actsandbills/DH_080211)
3. Italian Law no. 40, art. 4, 2005. (Access to the ART techniques.)
4. Levi Setti PE, Albani E, Cesana A, et al. Italian Constitutional Court modifications of a restrictive assisted reproduction technology law significantly improve pregnancy rate. *Hum Reprod* 2011; **26**: 376–381.
5. Landesgericht Berlin, May 2009. *Geschaftnummer* 512, 1Kap Js 1424/06 KLs (26/08).
6. ESHRE Task Force on Ethics and Law 1. The moral status of the pre-implantation embryo. *Hum Reprod* 2001; **16**: 1046–1047.
7. Dickens B. Interfaces of assisted reproduction, ethics and law. In: Shenfield F, Sureau C, eds. *Ethical Dilemmas in Assisted Reproduction*. New York, NY: Parthenon, 1997; 77–82.
8. Golombock S, Cook R, Bish A, Murray C. Families created by the new reproductive technologies: quality of parenting and social and emotional development of the children. *Child Dev* 1995; **66**: 285–298.
9. De Mouzon J, Goossens V, Bhattacharya S, et al. Results generated from European registers by ESHRE. *Hum Reprod* 2010; **25**: 1851–1862.
10. Vayena E, Peterson HB, Adamson D, Nygren KG. Art in developing countries: are we caring yet? *Fertil Steril* 2009; **92**: 413–416.
11. ESHRE Task Force on Ethics and Law 14. Equity of access to assisted reproductive technology. *Hum Reprod* 2008; **23**: 772–774.
12. Shenfield F, de Mouzon J, Pennings G, et al. Cross border reproductive care in six European countries. *Hum Reprod* 2010; **25**: 1361–1368.
13. ESHRE Task Force on Ethics and Law 17. Life-style related factors and access to medically assisted reproduction. *Hum Reprod* 2010; **25**: 578–583.
14. ESHRE Task Force on Ethics and Law 14. Welfare of the child in assisted reproduction. *Hum Reprod* 2007; **22**: 2585–2588.
15. Shenfield F, Steele SJ. What are the effects of anonymity and secrecy on the welfare of the child in gamete donation? *Hum Reprod* 1997; **12**: 392–395.
16. Shenfield F, Steele SJ. A gift is a gift is a gift, or why gametes donors should not be paid. *Hum Reprod* 1995; **10**: 253–254.
17. Commission directive 2006/86/EC, implementing Directive 2004/23/EC of the European Parliament and of the Council as regards traceability requirements, notification of serious adverse reactions and events and certain technical requirements for the coding, processing, reservation, storage and distribution of human tissues and cells. (Available at: http://eur-lex.europa.eu)
18. ESHRE Task Force on Ethics and Law 10. Surrogacy. *Hum Reprod* 2005; **10**: 2705–2707.
19. Pennings G. The double track policy for donor anonymity. *Hum Reprod* 1997; **12**: 2839–2844.
20. Golombok S, Tasker F, Murray C. Children raised in fatherless families from infancy: family relationships and the socioemotional development of children of lesbian and single heterosexual mothers. *J Child Psychol Psychiatry* 1997; **38**: 783–791.
21. Hyder N. Gay man and lesbian couple in custody battle. *Bionews* 2010; **584**: bionews.org.uk.
22. ESHRE Task Force on Ethics and Law 11. Posthumous assisted reproduction. *Hum Reprod* 2006; **21**: 3050–3053.
23. Greer DM, Styer AK, Toth TL, Kindregan CP, Romero JM. Case records of the Massachusetts General Hospital. Case 21–2010. A request for retrieval of oocytes from a 36-year-old woman with anoxic brain injury. *N Engl J Med* 2010; **363**: 276–283.
24. ESHRE Task Force on Ethics and Law 5. Preimplantation genetic diagnosis. *Hum Reprod* 2003; **18**: 649–651.
25. Testard J, Sele B. Towards an efficient medical eugenics: is the desirable always the feasible? *Hum Reprod* 1995; **11**: 3086–3090.
26. Shenfield F. Preimplantation genetic diagnosis for inherited breast cancer: legal and ethical issues. *Expert Rev Obstet Gynecol* 2008; **3**: 601–605.
27. ESHRE Task Force on Ethics and Law 9. The application of preimplantation genetic diagnosis for human leukocyte antigen typing of embryos. *Hum Reprod* 2005; **20**: 845–847.
28. Pennings G, Liebaers I. Creating a child to save another: HLA matching of siblings by means of preimplantation diagnosis. In: Shenfield F, Sureau C, eds. *Ethical Dilemmas in Human Reproduction*. New York, NY: Parthenon, 2002; 51–66.
29. Pennings G. Ethics of sex selection for family balancing. Family balancing as a morally acceptable application of sex selection. *Hum Reprod* 1996; **11**: 2339–2345.

30. Sen A. Missing women revisited. *BMJ* 2003; **327**: 1297–1298.

31. Wu Z, Viisainen K, Wang Y, Hemminki E. Perinatal mortality in rural China: retrospective cohort study. *BMJ* 2003; **327**: 1319–1322.

32. Sheth S. Missing female births in India. *Lancet* 2006; **367**: 185–186.

33. Shenfield F. Sex selection, why not! *Hum Reprod* 1994; **9**: 142.

34. ESHRE Task Force on Ethics and Law 6. Ethical issues related to multiple pregnancies in assisted reproduction. *Hum Reprod* 2006; **18**: 1–4.

35. McKelvey A, David AL, Shenfield F, Jauniaux ER. The impact of cross-border reproductive care or 'fertility tourism' on NHS maternity services. *BJOG* 2009; **116**: 1520–1523.

36. ESHRE Taskforce on Ethics and Law 15. Cross border reproductive care. *Hum Reprod* 2008; **23**: 2182–2184.

37. ESHRE Good clinical practice, http://www.eshre.eu.

38. ESHRE Task Force "Cross Border Reproductive Care" 2011, ESHRE Good practice guide for CBRC for centres and practitioners, doi: 10.1093/humrep/der090. [First published online: April 19, 2011.]

39. Jonas H. *The Imperative of Responsibility: in Search of an Ethics for the Technological Age*. Chicago, IL: Chicago University Press, 1984.

40. Nahman M. Nodes of desire. Romanian egg sellers, 'dignity' and feminist alliances in transnational ova exchange. *Eur J Women's Studies* 2008; **15**: 63–80.

Index

abdominal ectopic pregnancy
  management, 26
  ultrasound diagnosis, 23
access to ART, 183–184
acupuncture therapy, 61
adenomyosis, 69
adhesions, 26
adnexal torsion, 36
adrenoleukodystrophy, 9
alcohol abuse
  and access to ART, 184
ancient Egypt
  fertility testing, 1
Angelman syndrome, 102, 172–173
antepartum hemorrhage, 76, 83
anthracyclines, 131
antiphospholipid syndrome
  and early pregnancy failure, 55
antisperm antibodies, 93
  and early pregnancy failure, 55
anxiety
  and risk of early pregnancy failure, 56
artificial insemination
  early historical accounts, 1
  ethical issues, 1
artificial reproductive technology (ART)
  number of births per year, 4
  number of births to date, 4
aspirin therapy, 61
assisted hatching
  effects on early pregnancy failure, 59
Australia
  first IVF birth, 7
autoimmune disorders, 126
azoospermia, 93, 124, 126, 176
  sperm recovery techniques, 8

Barker hypothesis, 176, 178
Bavister, Barry, 6
Beckwith–Wiedemann syndrome, 102, 172–173
bicornuate uterus, 26
  risk of placenta previa, 69
biochemical markers
  of ectopic pregnancy, 23
  of pregnancy, 20
birth defects, 2
blastocyst sexing, 9
body mass index (BMI)
  and risk of early pregnancy failure, 55, 56
bone marrow failure
  stem cell transplantation, 10
breast cancer, 124, 131
  pregnancy after, 132
breech presentation, 26
  risk in ART pregnancies, 70
Brown, Louise, 168, 178
  first test-tube baby, 2, 6–7

cancer
  incidence of different types, 124
  therapeutic use of embryos, 2
cancer patients
  effects of chemotherapy on fertility, 125
  effects of radiotherapy, 125–126
  fertility preservation, 10, 124
  fertility preservation strategies, 126–129
  importance of fertility preservation, 124
  potential benefits of ovarian transplantation, 144
cancer patients tissue study
  ovarian transplantation, 140–145
cancer risk
  children born after ART, 103
cancer survivor pregnancy
  after breast cancer, 132
  after cervical cancer, 132
  incidence of low birth weight, 130–131
  incidence of preterm birth, 130–131
  miscarriage rates, 130–131
  prenatal advice for cancer survivors, 131
  risk of cardiotoxicity, 131
  risk of congenital malformations, 131
  risk of genetic disorders, 131
  spontaneous pregnancy rates, 129–130
cancer survivors
  ovarian transplantation results, 141–142
cancer treatment
  effects on fertility, 124–126
cerebral palsy, 85, 174
cervical cancer, 124
  pregnancy after, 132
cervical ectopic pregnancy
  management, 25
  ultrasound diagnosis, 22–23
cervical suture, 26
Cesarean scar, 14
Cesarean scar ectopic pregnancy
  management, 25
Cesarean scar pregnancy
  ultrasound diagnosis, 22–23
Cesarean section, 21, 83
  future risk of placenta previa, 69
  risk with ART, 76
Chang, Min Chueh, 5–6
chemotherapy
  effects on fertility, 125
  fertility preservation, 10
chemotherapy agents
  risk of cardiotoxicity, 131
childhood cancer
  in children born after ART, 175
children born after ART
  adult health outcomes, 176
  Angelman syndrome, 172–173
  antenatal and perinatal complications, 168–170
  Beckwith–Wiedemann syndrome, 172–173
  cerebral palsy, 174
  childhood cancer risk, 175
  congenital malformations, 170–172
  effects on their reproductive ability, 175–176
  emotional well-being, 176–177
  ethical considerations, 177–178
  filiation, 183
  imprinting disorders, 172–173
  inheritance of male infertility, 175–176
  long-term health implications, 174–177
  neurodevelopment, 173–174
  registers of data about, 168
  risk of birth defects, 170–172
chimerism, 9

chorionic villous sampling, 89
chorionicity
  multiple gestation pregnancy after ART, 17, 87–88
  ultrasound diagnosis, 17
chromosomal abnormalities
  and early pregnancy failure, 53
  and ICSI, 97–102
chronic illness
  risk factor in IVF, 66
chronic stress
  impact on ART outcome, 78
clinical pregnancy
  definition, 51
clomiphene citrate treatment, 88
  risk of early pregnancy failure, 57
color Doppler, 21
comparative genomic hybridization, 9–10
complications of ART
  associated with IVF treatment, 2–3
  early pregnancy complications, 72–75
  late pregnancy complications, 75–77
  management challenges, 32–33
  psychological complications, 77–78
  range of potential complications, 32–33
  ultrasound diagnosis, 29–32
  See also multiple gestation pregnancies; ovarian hyperstimulation syndrome.
congenital malformations
  in children born after ART, 170–172
  incidence with ICSI, 95–97
  risk after ART, 76–77
  risk in cancer survivor pregnancies, 131
congenital uterine anomalies, 26
cornual ectopic pregnancy
  ultrasound diagnosis, 22
corpus luteum
  ultrasound appearance, 21–22, 28
critical OHSS. *See* severe OHSS
cross-border reproductive care, 183–184, 188
cryopreservation
  and early pregnancy failure, 59
  cryotissue method, 139–140
  embryos, 8–9, 112–119, 127
  importance in ART, 108
  oocytes, 8–9, 108–112, 127–128
  ovarian tissue, 10, 128, 143
  slow freezing of ovarian tissue, 139
  slow-freeze protocols, 9
  sperm, 93, 128–129
  use for fertility preservation, 108
  vitrification method, 9, 59
  vitrification of ovarian tissue, 139–140
cyclophosphamide, 124
cystic fibrosis in ART offspring, 176

Darwin, Charles, 4
daunorubicin, 131
degenerative disorders
  therapeutic use of embryos, 2
depression
  impact of multiple pregnancies on parents, 77–78
  risk for men during ART, 78
dermoid cysts
  ultrasound diagnosis, 28
developmental plasticity in utero, 176
dimethyl sulfoxide (DMSO), 8
dizygotic (DZ) twin pregnancies, 87
dizygotic (DZ) twins, 16–17
DNA amplification, 9
DNA methylation defects
  and ICSI, 102–103
donation of oocytes, 9
donor anonymity/identity issue, 185
donor eggs, 1
donor insemination
  earliest record, 1
donor sperm, 1
Doppler examination, 28
Down's syndrome prenatal screening
  biochemical markers, 149–150
  factors affecting biochemical markers, 149–150
  first-trimester ultrasound assessment, 149
  high-order multiple pregnancy after ART, 160–163
  nasal bone ultrasound assessment, 149
  nuchal translucency test, 149
  singleton pregnancy after ART, 151–155
  twin pregnancies after ART, 155–160
doxorubicin, 131

early pregnancy complications, 72–75
  ectopic pregnancy risk after ART, 73–74
  heterotopic pregnancy risk after ART, 74–75
  miscarriage risk in ART, 72–73
  molar pregnancy risk after ART, 75
early pregnancy failure, 36
  acupuncture therapy, 61
  and antiphospholipid syndrome (APS), 55
  and antisperm antibodies, 55
  and ICSI, 58–59
  and in vitro techniques, 58–59
  and increased natural killer (NK) cells, 56
  and maternal age, 53
  and obesity, 55
  and polycystic ovarian syndrome (PCOS), 55
  and subfertility diagnosis, 53–55
  and thrombophilia, 55
  and thyroid antibodies, 55–56
  and uterine abnormalities, 55
  ART dependent factors, 56–59
  aspirin therapy, 61
  blastocyst stage embryo transfer, 60
  chromosome abnormalities, 53
  cleavage stage embryo transfer, 60
  clinical pregnancy, 51
  definition, 51
  due to natural causes, 52
  effects of anxiety, 56
  effects of assisted hatching, 59
  effects of GnRH analogues, 58
  effects of in vitro maturation (IVM) of oocytes, 59
  effects of ovarian stimulation agents, 57–58
  effects of ovarian stimulation/ovulation induction, 56–58
  embryo stage at transfer, 60
  embryonic factors, 59–60
  endometrioma surgery, 61
  endometriosis, 54–55
  ethicity risk factors, 56
  following ART, 52
  freshly fertilized embryos, 59
  frozen and thawed embryos, 59
  gamete intra-Fallopian transfer (GIFT), 58
  glucocorticoid treatment, 61
  heparin therapy, 61
  incidence following ART, 52–53
  interventions and therapies, 60–61
  luteal phase support, 58
  male factor subfertility, 55
  meiotic non-disjunction, 51
  metformin treatment, 61
  monitoring and predicting, 61–63
  number of embryo transfers, 60
  number of oocytes retrieved, 60
  patient-dependent factors, 53–56
  possible causes, 52
  preclinical (biochemical) pregnancy, 51
  predictors of future ART treatment success, 61–63
  preimplantation genetic diagosis (PGD), 60–61
  preimplantation genetic screening (PGS), 60–61
  quality of embryos, 59–60
  racial risk factors, 56

scale of preclinical pregnancy loss, 51
smoking risk factor, 56
weight risk factor, 56
zygote intra-Fallopian transfer (ZIFT), 58
See also miscarriage
ectopic pregnancy, 2, 6, 14, 21–26
associated with severe OHSS, 48–49
biochemical markers, 23
incidence in ART patients, 21
management, 73–74
management of abdominal pregnancy, 26
management of cervical pregnancy, 25
management of Cesarean scar pregnancy, 25
management of interstitial pregnancy, 25
management of ovarian pregnancy, 25
medical management of tubal ectopics, 25
risk after ART, 73–74
risk factors, 21
surgical intervention, 23–25
ultrasound diagnosis, 14, 21–23
Edinburgh Postnatal Depression Scale (EPDS), 78
Edwards, Robert
development of IVF treatment, 1–3, 6–7
Nobel Prize (2010), 2, 7, 182
preimplantation genetic diagnosis (PGD), 9
ejaculatory dysfunction, 93
embryo cryopreservation, 8–9, 112–119
fertility preservation strategy, 127
main benefits, 112
outcome studies, 112–119
process, 108–109, 112
slow-freezing method, 112
vitrification method, 112
embryo transfer
early experiments, 4–5
number of embryo transfers, 60
pressures for single embryo transfer, 83
regulation of number transferred, 82–83
stage of embryo at transfer, 60
embryonic diapause, 51
embryonic stem cell research, 2
embryos
effects of cryopreservation, 59
quality of, 59–60
emotional distress associated with ART, 77–78
endometrial cancer, 124
endometrial resection, 69
endometriomas
surgery, 61
ultrasound diagnosis, 28
endometriosis, 26
and early pregnancy failure, 54–55
endometritis, 69
epigenetic risks with ICSI, 102–103
epirubicin, 131
ethical issues
access to ART, 183–184
artificial insemination, 1
avoidance of multiple gestation pregnancies, 188
children born after ART, 177–178
controversy over IVF, 2
cross-border reproductive care, 183–184, 188
donor anonymity/identity, 185
gametes donation, 184–186
gender selection, 187–188
lifestyle factors and access to ART, 184
PGD uses and abuses, 186–188
posthumous reproduction, 185–186
responsibility principle applied to ART, 189–190
same-sex couples, 185
savior sibling, 186–187
social sex selection, 187–188
surrogacy, 184–186
use of donor eggs, 1
use of donor sperm, 1
ethnicity
and risk of early pregnancy failure, 56
eugenics debate, 2, 188
preimplantation genetic diagnosis (PGD), 186
EUROCAT (European Registry of Congenital Anomalies and Twins), 95

fertility
effects of cancer treatment, 124–126
effects of chemotherapy, 125
effects of radiotherapy, 125–126
emotional nature of, 124
implications for cancer survivors, 124
fertility preservation
cancer patients, 10, 124
cancer patients tissue study, 140–145
incidence of cancers, 124
indications for, 124
ovarian tissue cryopreservation, 10
potential use of ovarian transplantation, 144
spontaneous pregnancy in cancer survivors, 129–130
use of cryopreservation, 108
fertility preservation strategies
cryopreservation of embryos, 127
cryopreservation of oocytes, 127–128
cryopreservation of ovarian tissue, 128
cryopreservation of sperm, 128–129
for cancer patients, 126–129
gonadal suppression with GnRH agonists, 126
oophoropexy, 128
ovarian transposition, 128
fertility tourism, 83
fertilization
first observations of, 4
fetal malpresentation
risk in ART pregnancies, 70
fibroids, 26
fluorescence *insitu* hybridization (FISH), 9
follicle-stimulating hormone (FSH), 28
functional cysts, 26
functional ovarian cyst
ultrasound diagnosis, 28

gamete intra-Fallopian transfer (GIFT), 7–8
and early pregnancy failure, 58
gametes donation
ethical issues, 184–186
Gardner, Richard, 9
gender selection
ethical issues, 187–188
genital organ malformations in ART children, 96
genomic imprinting disorders, 172–173
risk with ICSI, 102–103
gestational diabetes, 36, 70, 77, 83
gestational hypertension, 83
glucocorticoid treatment, 61
gonadotrophic releasing hormone (GnRH)
gonadal suppression, 126
gonadotrophin releasing hormone (GnRH) analogues
and early pregnancy failure, 58

Heape, Walter, 4–5
hemoglobinopathies, 126
heparin therapy, 61
heterotopic pregnancy, 21
management, 74–75
risk after ART, 74–75
historical perspective
cryopreservation of oocytes and embryos, 8–9

historical perspective (cont.)
development of IVF treatment, 6–7
development of PGD, 9–10
earliest use of ART, 1
early accounts of artificial insemination, 1
fertility testing in ancient Egypt, 1
first artificial insemination, 4
first embryo transfer experiments, 4–5
first human fertilization in vitro, 6
first IVF birth in Australia, 7
first observations of fertilization, 4
first successful oocyte donation, 9
in vitro culture of eggs, 5–6
in vitro fertilization of human eggs, 5–6
in vitro maturation (IVM) of oocytes, 10
microscopic examination of human spermatozoa, 4
nature of fertilization, 4
ovarian tissue cryopreservation, 10
role of male and female gametes, 4
use of ovarian stimulation for IVF, 6, 7
work of Gregory Pincus, 5–6
work of John Hunter, 4
work of Min Chueh Chang, 5–6
work of Patrick Steptoe, 6–7
work of Robert Edwards, 6–7
work of Spallanzani, 4
work of van Leeuwenhoek, 4
work of Walter Heape, 4–5
worldwide application of IVF, 7
Hodgkin's disease, 130, 145
Hodgkin's lymphoma, 10, 124, 131
human chorionic gonadotrophin (β-hCG), 20, 51
human embryonic development, 2
Human Fertilisation and Embryology Authority (HFEA), UK, 16, 60, 168, 183
human leukocyte antigen (HLA) matching, 9
savior sibling, 186
Hunter, John, 1, 4
hydrosalpinges, 26
hydrothorax, 47
hyperandrogenemia, 55
hyperinsulinemia, 55
hypertension
associated with multiple gestation pregnancy, 76
hypospadias, 1
incidence in ICSI children, 95
hysteroscopic surgery, 69
idarubicin, 131
in vitro culture of eggs
early experiments, 5–6
in vitro fertilization
first human fertilization, 6
first successful experiments on human eggs, 5–6
See also IVF treatment
in vitro maturation (IVM) of oocytes, 10, 59
in vitro techniques
and early pregnancy failure, 58–59
induced labour, 69
infertility
prevalence of the problem, 1
psychological and social impacts, 1
risk factor for obstetric complications, 76
stigma associated with, 1
inflamed Fallopian tubes
ultrasound diagnosis, 32
insulin resistance, 55
International Committee for Monitoring Assisted Reproductive Technologies (ICMART), 4
international concerns about ART, 188–189
cross-border reproductive care, 188
multiple pregnancies, 188
interstitial ectopic pregnancy
management, 25
ultrasound diagnosis, 22
intracytoplasmic morphologically selected sperm injection (IMSI), 59
intracytoplasmic sperm injection (ICSI), 2, 8, 55, 108
and early pregnancy failure, 58–59
balancing risks and benefits, 103
concerns about safety, 93
epigenetic risks, 102–103
extent of use, 93
fertilization failure rate, 93
indications for use, 93
introduction of contaminants into the oocyte, 94
microbiological contamination of the oocyte, 94
potential to pass on male infertility, 175–176
rates of MZ twin pregnancy, 88
risk of chromosomal abnormalities, 97–102
safety concerns, 93
sperm retrieval methods, 93
use in severe male factor infertility, 93
See also pregnancy after ICSI
intratubal transfer procedures, 7–8
intrauterine death, 83
intrauterine growth restriction (IUGR), 83
IVF treatment
controversy over, 2
cost of medication, 10
cost of programs, 2
development by Robert Edwards, 6–7
ethical issues, 2
first test-tube baby, 2
incidence of multiple gestation pregnancy, 82
level of demand for, 2
National Health Service (U.K.) funding, 5
National Health Service (U.K.) provision, 2
possible complications, 2–3
risk of placenta accreta, 69
use of ovarian stimulation, 6, 7
work of Patrick Steptoe, 2
work of Robert Edwards, 1–3
worldwide application, 7

Jonas, Hans, 189

Klinefelter's syndrome, 175

laparoscopy technique of Steptoe, 6–7
Lasix, 44
late pregnancy complications, 75–77
congenital malformations, 76–77
infertility as a risk factor, 76
low birth weight, 76–77
perinatal mortality, 76–77
placenta previa, 76
pregnancy-induced hypertension, 76
preterm labor/birth, 76–77
risk of adverse events after AFT, 76–77
vaginal bleeding, 76
late-onset disorders
use of PGD, 186
legal issues
access to ART, 183–184
cross-border reproductive care, 183–184, 188
donor anonymity/identity, 185
filiation, 183
gametes donation, 184–186
posthumous reproduction, 185–186
same-sex couples, 185
social sex selection using PGD, 187–188
surrogacy, 184–186
leukemias, 124
lifestyle factors and access to ART, 184

low birth weight, 36, 76–77
and adult health issues, 176
risk in multiple gestations, 83
risk with ART, 66
luteal phase support
and early pregnancy failure, 58
luteinizing hormone (LH), 28

male factor infertility
use of ICSI, 93
male factor subfertility
and early pregnancy failure, 55
male infertility
transmission to offspring of AFT, 175–176
malignant ovarian tumors
ultrasound diagnosis, 28–29
Mantegazza, Paolo, 1
maternal age
and early pregnancy failure, 53
and multiple gestation pregnancy, 87
and risk of complications in pregnancy, 66, 69
Medical Research Council (U.K.), 2
meiotic non-disjunction
and pregnancy failure, 51
men
risk of depression during ART, 78
metformin, 61
microdeletions
transmission to ART offspring, 176
microsurgical epididymal sperm aspiration (MESA), 8, 93
miscarriage
in pregnancies following OHSS, 37–38
increased risk in multiple gestations, 83
management of, 20–21
risk in ART, 72–73
ultrasound diagnosis, 17–21
See also early pregnancy failure
mitoxantrone, 131
molar pregnancy risk after ART, 75
monogenic diseases
development of PGD for, 9–10
monozygotic (MZ) twin pregnancies
amnionicity, 87
chorionicity, 87
possible placentation configurations, 87, 88
rates of, 87
risk of adverse events, 87–88
monozygotic (MZ) twins, 16
ovarian transplantation between, 137
mucinous cystadenomas, 28
multifetal pregnancy reduction (MFPR) after ART, 88–89, 90, 188
screening before, 161–162
multiple gestation pregnancies, 36
and advanced maternal age, 87
ART patient awareness of risk, 82
ART patients' attitudes towards, 82
chorionicity after ART, 87–88
complication of ART, 2
Down's syndrome prenatal screening, 160–163
elective reduction after ART, 88–89, 90
financial implications, 83–84
impacts on parents, 83–84
incidence after IVF, 82
international concerns about, 188
medical and healthcare costs, 83–84
multifetal pregnancy reduction (MFPR) after ART, 88–89, 90, 161–162, 188
outcomes and consequences, 83–85
perinatal risks, 82
potential complication of ART, 66
pressures for single embryo transfer, 83
psychological impact on parents, 77–78
rate of MZ twinning after ART, 88
rates of MZ twin pregnancies, 87
reasons for high incidence after ART, 82
reasons to avoid, 188
responsibilities of ART centers, 90
risk associated with ART, 82
risk of adverse events in MZ twins, 87–88
risk of obstetric complications, 66
risks for mother and babies, 83
screening before fetal reduction, 161–162
serum screening, 160–161
twin–twin transfusion syndrome (TTTS), 87
ultrasound findings, 16–17
ultrasound screening, 161
vanishing twin after ART, 85–87
zygosity after ART, 87–88
myomectomy, 69

nasal bone
prenatal ultrasound assessment, 149
National Health Service (U.K.)
IVF treatment funding, 5
IVF treatment provision, 2
natural killer (NK) cells
and early pregnancy failure, 56
Nelson, Henry, 4
neonatal intensive care unit, 83, 84
neoplastic adnexal lesions, 26
neurodevelopment of children born after ART, 173–174
neurogenetic disorders
incidence after ART, 102
nuchal translucency test, 149, 158–160

obesity
and access to ART, 184
and early pregnancy failure, 55
risk of adverse pregnancy and birth outcomes, 69–70
obstructive azoospermia, 93
sperm recovery techniques, 8
oligospermia, 93, 124, 176
oligozoospermia, 102
oocyte collection
risks associated with, 2
oocyte cryopreservation, 8–9, 108–112
fertility preservation strategy, 127–128
outcome studies, 109–112
process, 108–109
slow-freezing method, 108–109
vitrification method, 109
oocyte donation, 9
preeclampsia risk factor, 69
oocyte retrieval
number retrieved, 60
oocytes
in vitro maturation (IVM), 10
oophoropexy
fertility preservation strategy, 128
oral contraceptive pill, 6
ovarian cysts
surgery for ruptured cysts, 48
ovarian ectopic pregnancy
management, 25
ultrasound diagnosis, 23
ovarian fibromas, 26
ovarian hyperstimulation, 172
ovarian hyperstimulation syndrome (OHSS), 2, 10
clinical features, 29, 36
complication of ART, 36
definition, 36
early and late pregnancy outcome, 37
early onset, 36–37
incidence, 36
late onset, 36–37
miscarriage rates in pregnancies following, 37–38
obstetric outcomes after, 38–40
potential effect on pregnancy outcome, 36
pregnancy rates, 36
ultrasound diagnosis, 29
See also severe OHSS
ovarian stimulation
for IVF treatment, 6, 7
ovarian stimulation agents
and early pregnancy failure, 57–58

ovarian tissue cryopreservation, 10, 128
slow-freezing method, 139
slow freezing vs. vitrification, 143
vitrification method, 139–140
ovarian tissue grafts, 137
long-term evaluation, 137
ovarian torsion
and severe OHSS, 48
clinical features, 31–32
management, 31–32
ultrasound diagnosis, 31–32
ovarian transplantation
between MZ twins, 137
cancer patients tissue study, 140–145
cancer survivor transplant results, 141–142
cryoinjury in preserved tissue, 143
frozen tissue transplants, 138
grafting technique, 137
patient population, 137
potential for clinical use, 146
potential for fertility preservation, 144
risk of ovarian metastasis in cancer patients, 145
surgery for fresh transplants, 137–138
ovarian transposition
fertility preservation strategy, 128
ovarian tumors, 26
ultrasound diagnosis, 28–29

paracentesis
for severe OHSS, 47
partial zona dissection (PZD), 8
pelvic hematoma or abscess, 26
pelvic infection
ultrasound diagnosis, 32
pelvic inflammatory disease, 26
pelvic surgery, 66
percutaneous epididymal sperm aspiration (PESA), 8, 93
pericarditis, 131
perinatal mortality, 66, 76–77
Pincus, Gregory, 5–6
placental abruption, 36
placenta accreta
postpartum hemorrhage, 69
risk factors, 69
placenta previa
risk after ART, 76
risk factors, 69
polar body testing for PGD, 9–10
polycystic ovarian syndrome (PCOS), 59, 66
and early pregnancy failure, 55
risk of adverse pregnancy and birth outcomes, 69–70
polymerase chain reaction (PCR), 9
posthumous reproduction, 185–186
postpartum hemorrhage, 77, 83
placenta accreta, 69
pouch of Douglas, 32
Prader–Willi syndrome, 102
pre-ART medical assessment, 70
preclinical (biochemical) pregnancy
definition, 51
preeclampsia, 76
risk factors, 70
pregnancy after ART
potential complications, 32–33
pregnancy after ICSI
balancing risks and benefits, 103
DNA-methylation defects, 102–103
epigenetic risks, 102–103
genomic imprinting disorders, 102–103
incidence of congenital abnormalities, 95–97
perinatal risks, 94–95
procedure-related risks, 94
risk of chromosomal abnormalities, 97–102
pregnancy-induced hypertension, 36, 69, 76, 83
pregnancy of unknown location (PUL), 20
preimplantation aneuploidy screening (PGS), 93
preimplantation genetic diagnosis (PGD), 2, 9–10, 60–61, 93
ethical dilemmas, 186
ethical issues, 186–188
eugenics debate, 186
gender selection, 187–188
late-onset disorders, 186
savior sibling, 186–187
social sex selection, 187–188
uses and abuses, 186–188
preimplantation genetic screening (PGS), 60–61
preimplantation HLA matching, 10
prematurity
risk in multiple gestations, 83
prenatal advice for cancer survivors, 131
prenatal screening
biochemical markers for Down's syndrome, 149
factors affecting biochemical markers, 149–150
first-trimester ultrasound assessment, 149
nasal bone ultrasound assessment, 149
nuchal translucency test, 149, 158–160
prenatal screening after ART
high-order multiple pregnancies, 160–163
singleton pregnancy, 151–155
twin pregnancies, 155–160
preterm delivery, 36, 76–77
risk in multiple gestation pregnancy, 83
risk with ART, 66
primiparity
risk factor for obstetric complications, 69
progesterone, 20
pseudosac
ultrasound diagnosis, 14–16
psychological complications of ART, 77–78
effects of chronic stress, 78
impact of multiple pregnancies, 77–78
pulmonary effusions, 47

race
and risk of early pregnancy failure, 56
radiotherapy
effects on fertility, 125–126
fertility preservation strategies, 128
use of ovarian transposition/ oophoropexy, 128
retinoblastoma
in children born after IVF, 103
retrograde ejaculation, 93
rheumatoid arthritis, 126
Royal Society, London, 1, 4, 7
ruptured cysts
ultrasound diagnosis, 32

salpingo-oophorectomy, 32
same-sex couples
access to ART, 185
savior sibling
ethical issues, 186–187
semen banking, 93
serous cystadenomas, 28
severe OHSS
and thrombophilia, 45–47
correction of circulatory volume, 40–43
diuretics, 44
dopamine treatment, 44–45
ectopic pregnancy associated with, 48–49
electrolyte replacement, 43
management considerations, 49
management of pregnancy following, 49
medical treatment, 40–47
ovarian torsion, 48
paracentesis, 47
surgery for ruptured cysts, 48
surgical treatment, 47–49
thromboembolism, 47

sex chromatin body, 9
sex-linked diseases, 9
sexing of blastocysts, 9
Silver–Russell syndrome, 102
Sims, James Marion, 1
single embryo transfer
  benefits of, 83
  increasing acceptance of, 83
singleton pregnancy after ART
  Down's syndrome screening, 151–155
  first-trimester screening, 153
  maternal age and risk of complications, 66
  maternal age risk factor, 69
  oocyte donation, 69
  perinatal outcome studies, 66–68
  preeclampsia risk factors, 69
  prenatal screening, 151–155
  previous Cesarean as risk factor, 69
  primiparity risk factor, 69
  risk factors for adverse outcome, 69–70
  risk of adverse perinatal outcome, 66
  risk of breech presentation, 70
  risk of complications, 66
  risk of fetal malpresentation, 70
  risk of placenta accreta, 69
  risk of placenta previa, 69
  risk of stillbirth, 70
  risks associated with obesity, 69–70
  risks associated with PCOS, 69–70
  second-trimester screening, 151–153
  sequential screening, 153–155
small for gestational age (SGA) babies, 83
smoking
  and access to ART, 184
  and risk of early pregnancy failure, 56
social sex selection
  ethical issues, 187–188
Spallanzani, Lazzaro, 4
sperm cryopreservation, 128–129
sperm impairment
  intracytoplasmic sperm injection (ICSI), 8
sperm retrieval methods, 8, 93
stem cell research, 2, 9
stem cell transplantation, 10
Steptoe, Patrick, 2
  laparoscopy technique, 6–7
  work on IVF, 6–7
stillbirth risk with ART, 70
stress
  associated with ART, 77–78
  impact on ART outcome, 78
subfertility diagnosis
  and early pregnancy failure, 53–55
submucous fibroids, 69
subzonal insemination (SUZI), 8
surrogacy
  ethical issues, 184–186

testicular biopsy (TESE), 8
testicular cancer, 124, 126
testicular sperm aspiration (TESA), 93
testicular sperm extraction (TESE), 93
testis
  sensitivity to chemotherapy, 125
test-tube babies
  first test-tube baby, 6–7
  Louise Brown, 2, 6–7
thoracocentesis, 47
thromboembolism
  and OHSS, 47
thrombophilia
  and early pregnancy failure, 55
  and OHSS, 45–47
thyroid antibodies
  and early pregnancy failure, 55–56
thyroid disorders, 66
tubo-ovarian pathology
  ultrasound diagnosis, 26–29
twin pregnancies after ART
  combined NT and serum markers, 158–160
  Down's syndrome screening, 155–160
  first-trimester screening, 156–158
  second-trimester screening, 155–156
twin–twin transfusion syndrome (TTTS), 87

ultrasound diagnosis
  appearance of the corpus luteum, 21–22, 28
  complications of ART, 29–32
  dermoid cysts, 28
  ectopic pregnancy, 14, 21–23
  endometriomas, 28
  evaluation of ultrasound characteristics, 26–27
  functional ovarian cyst, 28
  inflamed Fallopian tubes, 32
  malignant ovarian tumors, 28–29
  miscarriage, 17–21
  mucinous cystadenomas, 28
  ovarian hyperstimulation syndrome (OHSS), 29
  ovarian torsion, 31–32
  pattern recognition, 26–27
  pelvic infection, 32
  pseudosac, 14–16
  ruptured cysts, 32
  serous cystadenomas, 28
  tubo-ovarian pathology, 26–29
  use in obstetrics and gynecology, 14
  uterine fibroids, 26
  uterine pathology, 26
ultrasound in normal pregnancy
  amnionicity of multiple pregnancies, 17
  chorionicity of multiple pregnancies, 17
  development in early pregnancy, 14–16
  first scan after conception, 14–16
  multiple pregnancies, 16–17
  transvaginal approach, 14
ultrasound prenatal screening
  first-trimester assessment, 149
  nasal bone assessment, 149
  nuchal translucency test, 149
ultrasound screening
  multiple gestations after ART, 161
unicornuate uterus, 26
uterine abnormalities
  and early pregnancy failure, 55
uterine fibroids, 26
uterine pathology
  bicornuate uterus, 26
  congenital uterine anomalies, 26
  fibroids, 26
  ultrasound diagnosis, 26
  unicornuate uterus, 26

vaginal bleeding
  pregnancy complication, 76
van Leeuwenhoek, Anton Philips, 4
vanishing twin after ART, 85–87
vasectomy
  semen banking prior to, 93
Vatican
  objection to IVF, 2, 7
vitrification method, 9, 59
  embryo cryopreservation, 112
  oocyte cryopreservation, 109
  ovarian tissue cryopreservation, 139–140

weight, and risk of early pregnancy failure, 56
Wilms' tumor, 130, 131
Wood, Carl
  Monash research team, 6

X-linked mental retardation, 9

zona pellucida, 8, 59
zygosity
  multiple gestation pregnancy after ART, 87–88
zygote intra-Fallopian transfer (ZIFT), 7–8
  and early pregnancy failure, 58